ADVANCES IN ANTENNA, SIGNAL PROCESSING, AND MICROELECTRONICS ENGINEERING

ADVANCES IN ANTENNA, SIGNAL PROCESSING, AND MICROELECTRONICS ENGINEERING

Edited by

Devendra Kumar Sharma, PhD
Rohit Sharma, PhD
Bhadra Pokharel, PhD
Vinod Kumar, PhD
Raghvendra Kumar, PhD

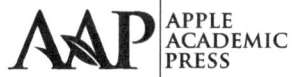

First edition published 2021

Apple Academic Press Inc.
1265 Goldenrod Circle, NE,
Palm Bay, FL 32905 USA
4164 Lakeshore Road, Burlington,
ON, L7L 1A4 Canada

CRC Press
6000 Broken Sound Parkway NW,
Suite 300, Boca Raton, FL 33487-2742 USA
2 Park Square, Milton Park,
Abingdon, Oxon, OX14 4RN UK

© 2021 Apple Academic Press, Inc.

Apple Academic Press exclusively co-publishes with CRC Press, an imprint of Taylor & Francis Group, LLC

Reasonable efforts have been made to publish reliable data and information, but the authors, editors, and publisher cannot assume responsibility for the validity of all materials or the consequences of their use. The authors, editors, and publishers have attempted to trace the copyright holders of all material reproduced in this publication and apologize to copyright holders if permission to publish in this form has not been obtained. If any copyright material has not been acknowledged, please write and let us know so we may rectify in any future reprint.

Except as permitted under U.S. Copyright Law, no part of this book may be reprinted, reproduced, transmitted, or utilized in any form by any electronic, mechanical, or other means, now known or hereafter invented, including photocopying, microfilming, and recording, or in any information storage or retrieval system, without written permission from the publishers.

For permission to photocopy or use material electronically from this work, access www.copyright.com or contact the Copyright Clearance Center, Inc. (CCC), 222 Rosewood Drive, Danvers, MA 01923, 978-750-8400. For works that are not available on CCC please contact mpkbookspermissions@tandf.co.uk

Trademark notice: Product or corporate names may be trademarks or registered trademarks and are used only for identification and explanation without intent to infringe.

Library and Archives Canada Cataloguing in Publication

Title: Advances in antenna, signal processing, and microelectronics engineering / edited by Devendra Kumar Sharma, PhD, Rohit Sharma, PhD, Bhadra Pokharel, PhD, Vinod Kumar, PhD, Raghvendra Kumar, PhD.
Names: Sharma, Devendra Kumar, editor. | Sharma, Rohit (Assistant professor of electronics), editor. | Pokharel, Bhadra Prasad, editor. | Kumar, Vinod (Associate professor of electronics), editor. | Kumar, Raghvendra, 1987- editor.
Description: Includes bibliographical references and index.
Identifiers: Canadiana (print) 20200335014 | Canadiana (ebook) 2020033512X | ISBN 9781771888837 (hardcover) | ISBN 9781003006190 (ebook)
Subjects: LCSH: Antennas (Electronics) | LCSH: Signal processing. | LCSH: Microelectronics.
Classification: LCC TK7871.6 .A38 2021 | DDC 621.382/4—dc23

Library of Congress Cataloging-in-Publication Data

Names: Sharma, Devendra Kumar, editor. | Sharma, Rohit (Assistant professor of electronics), editor. | Pokharel, Bhadra Prasad, editor. | Kumar, Vinod (Associate professor of electronics), editor. | Kumar, Raghvendra, 1987- editor.
Title: Advances in antenna, signal processing, and microelectronics engineering / edited by Devendra Kumar Sharma, Rohit Sharma, Bhadra Pokharel, Vinod Kumar, Raghvendra Kumar.
Description: Palm Bay, FL : Apple Academic Press, 2021. | Includes bibliographical references and index. | Summary: "With the rapid growth of wireless communications, this book meets a strong demand for information and new research in the area of antenna, signal processing, and microelectronics engineering. Providing an interdisciplinary platform for discussing innovations, trends, and advances as well as the challenges encountered in this field, Advances in Antenna, Signal Processing, and Microelectronics Engineering brings together leading academicians, scientists, and researchers to share their knowledge and research in the area. The chapters in this volume address the functional framework in the area of antenna, signal processing, and microelectronics engineering and explore the concepts from the basic to advanced level. The diverse topics include estimation of diversity and muliple-input multiple-output parameters of multiple-element printed inverted F-antenna in the presence of the human body; the design of reversible combinational and sequential circuits using qualitative comparative analysis; the use of carbon-generated materials in new devices that interconnects technologies and nano-antennas in microelectronics; use of deep learning process for introducing the theoretical and practical aspects of cellular neural networks; monolithic microwave integrated circuit antennas; a new approach for deriving analytical models for front and back gate threshold voltages by solving Laplace and Poisson's equation in multilayer structure of FD SOI MOSFETs; robot navigation in incoherent environments; sensor architecture, and much more. Key features: Addresses the functional framework in the area of antenna, signal processing, and microelectronics engineering Explores the concepts from the basic to advanced level Covers the major challenges, issues, and advances in antennas, signal processing, and microelectronics engineering Explores optimization techniques for smart antenna and microelectronics for different applications Explores different materials and design techniques in the area of antennas and microelectronics"-- Provided by publisher.
Identifiers: LCCN 2020042151 (print) | LCCN 2020042152 (ebook) | ISBN 9781771888837 (hardcover) | ISBN 9781003006190 (ebook)
Subjects: MESH: Electronics, Medical--trends | Signal Processing, Computer-Assisted--instrumentation | Wireless Technology
Classification: LCC R855.3 (print) | LCC R855.3 (ebook) | NLM QT 36.2 | DDC 610.285--dc23
LC record available at https://lccn.loc.gov/2020042151
LC ebook record available at https://lccn.loc.gov/2020042152

ISBN: 978-1-77188-883-7 (hbk)
ISBN: 978-1-77463-784-5 (pbk)
ISBN: 978-1-00300-619-0 (ebk)

About the Editors

Devendra Kumar Sharma, PhD, is currently a Professor and Dean of the SRM Institute of Science and Technology, Delhi-NCR Campus, Ghaziabad, India. Dr. Sharma has authored many papers in reputed journals and conferences. His research interests are in VLSI interconnects, electronic circuits, digital design, testing, and signal processing. He is member of several professional bodies and is reviewer of many international journals and conferences. Dr Sharma has participated in many international and national conferences as session chair and as member of steering, advisory, and technical program committees. He received his BE degree in Electronics Engineering from M.N.R. Engineering College, Allahabad, his ME degree from the University of Roorkee, and his PhD from NIT Kurukshetra, India. He served PSU in different positions for more than eight years in Q.A. & Testing/R&D departments.

Rohit Sharma, PhD, is an Assistant Professor in the Department of Electronics and Communication Engineering at the SRM Institute of Science and Technology, Delhi–NCR Campus, Ghaziabad, India. He is an active member of many organizations, including the Indian Society for Technical Education (ISTE), IEEE, ICS, International Association of Engineers (IAENG), and International Association of Computer Science and Information Technology (IACSIT). He is an editorial board member and reviewer for more than eight international journals and conferences. He has published about over 35 research papers in international and national journals and about nine research papers at international and national conferences. Dr. Sharma has participated in many international and national conferences as session chair and as a member in the steering, advisory, or international program committees. He earned his PhD from Teerthanker Mahaveer University, Moradabad, India.

Bhadra Pokharel, PhD, currently works at the Materials Science and Engineering Program and Department of Physics, Pulchowk Campus, Institute of Engineering, Tribhuvan University, India. He is currently working on two research projects: 1. Phase Transition Behaviour in Ferroelectric Ceramics, and 2. Nano-porous Activated Carbon. He earned his PhD from Banaras Hindu University, School of Material & Technology, Varanasi, India.

Vinod Kumar, PhD, is an Associate Professor in the Department of Electronics and Communication Engineering at SRMIST, Ghaziabad, India. His research area of interest includes MOS sensors, plasma-processed materials and devices, photo detectors, thin film devices, organic field-effect transistor (OFET), etc. Dr Kumar has authored many journal papers that have been indexed in SCOPUS/SCI and in international conferences. Dr. Kumar has more than 21 years of experience in the field of teaching, research, and industry. He is a member of professional societies, including IEEE and the Indian Society for Technical Education (ISTE), and he is reviewer for many international journals and conferences. Dr Kumar has organized and participated in many international and national conferences as a member of the steering, advisory, or international program committees. He received his BE degree in Electronics Engineering from Y.C.C.E, Nagpur University, Nagpur, India. He received his MTech (Microelectronics) and his PhD degree from the Department of Electronics Engineering at the Indian Institute of Technology (BHU), Varanasi, India.

Raghvendra Kumar, PhD, is an Associate Professor in the Computer Science and Engineering Department at the Gandhi Institute of Engineering and Technology University (GIET), Gunupur, Odisha, India. He also serves as Director of the IT and Data Science Department at the Vietnam Center of Research in Economics, Management, Environment, Hanoi, Viet Nam. Dr. Kumar serves as editor of the book series Internet of Everything: Security and Privacy Paradigm (CRC Press/Taylor & Francis Group) and the book series Biomedical Engineering: Techniques and Applications (Apple Academic Press). He has published a number of research papers in international journals and conferences and authored and edited about 20 computer science books in field of Internet of Things, data mining, biomedical engineering, big data, robotics, graph theory, and Turing machines. He is the Managing Editor of the *International Journal of Machine Learning and Networked Collaborative Engineering* and also served as a guest editor for many special issues of reputed journals. He received a best paper award at the IEEE Conference 2013 and Young Achiever Award–2016 by IEAE Association for his research work in the field of distributed database. Dr Kumar has been active in many roles for international and national conferences, including organizing chair, volume editor, publication chair, keynote speaker, session chair or co-chair, publicity chair, advisory board member, and technical program committee member. His research areas are computer science-cloud computing, big data and database, security and privacy, multimedia system, machine learning, computational intelligence, and image processing.

Dr Kumar received his BTech in Computer Science and Engineering from SRM University Chennai (Tamil Nadu), India, his MTech in Computer Science and Engineering from KIIT University, Bhubaneswar, (Odisha) India, and his PhD in Computer Science and Engineering from Jodhpur National University, Jodhpur (Rajasthan), India.

Contents

Contributors .... *xi*

Abbreviations .... *xiii*

Preface .... *xvii*

1. **Estimation of Diversity and MIMO Parameters of Multiple Planar-Inverted F-Antenna in the Presence of Users' Body** 1
   Hari Shankar Singh

2. **Reversible Logic Design Using QCA: Challenges and Future Aspects** 31
   Rupali Singh, and Devendra Kumar Sharma

3. **An Introduction to a New Era of Microelectronics Devices and Interconnects** 61
   Vangmayee Sharda

4. **Deep CNN Framework for Classification and Feature Extraction** 83
   Shivkaran Ravidas, and M. A. Ansari

5. **Prospects of MMIC Antennas** 99
   Satya Sai Srikant, Saptarshi Gupta, and Atul Kumar Pandey

6. **A 3D Analytic Modeling of Threshold Voltages of FD SOI MOSFET** 121
   Krishna Meel, Ram Gopal, and Deepak Bhatnagar

7. **Fuzzy-Based Stratagem for Teleoperation of Robots in Incoherent Environments** 149
   Sriparna Saha, Rimita Lahiri, and Amit Konar

8. **Sensor Architecture, Coverage, and Connectivity: A Comprehensive Study** 185
   Sushree B. B. Priyadarshini, D. Singh, and R. Sharma

9. **Smart Antennas for Contemporary Wireless Communication Systems: Concepts, Challenges, and Performance** 205
   Garima Srivastava, Neeta Singh, and Sachin Kumar

10. Introduction to Metamaterials 221
   Ragini Sharma, Vandana Niranjan, and Vibhav K. Sachan

Index 241

Contributors

M. A. Ansari
Department of Electrical Engineering, School of Engineering, Gautam Buddha University, Greater Noida, Uttar Pradesh, India

Deepak Bhatnagar
Department of Physics, University of Rajasthan, Jaipur, Rajasthan, India

Ram Gopal
CSIR—Central Electronics Engineering Research Institute, Pilani, Rajasthan, India

Saptarshi Gupta
SRM Institute of Science and Technology, Modinagar, Uttar Pradesh, India

Amit Konar
Department of Electronics and Telecommunication Engineering, Jadavpur University, West Bengal, India

Sachin Kumar
School of Electronics Engineering, Kyungpook National University, Daegu, Republic of Korea

Rimita Lahiri
Department of Electronics and Telecommunication Engineering, Jadavpur University, India

Krishna Meel
Department of Science and Humanities, BK Birla Institute of Engineering and Technology, Pilani, Rajasthan, India

Vandana Niranjan
Indira Gandhi Delhi Technical University for Women, Delhi, India

Atul Kumar Pandey
DRDO-SSPL, Delhi, India

Sushree B. B. Priyadarshini
Department of Computer Science and Information Technology, Institute of Technical Education and Research, Siksha 'O' Anusandhan (Deemed to be University), Bhubaneswar, Odisha, India

Shivkaran Ravidas
Department of Electrical Engineering, School of Engineering, Gautam Buddha University, Greater Noida, Uttar Pradesh, India

Vibhav K. Sachan
KIET Group of Institutions, Ghaziabad, Uttar Pradesh, India

Sriparna Saha
Department of Computer Science and Engineering, Maulana Abul Kalam Azad University of Technology, West Bengal, India

Vangmayee Sharda
Amity University, Uttar Pradesh, India

Devendra Kumar Sharma
Department of Electronics and Communication Engineering, SRM Institute of Science and Technology, Ghaziabad, Uttar Pradesh, India

Ragini Sharma
KIET Group of Institutions, Ghaziabad, Uttar Pradesh, India

R. Sharma
Department of Electronics and Communication Engineering, SRM University, NCR Campus, Ghaziabad, Uttar Pradesh, India

D. Singh
Department of Computer Science and Information Technology, Institute of Technical Education and Research, Siksha 'O' Anusandhan (Deemed to be University), Bhubaneswar, Odisha, India

Hari Shankar Singh
Department of Electronics and Communication Engineering, Thapar Institute of Engineering and Technology, Patiala 147 001, Punjab, India

Neeta Singh
Department of Electronics and Communication Engineering, Ambedkar Institute of Advanced Communication Technologies and Research, Delhi, India

Rupali Singh
Department of Electronics and Communication Engineering, SRM Institute of Science and Technology, Ghaziabad, Uttar Pradesh, India

Satya Sai Srikant
SRM Institute of Science and Technology, Modinagar, Uttar Pradesh, India

Garima Srivastava
Department of Electronics and Communication Engineering,
Ambedkar Institute of Advanced Communication Technologies and Research, Delhi, India

Abbreviations

ADG	apparent diversity gain
ALUs	arithmetic and logic units
ANN	artificial neural network
BS	base station
BCB	benzocyclobutene
BSIM	Berkeley short-channel IGFET Model
BDS	binary disk sensing
BOR	body of revolution
CLS	capacitance-loaded strip
CNTFET	carbon nanotube FET
CNTs	carbon nanotubes
CTIA	Cellular Telecommunications Industry Association
CP	central point
CH	cluster head
CDMA	code division multiple access
CMOS	complementary metal–oxide–semiconductor
CST MWS	computer simulation technology microwave studio
CNNs	convolutional neural networks
CPW	coplanar waveguide
CD	critical difference
CPR	cross-polarization ratio
DoF	depth of field
DSP	digital signal processing
DOA	direction of arrival
DCA-SC	Distributed Collaborative Camera Actuation based on Scalar Count
DNG	double-negative
DPS	double-positive
DA	drive with acceleration
DKCS	dynamic k-coverage scheduling scheme
EDG	effective diversity gain
EiRP	effective isotropic radiated power
EM	electromagnetic
ED	ensemble decision tree

ECG	envelope correlation coefficient
ENG	epsilon negative
EB	event boundary
XOR	eXclusive OR
FCC	Federal Communications Commission
FoV	field of view
FIR	finite impulse response
FD	fully depleted
GAAFET	gate-all-around FET
GNR	graphene nanoribbon
GNR SBFET	graphene nanoribbon Schottky barrier FET
IR	infrared
ICs	integrated circuits
kNN	k-nearest neighbor
LHM	left-handed metamaterial
LMA-NN	Levenberg–Marquardt algorithm induced neural network
LMF	lower membership function
MEG	mean effective gain
MOSFETs	metal–oxide–semiconductor field-effect transistors
MIC	microwave integrated circuits
MMIC	monolithic microwave integrated circuit
MLP	multilayer perceptron
MIMO	multiple-input multiple-output
ME	multiplexing efficiency
MWCNT	multiwalled carbon nanotube
MNG	Mu-negative
PDA	personal digital assistant
PIFA	planar inverted-F antenna
PCB	printed circuit board
PMOS	p-type metal-oxide semiconductor
QoS	quality of service
QCA	quantum-dot cellular automata
RF	radio frequency
ROC	receiver operating curves
RCs	redundancy cells
RHM	right-handed materials
ROS	robot operating system
SPLSR	SAR to peak location spacing ratio
SC	scalar count

SP	scalar premiere
SISO	serial in serial out
SNR	signal-to-noise ratio
SOI	silicon-on-insulator
SET	single-electron transistor
SIMO	single-input and multiple-output
SWCNT	single-walled carbon nanotube
SDK	software development kit
SDMA	spatial division multiple access
SAR	specific absorption rate
SRR	split ring resonator
SWR	standing wave ratio
SVM	support vector machine
TW	thin wire
TDMA	time division multiple access
TRP	total radiated power
TE	transverse electric
TEM	transverse electromagnetic
TM	transverse magnetic
TEFT	tunnel field effect transistor
ULSI	ultra large-scale integration
UMF	upper membership function
VLSI	very large-scale integration
VSWR	voltage standing wave ratio
WSN	wireless sensor network
WN	working node

Preface

This book brings together leading academicians, scientists, and researchers to exchange and share their ideas and research in the area of antennas, signal processing, and microelectronics engineering. It also provides an interdisciplinary platform for researchers, practitioners, and educators to present and discuss the innovations, trends, and concerns, as well as the challenges encountered in the specified and related domain.

ORGANIZATION OF THE BOOK

The book is organized into 10 chapters. A brief description of each of the chapters follows.

Chapter 1 carried out the estimation of "diversity and MIMO parameters" of multiple-element printed inverted F-antennas in the presence of the human body. In this chapter, the diversity parameters such as MEG, ECC, and EDG for multiple-element printed inverted F-antennas are explored.

Chapter 2 focuses on the major aspects of reversible quantum circuits, including basic to the complex structures with their comprehensive analyses. This chapter targets the design of reversible combinational and sequential circuits using QCA.

Chapter 3 deals with the use of carbon-generated materials to introduce new devices, interconnects technologies, and nanoantenna in microelectronics. This chapter also addresses the different interconnect technologies that would allow the rapid transmission of information.

Chapter 4 presents the use of the deep learning process for introducing the theoretical and practical aspects of CNNs. It is pointed out that profound CNNs can be utilized for classification as well as for object detection and can also be extended for face detection and face recognition.

Chapter 5 investigates the development of various MMIC antennas and their interface with the active microwave circuit components for millimeter and submillimeter wave applications.

Chapter 6 presents a new approach for deriving analytical models for front- and back-gate threshold voltages by solving Laplace and Poisson's equations in a multilayer structure of FD SOI MOSFETs.

Chapter 7 deals with a novel purpose of robot navigation in incoherent environments, which are inaccessible to human beings. In this chapter, the authors proposed a system that has propitious potential for upcoming applications of robot maneuvers based on well-accepted performance metrics.

Chapter 8 discusses various concepts of smart sensors such as area coverage, barrier coverage, point coverage, target coverage, and k-coverage. In particular, the chapter also identifies the ambient energy harvesting process that utilizes the energy from the environment such as solar, thermal, and RF energy.

Chapter 9 describes the main functions of smart antennas such as the beam forming and direction of arrival estimation. This chapter also presents the applications of smart antennas for satellite, radars, acoustic signal processing, cellular systems, and GPS/Wi-Fi/WLAN/Wi-MAX.

Chapter 10 illustrates the history, basic concepts, and applications of metamaterials. This chapter also describes the simulation, characterization, incorporation and fabrication of metamaterials with the help of several examples.

—**Devendra Kumar Sharma**
Rohit Sharma
Bhadra Pokharel
Vinod Kumar
Raghvendra Kumar

CHAPTER 1

Estimation of Diversity and MIMO Parameters of Multiple Planar-Inverted F-Antenna in the Presence of Users' Body

HARI SHANKAR SINGH

Department of Electronics and Communication Engineering, Thapar Institute of Engineering and Technology, Patiala 147001, Punjab, India

ABSTARCT

In this chapter, the estimation of diversity and multiple-input multiple-output (MIMO) parameters is carried out in the presence of the users' body. The diversity parameters such as mean effective gain, envelope correlation coefficient, and effective diversity gain are calculated. Further, MIMO parameters such as channel capacity and multiplexing efficiency are also estimated in a mobile environment and human body. The design of the antenna is considered from the published article of the same author. Mainly, the antenna is designed for MIMO applications, and study has been carried out in the free space only. The published antenna design cannot be applicable on the real-time platform until and unless its diversity and MIMO parameters should follow the defined criteria of the Cellular Telecommunications Industry Association (CTIA). In this study, three common user modes of the mobile phone are taken named as "specific anthropomorphic mannequin head and personal digital assistant (PDA) hand (voice position)," "PDA hand (data position)," and "dual hands (read position)." The estimation of diversity and MIMO parameters is done for three different user positions. All the parameters are estimated by positioning the antenna at the top and bottom of a printed circuit board (PCB). This study was carried out to check the optimum location of the antennas on the mobile phone PCB. Moreover, the specific absorption rate (SAR) will be a crucial parameter when we consider the case of a mobile phone. Therefore, the designed antenna should follow the guidelines of the SAR limit on the actual platform. Hence, in this chapter, the calculation of

SAR for the proposed antenna is carried out and tabulated. In the case of a MIMO antenna, SAR of one antenna may affect the SAR of another antenna. Therefore, SAR of a MIMO antenna can be estimated in terms of SAR to peak location spacing ratio, and it should be less than 0.3 according to the Federal Communications Commission. Furthermore, the amount of power loss plays a vital role in the close proximity of human body to estimate the performance of the MIMO antenna. Therefore, the parameters, that is, total radiated power and power loss are also estimated in the user's body. Based on the above study and estimated parameters, it can be concluded that the designed antenna will be suitable for the real-time application because all the estimated parameters should follow the critical standard limit of CTIA.

1.1 INTRODUCTION

Nowadays, there is a growing demand for high-speed communication in mobile phones. Moreover, public demands a high degree of quality along with high-speed data transmission and reception that driving the force in the rapid development of wireless technology. The high quality of services includes good audio/video communication, high-speed data transmission and reception, reduction in multipath fading, and most importantly, better user proximity performances. The installation of multiple-input multiple-output (MIMO) systems can provide the solution of data speed and quality of communication [1]. However, the performances of multi-antenna systems in a compact device may change due to the nearby components and user's body. The antenna network parameters and the radiation parameters may change due to the proximity environment. In addition to the performance of the antenna, the diversity and parameters of MIMO antenna systems may also vary due to the proximity environment. Therefore, the fixed boundaries of space and positing of multi-antenna systems in a mobile phone are a big challenge for antenna developers to restrict the interaction of antenna systems with proximity components. Moreover, the additional challenges are to maintain the diversity and MIMO performances of multi-antenna systems when the mobile phone will be placed in the user proximity [2–4]. Lots of research have been carried out over the diversity and MIMO parameters in the presence of user proximity [5–11]. Zervos et al. [5] in 2004 investigated about the radiation efficiency of antenna, which is installed inside a mobile handset. In this study, the theoretical results are compared with the measured one. Thereafter, work is carried out by Villanen et al. [6] in 2006, which is concentrated on to reduce the size of the mobile antenna by creating the radiation of the currents on the mobile phone chassis. In 2008, Okada et al.

[7] investigated an unbalanced fed dipole antenna, and Huan et al. [8], in 2009, investigated antenna performance in the presence of a human hand. Soon after, in 2011, Ilvonen et al. [9] performed the systematic investigation of the size and location of an antenna on the ground plane in the user proximity. In this study, the size of the antenna and their location on the ground plane are studied in the presence of a user's hand phantom. Just after a year, in 2012, Montaser et al. [10] investigated a mobile handset planar inverted-F antenna (PIFA) array by putting close to the head and hand phantom at the 1.9 GHz band. Furthermore, Shi et al. [11], in 2014, evaluated a method to compare the obtained specific absorption rate (SAR) from four different antenna package. In this study, antenna performance is noted in the presence of a human tissue. In all the above literature, the discussion has been carried out over a single antenna installed within mobile handsets. However, in the recent days, the expectations in terms of the quality of services cannot meet with the single antenna element. Therefore, multi-antenna technology is required to enhance the quality of services. However, the interaction of the user's body with multi-antenna systems degrades the diversity and MIMO performance. Some of the studies have been done so far over multi-antenna elements in the presence of human body [12–19]. Plicanic et al. [12–13], in 2008 and 2009, investigated the performance of a multifunctional diversity antenna by putting near to the hand and head phantom. In their study, a single fixed position of antenna systems over a mobile phone's printed circuit board (PCB) was taken for investigation. Similarly, Buskgaard et al. [14] discussed the diversity performance of an antenna in the user proximity. Moreover, Zhang et al. [15], in 2013, illustrated an adaptive method to investigate the performance of multi-antenna systems in human body vicinity. Thereafter, Singh et al. [16–19] investigated the network and radiation parameters of multiple antenna elements in the mobile environment and user proximity. Moreover, the performance of an antenna was also analyzed by pasting the antenna top and bottom of a mobile phone's PCB. In view of the above discussion, the estimation of diversity and channel performance of the multiple antenna elements in the user proximity is still a scope of discussion.

In this chapter, the MIMO and diversity parameters are calculated in the presence of the mobile phone and user's body. In this study, three common user cases of the mobile phone are considered named, respectively, as voice position, data position, and read position. The estimation of the diversity and MIMO parameters is done for three different common user modes. All the parameters are calculated for the top and bottom located antenna elements. Moreover, SAR is estimated in accordance with the Federal Communications Commission (FCC) and European standards. However, in the case of the MIMO antenna, SAR of one antenna may affect the SAR of another antenna. Therefore, SAR of the MIMO antenna is estimated in terms of SAR to peak location spacing ratio (SPLSR) and found less than 0.3, which satisfies the criteria of FCC. Moreover, in the proximity of mobile phone and human body, total radiated power (TRP) and loss of power (in dBm) are also estimated and found within the operational limit. All the modeling and setup for simulations have been done in the finite integration numerical technique-based computer simulation technology microwave studio (CST MWS).

1.2 FREE SPACE AND USER PROXIMITY SIMULATION SETUP

The design of the antenna is considered from [20]. The antenna covers 1740–1885 MHz and 3250–3805 MHz frequency bands. The application platform of the designed antenna is GSM1800 and WiMAX for mobile terminals. PIFAs are placed back to back on the PCB. Each element is constructed with L- and J-shaped slots. The details of antenna in free space are given in [20].

All the investigations have been carried out in the free space, although the analysis of the antenna in the presence of the user proximity, that is, the mobile phone configuration and human body is equally important. Therefore, the mobile phone configurations such as liquid crystal display, connectors, battery, buttons, speaker, plastic body housing, camera, and microphones are created in the vicinity of the designed antenna. The antenna design along with mobile phone components is shown in Figure 1.1. In the simulations, major components of the mobile phones considered are metal. The mobile housing is considered a plastic box. The mobile phone is covered inside a plastic box made up of a material with a dielectric constant of 3, a loss tangent of 0.06, and a conductivity of 0.24 S/m. Moreover, the actual scenario of the user proximity will be presented once the mobile handset is integrated with the human body. The user proximity consists of a designed antenna, mobile handset configurations, and a human body. Mobile phone consumers use their phones in different ways, that is, voice position, data position, and read position. In the data position, only the personal digital assistant (PDA) hand phantom is used to hold the mobile phone, whereas in the voice position, hand phantom along with human head (specific anthropomorphic mannequin head) is used. In the voice position, the mobile phone is held near the human head phantom at the distance of ~5 mm from human cheeks to maintain the criteria defined by the Cellular Telecommunications Industry Association (CTIA) [21]. However, the read position uses the dual hand phantom to hold the handset. The diversity parameters are estimated in three different user proximity scenarios, that is, voice position, data position, and read

Estimation of Diversity and MIMO Parameters 5

position, by keeping the antenna at the top and bottom locations of the PCB. The simulation setup of the user proximity is designed in CST MWS. The holding rule of the mobile handset by the user is considered according to the CTIA standard. Moreover, in general practice of voice position, human uses either the left or the right hand to hold the mobile handset. In view of this, antenna elements of MIMO systems will not be symmetrical with respect to the human hand in proximity to the head. In the simulation, the setup is created by considering the right hand of the human to hold the mobile phone because most users use their right hands only. However, the same scenario will be applicable to the left-hand holding position. In addition to the holding of the mobile phone by the hand phantom, the placement near the human head is very important. In the voice position, the distance between the head phantom to hold the mobile phone is nearly 5 mm. The voice position user proximity is shown in Figure 1.2(a). Further, data position is the same as voice position, except the absence of the human head phantom in the former. In the data position, the head phantom is not considered in the simulation; rest all scenarios are the same as those in the voice position. The data position user proximity is shown in Figure 1.2(b). Furthermore, there is no specific rule to hold the mobile phone in the read position (dual hand). In

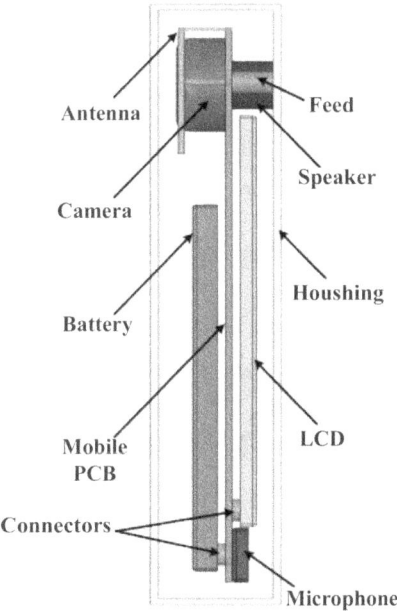

FIGURE 1.1 Mobile phone configuration with designed PIFA.

the simulation, the left- and right-hand phantom is used to hold the phone. The read position user proximity is shown in Figure 1.2(c).

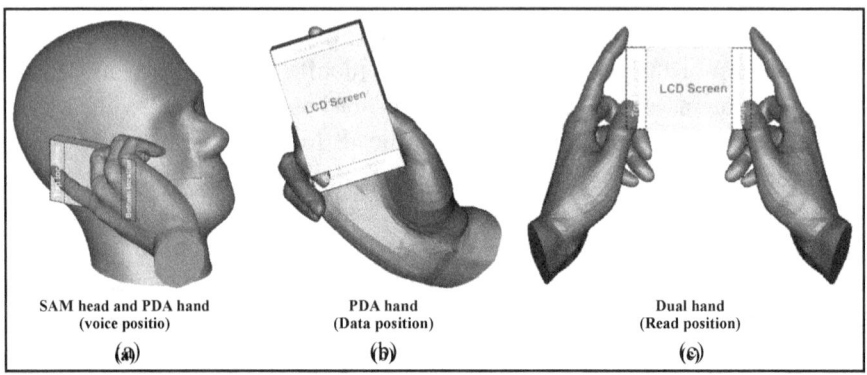

FIGURE 1.2 (A) Voice position, (B) data position, and (C) read position.

In the simulations, the human body phantom is considered as layers of dielectric materials. The human head is modeled as a homogeneous layer of fluid and shells. The fluids are the inner layer, whereas the shells are the outer layer, that is, the fluid is confined within the shells. Moreover, the hand phantom is considered as a single layer of dielectric materials. The permittivity and conductivity of the material used in a human body phantom are given in [22]. The dielectric constant of the head phantom (fluids and shells) and hand phantom are tabulated in Table 1.1.

TABLE 1.1 Dielectric Constant of a Human Head and Hand

User's Body	Tissues	Frequency (MHz)	Permittivity (ε_r)	Conductivity (σ)
Head phantom	Shells	1800 and 3500	3.69	0.00165
	Fluids	1800	41.5	0.97
		3500	38.5	1.8
Hand phantom		1800	32.6	1.26
		3500	29.8	1.79

1.3 SIMULATION RESULTS AND ANALYSIS

CST MWS is used for design, simulation, and optimization of an antenna. The free space and user proximity analysis are carried out to estimate the diversity and MIMO parameters of an antenna. Further, TRP and SAR are estimated to investigate the suitability of the antenna on a real-time platform. In this section, all the results are presented and discussed.

1.3.1 EFFECT OF MOBILE ENVIRONMENT AND USER PROXIMITY ON S-PARAMETERS

The designed antenna covers the 1740–1885 MHz and 3250–3805 MHz frequency bands. The antenna can be deployed on the real-time platform for GSM1800 and WiMAX. Further, to check the robustness of a design antenna, the actual scenario of a mobile phone along with the mode of operation (voice, data, and read) of the phone needs to be created. Figure 1.3 shows the variation of the reflection coefficient in a mobile environment and human body. It is observed that the effect of the nearby proximity (mobile phone components and human body) is insignificant. In the case of a mobile environment, the reflection coefficient is closely matched with free space, which means that the designed antenna provides the same operating frequency band as in the free space. Moreover, the reflection coefficient for the top located antenna is still stable if it is put near the human body as shown in Figure 1.3(a). The good impedance matching and the stable reflection coefficient of the MIMO antenna in the proximity of the end user will provide a better result on the actual platform.

Moreover, the reflection coefficient of the designed antenna is also tested by keeping the PIFA at the bottom of the PCB. Figure 1.3(b) shows the variation of the reflection coefficient when the antenna is positioned at the bottom of the PCB. The variation of the reflection coefficient is slightly higher than the top-located PIFA because the larger area of the antenna is covered by the human hand phantom. However, the antenna operates over the desired frequency bands based on the -6 dB reflection coefficient in the presence of a human body.

1.3.2 DIVERSITY PARAMETER ESTIMATION

In this section, diversity parameters, that is, the mean effective gain (MEG), envelope correlation coefficient (ECC), and effective diversity gain (EDG) are estimated in the actual scenario of a mobile phone (mobile phone components) and user's body. All the diversity parameters are calculated using CST MWS. In the case of mobile communication, highly faded signals are received at the terminal. Therefore, the multiple antennas will be used either in the diversity mode or in the MIMO mode based on the signal-to-noise ratio (SNR) strength [15]. In the fading environment, if SNR is high, the high data rate can be achieved by selecting the MIMO mode. Then relevant MIMO parameters are estimated. Moreover, if the faded environment is having a low SNR, then the diversity mode will be selected to achieve a high speed of data transfer. In this case, diversity parameters will be evaluated.

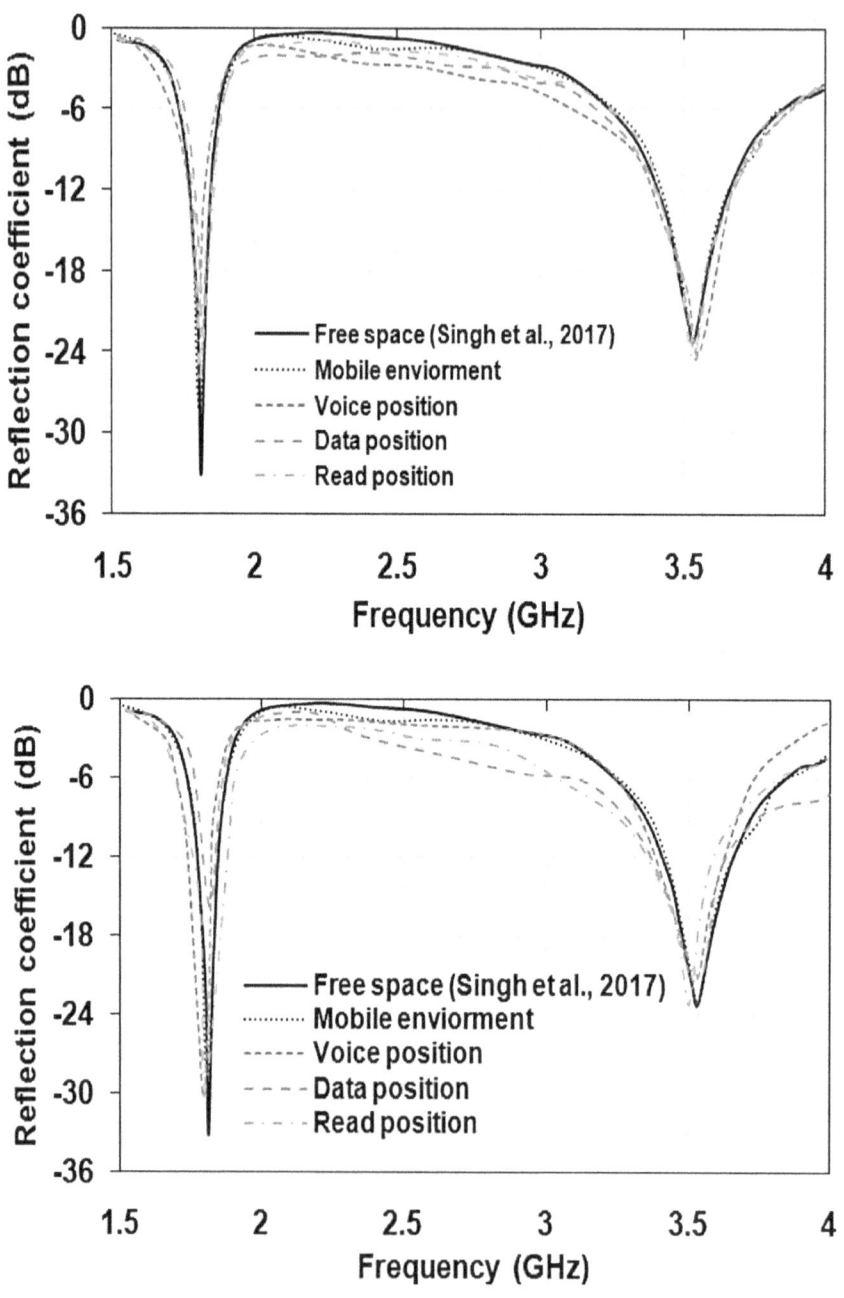

FIGURE 1.3 Effect of the mobile environment and human body on the reflection coefficient for (A) top-located MIMO and (B) bottom-located MIMO.

Estimation of Diversity and MIMO Parameters

Since we have assumed the case of mobile phone communication, we need to estimate diversity and MIMO parameters one by one in free space along with the user proximity.

1.3.2.1 MEAN EFFECTIVE GAIN

MEG is one of the diversity parameters in the fading environment which is defined as the ratio of the mean received power from a random route to the total mean incident power to the antenna. It is defined as [23]

$$MEG = \int_0^{2\pi}\int_0^{\pi}\left[\frac{XPR}{1+XPR}G_\theta(\theta,\phi)P\theta(\theta,\phi)+\frac{1}{1+XPR}G_\phi(\theta,\phi)P\phi(\theta,\phi)\right]\sin\theta\,d\theta\,d\phi \quad (1.1)$$

where XPR is the ratio of horizontal to vertical power (cross-polarization ratio), G_θ and G_ϕ are the θ-direction power gain and ϕ-direction power gain, respectively, and P_θ and P_ϕ are the θ-direction and ϕ-direction angular density functions of incident power, respectively. In the case of a mobile phone, the user movement will be randomly in the given area; therefore, the incoming signal at the user end can arise from any direction in the azimuth plane with an equal probability. While in the case of the elevation direction, we cannot predict such scenario. In such cases, several models have been given to predict the power in the θ-direction and ϕ-direction [24, 25]. Since the angular power density can be changed due to the nearby environment of the mobile user, different statistical models and their parameters can be considered according to the indoor, outdoor, and isotropic environments [26]. The distribution of the angular power density function (P_θ and P_ϕ) is assumed as the Gaussian in the elevation and azimuth directions, respectively, which is given as

$$P_\theta(\theta,\phi) = A_\theta \exp\left[\frac{-\left\{\theta-\left(\frac{\pi}{2}-m_v\right)\right\}^2}{2\sigma_v^2}\right], (0 \leq \theta \leq \pi) \quad (1.2)$$

$$P_\phi(\theta,\phi) = A_\phi \exp\left[\frac{-\left\{\theta-\left(\frac{\pi}{2}-m_H\right)\right\}^2}{2\sigma_H^2}\right], (0 \leq \theta \leq \pi) \quad (1.3)$$

where m_v and m_H are the mean elevation angles from the vertical and horizontal directions, respectively; σ_v and σ_H are the standard deviations of the

θ-direction and ϕ-direction wave distributions, respectively. Moreover, the constants A_θ and A_ϕ are calculated as

$$\int_0^{2\pi}\int_0^\pi P_\theta(\theta,\phi)\sin\theta d\theta d\phi = \int_0^{2\pi}\int_0^\pi P\phi(\theta,\phi)\sin\theta d\theta d\phi = 1 \qquad (1.4)$$

XPR is considered as 10 dB for the indoor environment, 1 dB for the outdoor environment, and 0 dB for the isotropic environment. To calculate the MEG in a different environment of user proximity, that is, mobile environment, voice position, data position, read position along with free space, the mean elevation angles $m_v = 10°$, $m_H = 10°$, and the standard deviations $\sigma_v = 15°$ and $\sigma_H = 15°$ are considered. The calculated values of MEG are given in Table 1.2. It is noted that the calculated values of MEG of free space are less than the user proximity. The MEGs of top-located PIFAs are higher than that of the bottom-located PIFAs. Moreover, the MEGs of the mobile phone are slightly higher than that in the presence of the human body. It is noticed that when PIFAs are placed at the top location of the mobile phone PCB, the maximum drop values in the MEGs are 8 dBi, 9 dBi, and 6 dBi in the indoor environment (XPR = 10 dB), outdoor environment (XPR = 1 dB), and isotropic environment (XPR = 0 dB), respectively, at 1.8 GHz, whereas the maximum drop values in MEGs are approximately 7 dBi, 6 dBi, and 5 dBi in the indoor environment, outdoor environment, and isotropic environment, respectively, at 3.5 GHz. However, the ratio of MEGs in the different faded scenario and the user proximity environment is near unity, which fulfilled the criteria of the MIMO system. Further, for the bottom-located PIFAs at PCB, the maximum drop values of MEG are approximately 8 dBi, 8 dBi, and 7 dBi in the indoor environment, outdoor environment, and isotropic environment, respectively, at 1.8 GHz, whereas at 3.5 GHz, the maximum drop values are 7 dBi, 6 dBi, and 5 dBi in the indoor environment, outdoor environment, and isotropic environment, respectively. However, the ratio of MEG-1 and MEG-2 at a different frequency and in a different user proximity is close to unity, which met the condition of MIMO systems to make the robust communication in the fading environment.

1.3.2.2 ENVELOPE CORRELATION COEFFICIENT

The approach to calculate the ECC will be based on either S-parameter data or far-field data. However, the S-parameter-based method includes some assumptions such as the antenna systems must be lossless; only one port of the multi-antenna systems is fed, whereas the other port will be matched terminated with 50 Ω; and there must not be any fading environment (only a

TABLE 1.2 Calculated MEGs for Different XPRs in Different User Proximity

Frequency (GHz)	User Proximity	Indoor		Outdoor		Isotropic	
		MEG-1 (dBi)	MEG-2 (dBi)	MEG-1 (dBi)	MEG-2 (dBi)	MEG-1 (dBi)	MEG-2 (dBi)
PIFAs at the Top Location of the PCB							
1.8	Free space	−12.5	−12.5	−10.6	−10.6	−8.9	−8.9
	Mobile phone	−9.4	−9.4	−7.4	−7.4	−6.2	−6.2
	Voice position	−8.01	−7.9	−6.04	−6.04	−5.02	−5.02
	Data position	−6.4	−6.09	−4.18	−4.21	−3.94	−4.01
	Read position	−4.1	−3.98	−3.01	−3.5	−1.89	−1.56
3.5	Free space	−10.02	−10.02	−8.61	−8.61	−7.52	−7.52
	Mobile phone	−8.65	−8.65	−9.69	−9.74	−5.47	−5.88
	Voice position	−6.49	−5.99	−6.01	−5.99	−3.26	−3.26
	Data position	−4.87	−5.01	−3.16	−3.16	−2.01	−2.18
	Read position	−3.01	−3.01	−2.15	−2.61	−1.89	−2.01
PIFAs at the Bottom Location of the PCB							
1.8	Free space	−12.5	−12.5	−10.6	−10.6	−8.9	−8.9
	Mobile phone	−8.31	−8.95	−6.24	−6.32	−5.61	−5.99
	Voice position	−6.62	−6.02	−5.97	−6.02	−4.16	−4.01
	Data position	−5.01	−5.99	−4.03	−3.99	−3.47	−3.01
	Read position	−4.87	−4.01	−2.89	−3.01	−1.02	−1.66
3.5	Free space	−9.21	−9.21	−8.12	−8.01	−6.49	−6.88
	Mobile phone	−7.42	−7.42	−6.45	−6.95	−4.58	−4.05
	Voice position	−5.31	−5.02	−4.83	−4.99	−3.61	−3.01
	Data position	−3.12	−3.61	−3.03	−2.95	−1.94	−1.89
	Read position	−2.89	−2.15	−2.62	−2.01	−1.05	−1.52

uniform scattering environment). The empirical formula of the ECC in terms of S-parameters is given by [27]

$$\rho_e = \frac{\left|S_{11}^* S_{12} + S_{21}^* S_{22}\right|^2}{\left(1-\left(\left|S_{11}^2\right|+\left|S_{21}^2\right|\right)\right)\left(1-\left(\left|S_{22}^2\right|+\left|S_{12}^2\right|\right)\right)} \quad (1.5)$$

In the multipath fading environment, uniform scattering uniform cannot be predicted. Moreover, the practical antenna structure will not be predicted as a completely lossless structure. Therefore, two assumptions out of three did not satisfy by the above equation. Hence, this equation failed to estimate the accurate ECC in the actual scenario of the mobile phone. Therefore, an alternate way to calculate the ECC is the far-field data approach. The ECC (ρ_e) is calculated using far-field data in terms of complex cross-correlation (ρ_c)

$$\rho_e \approx \left|\rho_c\right|^2 \quad (1.6)$$

Moreover, the complex cross-correlation (ρ_c) is calculated in terms of field patterns [28], which is given by

$$\rho_c = \frac{\int_0^{2\pi} A_{12}(\phi) d\phi}{\left[\int_0^{2\pi} A_{11}(\phi) d\phi \int_0^{2\pi} A_{22}(\phi) d\phi\right]^{1/2}} \quad (1.7)$$

where $A_{pq}(\phi) = XPR * E_{\theta p}\left(\frac{\pi}{2},\phi\right) E_{\theta q}^*\left(\frac{\pi}{2},\phi\right) + E_{\phi p}\left(\frac{\pi}{2},\phi\right) E_{\phi q}^*\left(\frac{\pi}{2},\phi\right)$ and $\bar{E}_p(\theta,\phi)$ $= E_{\theta p}(\theta,\phi)\hat{\theta} + E_{\phi p}(\theta,\phi)\hat{\phi}$ are the field patterns of the antenna, where p and $q = 1$ and 2.

The calculated values of ECC in the presence of the mobile environment and the human body for the top- and bottom-located PIFA over PCB are given in Figures 1.4(a) and (b). It is observed that the ECC for the bottom-located antenna is higher than that for the top-located multi-element PIFA. Since the area covered by the human body for the bottom-placed antenna is more, reflection occurred heavily. The received reflected wave provides a high correlation factor result in high ECC achieved for the bottom position of the antenna.

In the read mode, hands of the mobile phone user located symmetrically for the top- and bottom-located multi-element systems; therefore, ECC is approximately the same in this case. However, calculated values of ECC are well below the standard limit of 0.5. To avoid the signal degradation, the antenna is placed either at the top or bottom location of PCB.

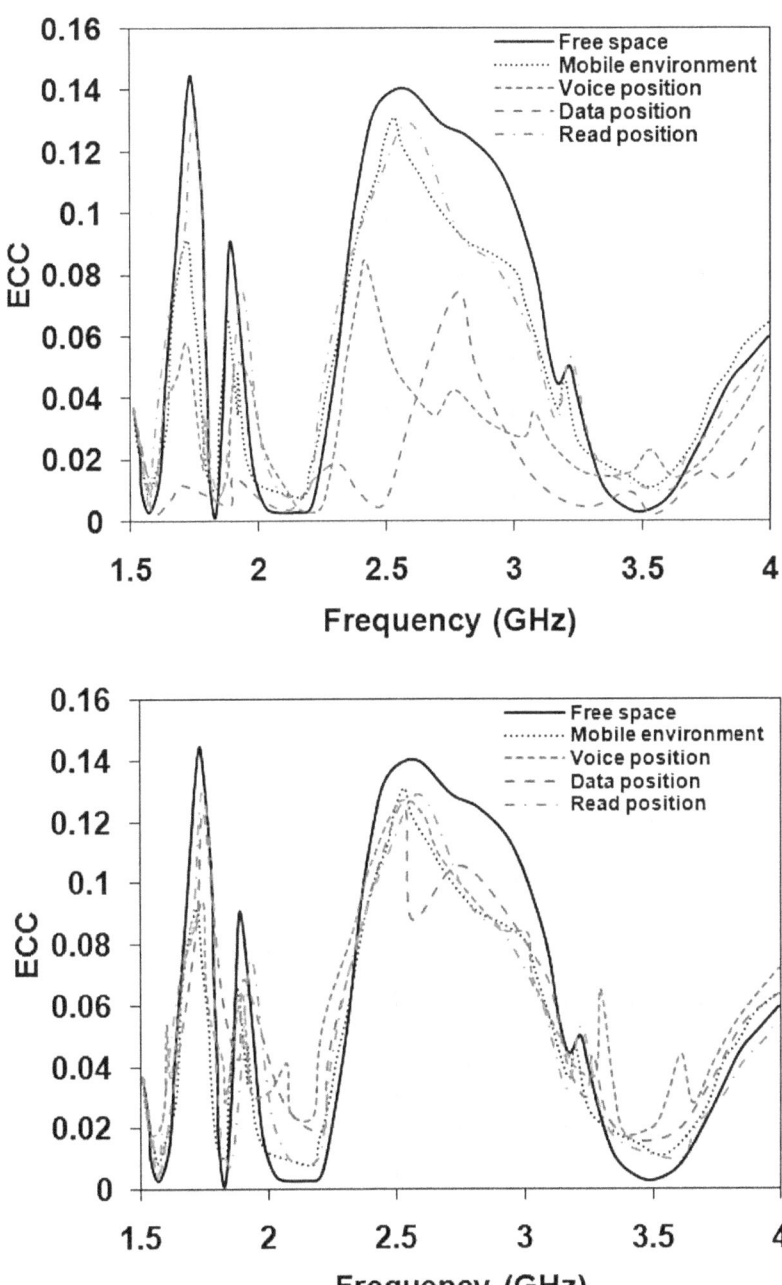

FIGURE 1.4 ECC vs. frequency in a mobile environment and human body for (A) top-located MIMO and (B) bottom-located MIMO.

1.3.2.3 EFFECTIVE DIVERSITY GAIN

Furthermore, one more important diversity parameter, that is, EDG is required to investigate. EDG is obtained by the multiplication of the apparent diversity gain (ADG) and total antenna efficiency. However, ADG (G_{app}) is defined in terms of the correlation coefficient, which is given by [29]

$$G_{app} = 10^*_{e\rho} \qquad (1.8)$$

In Equation (1.8), factor 10 indicates that ADG is maximum if the probability of selection will be 1% and e_ρ is the correlation factor that reduces ADG. e_ρ is written as [29]

$$e_\rho = \sqrt{1-|\rho_e|^2}$$

The effectiveness of diversity is calculated using EDG which is obtained by multiplying ADG and total antenna efficiency. The total efficiency accounted mismatch losses due to the mismatching between the coaxial probe and antenna, dielectric losses, and conduction or ohmic losses. The mathematical formula of the total antenna efficiency is given by [30]

$$\eta_{total} = \eta_{rad}\left(1-|S_{11}|^2-|S_{21}|^2\right) \qquad (1.9)$$

And EDG is given by

$$EDG\left(G_{effective}\right) = G_{app} \times \eta_{total} \qquad (1.10)$$

The calculated values of EDG in the free space, mobile environment, voice position, data position, and read position are tabulated in Table 1.3. EDG is directly related to the total antenna efficiency; therefore, EDG is lower in the presence of the user body and mobile environment than that in the free space. Moreover, ADG is also lower in the user proximity than that in the free space. The lower ADG in a user proximity is due to the high correlation factor and a high degree of reflection. However, the total antenna efficiency reduces by approximately 20%–30% in the user proximity in comparison to the free space at both 1.8 and 3.5 GHz when multiband PIFAs are placed at the top position of the mobile phone PCB. EDG also reduces simultaneously. Hence, overall EDG reduces in the actual scenario (mobile environment and the human body) as compared to the free space due to lower G_{app} and total efficiency. The estimated values of EDG varied between 8 and 9 in free space and 4 to 7 in user proximity when the antenna is at the top position. On the other way, the EDG is 8 in free space and 3 and 7 in the user proximity when the antenna is at the bottom position. In the user proximity, the minimum value of EDG is 3 in the case of talk position when the antenna is placed at the bottom of PCB. Therefore, the trade-off of EDG and other performance parameters of the antenna can provide the information about the suitable location of the antenna over PCB.

TABLE 1.3 Calculated Values of EDG in Different User Proximity

Frequency (GHz)	User Proximity	ADG, G_{app}	TotalEfficiency, η_{total}	EDG, $G_{effective}$
PIFAs at the Top Location of the PCB				
1.8	Free space	9.998	90.6	9.06
	Mobile phone	9.594	80.2	7.67
	Voice position	8.995	62.1	5.58
	Data position	9.164	66.2	6.07
	Read position	9.265	66.7	6.18
3.5	Free space	9.996	89.5	8.95
	Mobile phone	9.758	77.5	7.56
	Voice position	8.458	58.4	4.94
	Data position	9.016	64.8	5.84
	Read position	9.425	62.1	5.85
PIFAs at the Bottom Location of the PCB				
1.8	Free space	9.999	86.1	8.61
	Mobile phone	9.659	78.6	7.59
	Voice position	7.954	56.2	4.47
	Data position	8.957	57.3	5.13
	Read position	8.999	59.4	5.34
3.5	Free space	9.999	85.1	8.51
	Mobile phone	9.715	72.4	7.03
	Voice position	7.126	53.7	3.83
	Data position	8.125	54.2	4.40
	Read position	8.485	58.4	4.69

1.3.3 MIMO PARAMETER ESTIMATION

In the above analysis, the diversity parameters are estimated by assuming that the SNR is lower. Moreover, if the faded environment having high SNR values, then the high data rate can be achieved by selecting the MIMO mode. Then relevant MIMO parameters are thus estimated. In this section, MIMO parameters such as multiplexing efficiency (ME) and channel capacity are investigated in a free space and a real scenario. Similarly, the simulations have been done in CST MWS to calculate the parameters.

1.3.3.1 MULTIPLEXING EFFICIENCY

ME is calculated by assuming a high SNR under the isotropic condition. ME is simply calculated to estimate the MIMO channel performances. It can be calculated using ECC and total antenna efficiency of the multi-antenna systems. The mathematical equation of ME is [31]

$$\text{Multiplexing Efficiency (ME)} = \sqrt{(1-\rho_e)\eta_1\eta_2} \qquad (1.11)$$

where η_1 and η_2 are the total antenna efficiencies of the antenna elements 1 and 2 of the MIMO systems, respectively, and ρ_e is the ECC between multi-antenna elements.

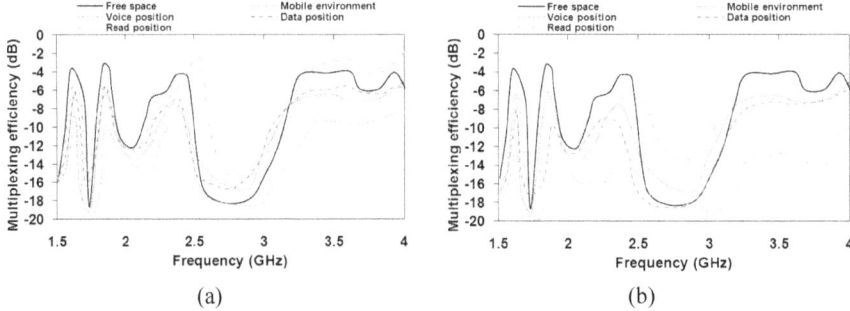

FIGURE 1.5 ECC vs. frequency in a mobile environment and human body for (A) top-located MIMO and (B) bottom-located MIMO.

The calculated MEs for top-positioned multi-antenna elements and bottom-positioned multi-antenna elements are depicted in Figures 1.5(a) and (b), respectively. It has already been observed that the top-positioned antenna provides better efficiency and a lower correlation than the bottom-positioned antenna. Therefore, ME is better at the top position. When the antenna is positioned at top of the mobile phone PCB, ME degrades 3 dB, 7 dB, 3.2 dB, and 3.2 dB for the mobile phone environment, talk position, data position, and read position, respectively, at a lower operating frequency and 3 dB, 6 dB, and 3 dB for the mobile phone environment, talk position, data position, respectively, at a higher operating frequency. On the other hand, for the bottom-positioned antenna over mobile PCB, ME degrades 6 dB, 13 dB, 7 dB, and 5 dB for the mobile phone environment, talk position, data position, and read position, respectively, at a lower operating frequency and 3 dB, 10 dB, 3 dB, and 1 dB for the mobile phone environment, talk position, data position, and read position, respectively, at a higher operating frequency. It is clearly noted that bottom-positioned multi-elements provide higher losses and lower efficiencies, and a high degree of correlation resulting in the maximum degradation in ME is observed.

1.3.3.2 CHANNEL CAPACITY

In this study, we use multiple antennas at both the transmitter and receiver terminals. For considering the ideal case, we put a dipole antenna at the transmitter terminal and a designed antenna at the receiver terminal for receiving the signals so that the channel is modeled with two transmitters (dipole antenna as a transmitting antenna, $N_T = 2$) and two receivers (design antenna as a receiving antenna, $N_R = 2$) as shown in Figure 1.6. The transmitting and receiving signals are related as [32]

$$y = H_x + n \tag{1.12}$$

where the input signal vector x and output signal vector y are connected through channel matrix H with the addition of the additive white Gaussian noise vector n.

The four channel elements, that is, h_{11}, h_{12}, h_{21}, and h_{22} formed in the channel matrix H are known as the channel coefficients. Each channel coefficient of H is related to the transmission coefficients between the transmitting and the receiving antennas of the system [31]. It is estimated for the case of 2×2 MIMO systems as

$$H = \begin{bmatrix} h_{11} & h_{12} \\ h_{21} & h_{22} \end{bmatrix} \tag{1.13}$$

All four channel elements, that is, h_{11}, h_{12}, h_{21}, and h_{22} in the channel matrix H are constructed from the transmission coefficients between the transmitter and receiver from

$$h_{ij} = S_{ij} \tag{1.14}$$

$$S_{ij} = S_{ij}^d + S_{ij}^m \tag{1.15}$$

where S_{ij} is the complex transmission coefficient between the jth transmitting antenna and ith receiving antenna, S_{ij}^d is the direct component, and S_{ij}^m is the superposition of all multipath components. The modeling of the channel matrix can be done on the numerical simulator CST MWS. The channel matrix is computed using Equations (1.13)–(1.15). If there is no channel-state information at the transmitter, then optimally allocate equal power over all antennas.

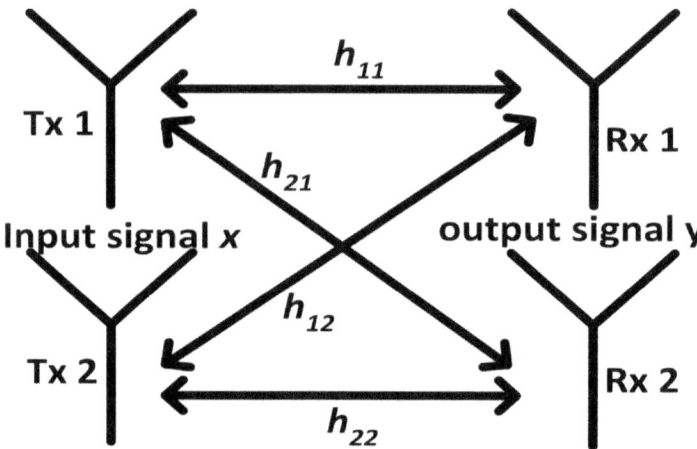

FIGURE 1.6 Modeling of channel capacity (two transmitting and two receiving antennas).

The total transmitted power is constrained by the covariance matrix Tr $(R_{xx}) = P_t$. The convenient general capacity expression is given by [33]

$$C = \log_2 \left\{ \left| I + \frac{SNR}{N_T} HH^T \right| \right\} \quad (1.16)$$

where I is an $N_R \times N_R$ identity matrix, N_T is the number of the transmitter, H^T is the conjugate transpose of the channel matrix H, and SNR is the transmitter's signal-to-noise ratio.

Figures 1.7(a) and (b) depict the computed channel capacity at two operating frequencies, that is, 1.8 and 3.5 GHz. Figures 1.7(a) and (b) consist of two graphs for top-located multi-element PIFAs and bottom-located multi-element PIFAs. The channel capacity is estimated and compared for single-input and multiple-output (SIMO) and MIMO systems. In the case of SIMO, only one dipole at the transmitting terminal and the designed MIMO

Estimation of Diversity and MIMO Parameters 19

at the receiver terminal are considered. Similarly, in the case of MIMO, two transmitters (dipole) and two receivers (designed MIMO antenna) are considered. Further, the channel capacity is also calculated by putting the designed MIMO antenna in the mobile environment and the human body. From Figure 1.7(a), it is observed that the channel capacity is high for higher SNRs in the free space, while at lower SNRs, diversity shows better performances. The channel capacity is unaffected for free space and the mobile environment irrespective of whether the antenna is located at the top or bottom of the mobile PCB at both operating frequencies. Moreover, the channel capacity reduces in the mobile environment as compared to that in the free space due to a small change in radiation patterns in the presence of heavy metallic components of a mobile phone, whereas it becomes better than that in the SIMO systems. In the case of talk position, data position, and ready position, the radiation patterns of the antenna changed, resulting in loss in some dominant lobes of the pattern. For the bottom-located antenna, a larger area of PIFAs is covered by the human body than that in the top position; therefore, lobes of the radiation pattern of the PIFA are heavily affected. Therefore, the lower channel capacity is noticed for the bottom-located antenna over PCB in the user body at both operating frequencies. Moreover, it is clearly noted that the channel capacity of MIMO in talk and data positions is lower than that in the SIMO at 3.5 GHz due to the loss of multiple lobes of the pattern in the presence of the human body for the bottom position. Finally, it can be concluded that the channel capacity is better at the top position than at the bottom position of the antenna at both the operating frequencies.

1.3.4 TOTAL RADIATED POWER ESTIMATION

TRP is explained as the sum of all power radiated by the antenna, regardless of the direction of polarization as shown in Figure 1.8. If the antenna is enclosed by a perfect absorbing material, then TRP would be the power absorbed by the sphere. It is directly related to power delivered to the antenna and antenna radiation efficiency, which is given by [21]

$$TRP = P_A \cdot \eta_{\text{Rad Eff}} \tag{1.17}$$

where $\eta_{\text{Rad Eff}}$ is the radiation efficiency of antenna and P_A is the power delivered to the antenna. The TRP from the antenna is

$$TRP = \oint U(\theta,\phi) \, d\Omega$$

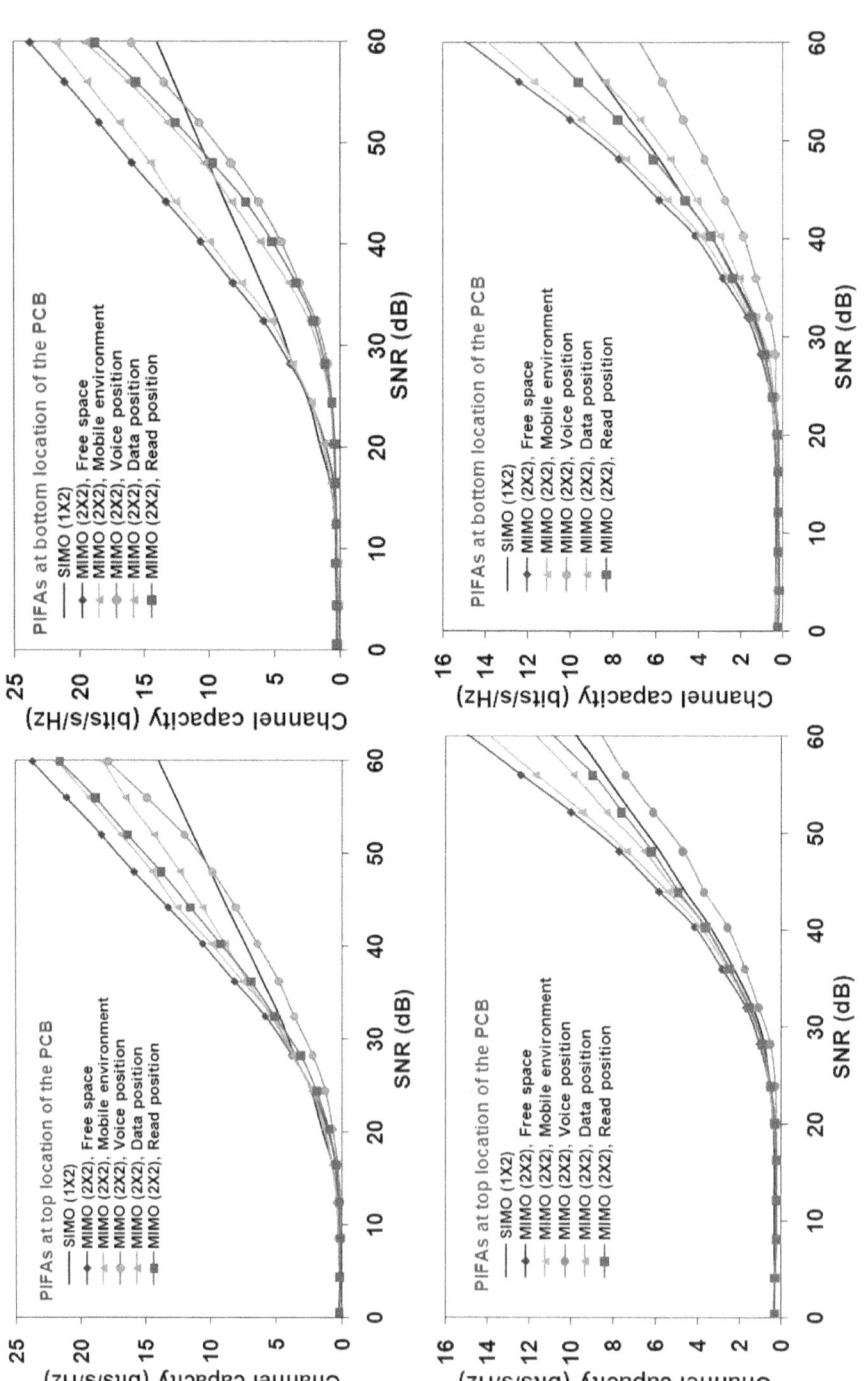

FIGURE 1.7 (A) Computed channel capacity at 1.8 GHz and (B) computed channel capacity at 3.5 GHz.

where $U(\theta,\phi)$ is the radiation intensity in Watt/steradian and $d\Omega = \sin(\theta) d\theta d\phi$. The effective isotropic radiated power (EiRP) is written in the form of radiation intensity as

$$EiRP(\theta,\phi) = P_T G_T(\theta,\phi) = 4\pi U(\theta,\phi)$$

where $P_T G_T$ is the product of the power delivered to the antenna and the antenna power gain. Therefore,

$$U(\theta,\phi) = \frac{EiRP(\theta,\phi)}{4\pi}$$

Hence, the integral formula of TRP is given by

$$TRP = \frac{1}{4\pi} \int_{\theta=0}^{\pi} \int_{\phi=0}^{2\pi} EiRP(\theta,\phi) \sin(\theta) d\theta d\phi \qquad (1.18)$$

Furthermore, the simplified formula of TRP is

$$TRP = Conducted\ Power\ (W) \times E_{miss} \times E_{rad} \qquad (1.19)$$

where E_{miss} is the mismatch efficiency and E_{rad} is the radiation efficiency of the antenna. All the transmitted power is assumed as the conducted power. The conducted power is considered as 1 W or 30 dBm in this study.

In the case of multiple antenna systems, TRP of the antenna element 1 is named TRP-1 and TRP of the antenna element 2 is named TRP-2. The estimated TRP is tabulated in Table 1.4. It is observed that TRP in free space is higher than that in the user environment. When the antenna is positioned at the top of PCB, TRP decreases to 1.2, 9.5, and 8.1 dBm (for antenna 1 and antenna 2, respectively), 7.7 and 7.5 dBm (for antenna 1 and antenna 2, respectively), and 6.4 and 6.8 dBm (for antenna 1 and antenna 2, respectively), for mobile phone, voice position, data position, and read position, respectively, in comparison to the free space at 1.8 GHz, whereas decreases 0.9, 7.9, and 7.4 dBm (for antenna 1 and antenna 2, respectively), 6.4 and 6.1dBm (for antenna 1 and antenna 2, respectively), and 2.7 and 2.3 dBm (for antenna 1 and antenna 2, respectively), for the mobile phone, voice position, data position, and read position, respectively, in comparison to the free space at 3.5 GHz. For the bottom-located PIFAs over mobile PCB, the power loss is high compared to the top position because the bottom-placed antenna elements suffer from the maximum reflection and higher losses from the mobile environment and human body. Moreover, the bar graph of Figure 1.9 clearly describes about the loss of power in the mobile environment and human body. It is noticed that at 1.8 GHz, the loss of power varies between

6 and 9.5 dBm for the top-positioned antenna over the mobile phone PCB, whereas it varies between 8 and 12 dBm in the case of the bottom-positioned antenna over PCB. It is clearly noticed that the power loss is maximum when the antenna is positioned at the bottom. Furthermore, at 3.5 GHz, the power loss varies between 2.5 and 8 dBm in the case of the top-placed PIFAs and varies between 6.9 and 10 dBm in the case of the bottom-placed PIFAs. Therefore, the overall conclusion is that the maximum power loss occurred for the bottom-placed antenna over PCB irrespective of the frequency of operation.

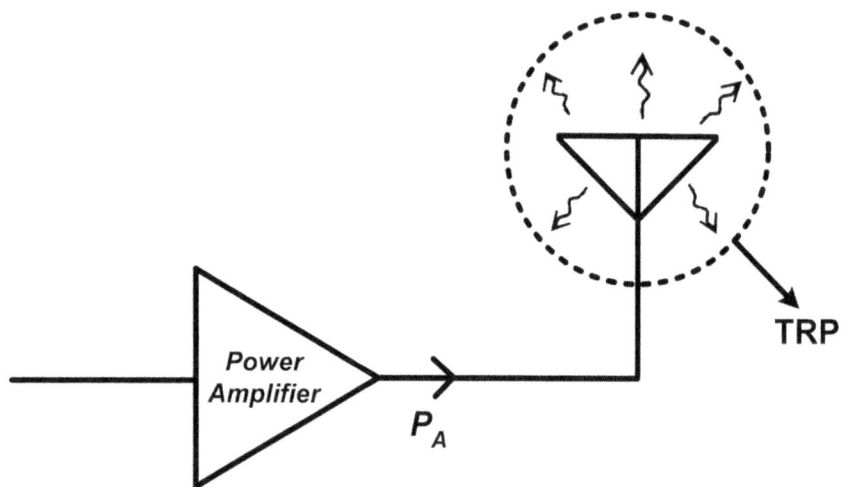

FIGURE 1.8 Total radiated power from the antenna.

1.3.5 SPECIFIC ABSORPTION RATE AND SAR TO PEAK LOCATION SPACING RATIO ESTIMATION

In the case of the point SAR, it is defined as the rate of change of energy transferred to the charged particle in an infinitesimal volume at that point divided by the mass of the infinitesimal volume as [34]

$$SAR = (\partial W_c / \partial t)/\rho_m \qquad (20)$$

where ρ_m is the mass density at the point. This is also called the local SAR. However, the average SAR is defined as the ratio of the total energy transferred to the human head tissue to the total mass of the head tissue. The average SAR is defined as

$$\text{Average SAR} = \int \langle P_c \rangle \, dv / M \tag{21}$$

In the case of the mobile phone, we need to estimate the average SAR. The simulation setup to estimate SAR is shown in Figure 1.10. This simulation setup is created as per the guidelines given by CTIA [35].

TABLE 1.4 Calculated Values of TRP in Different User Proximity

Frequency (GHz)	User Proximity	TRP-1 (dBm)	TRP-2 (dBm)
PIFAs at the Top Location of the PCB			
1.8	Free space	25	25
	Mobile phone	23.8	23.8
	Voice position	15.5	16.9
	Data position	17.3	17.5
	Read position	18.6	18.2
3.5	Free space	23	23
	Mobile phone	22.1	22.1
	Voice position	15.1	15.6
	Data position	18.6	18.9
	Read position	20.3	20.7
PIFAs at the bottom Location of the PCB			
1.8	Free space	25	25
	Mobile phone	23.8	23.8
	Voice position	13.4	13.7
	Data position	15.9	16.1
	Read position	16.5	16.7
3.5	Free space	23	23
	Mobile phone	22.1	22.1
	Voice position	13.2	12.8
	Data position	14.6	15.1
	Read position	16.3	15.8

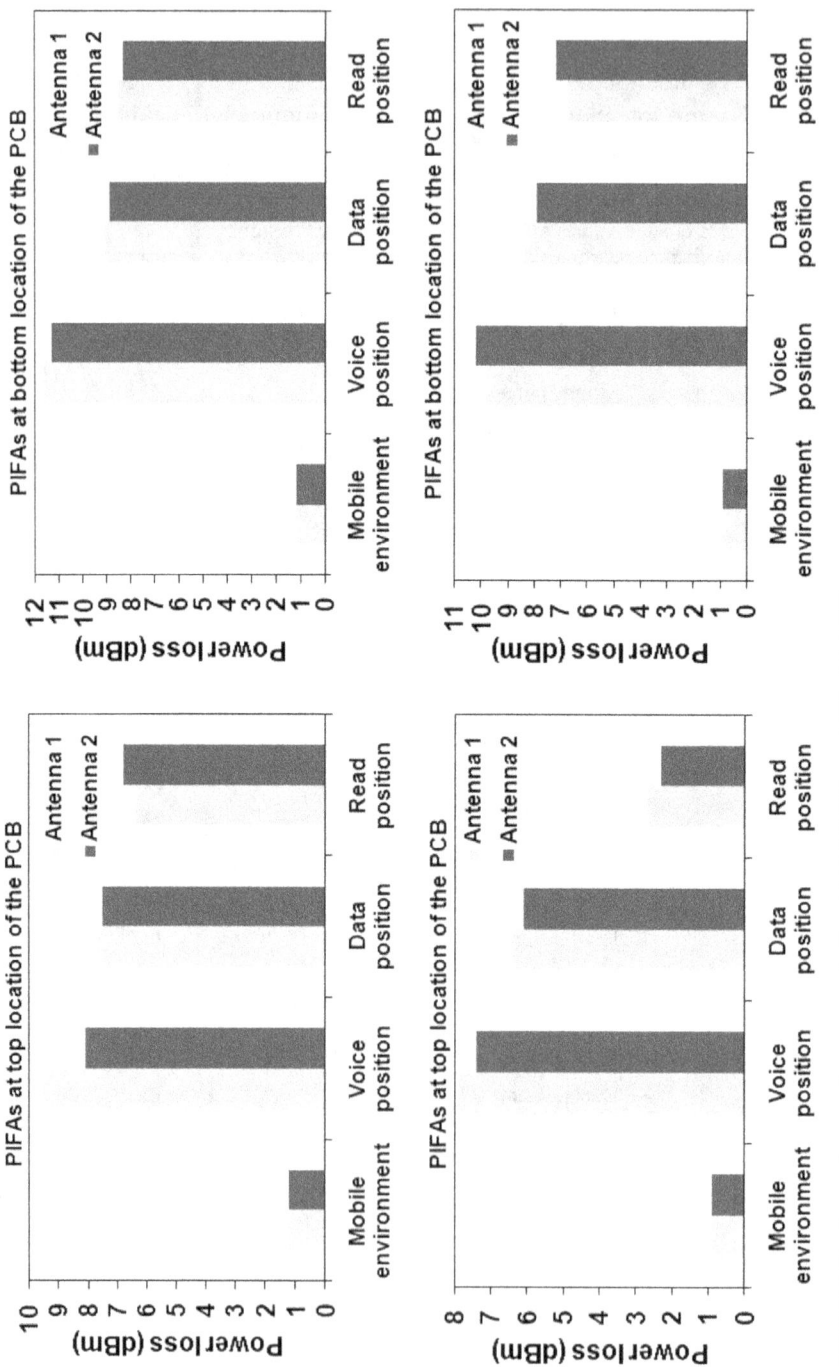

FIGURE 1.9 Loss of power in user proximity at (A) 1.8 GHz and (B) at 3.5 GHz.

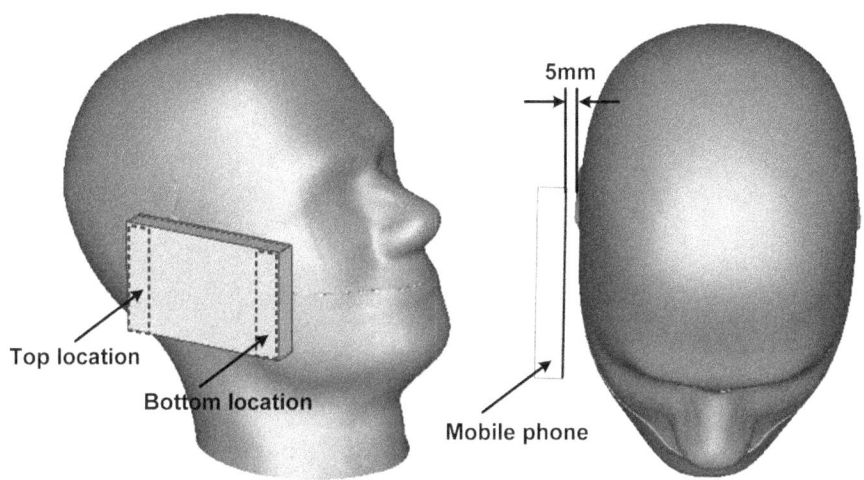

FIGURE 1.10 SAR simulation setup.

However, the existing equipment fails to measure the average SAR inside the human tissue when multiple elements operate simultaneously. Therefore, SPLSR is used to estimate the distribution of SAR [36], which is given by

$$SPLSR = (SAR_1 + SAR_2)/D \tag{1.22}$$

where SAR_1 and SAR_2 are the average values of SAR (W/kg) for the antenna-1 and antenna-2, respectively, and D (in cm) is the distance between the two peaks of SAR. The calculated values of SPLSR are tabulated in Table 1.5. SPLSR over 1 and 10 g tissues are well below the defined limit. SPLSR of the bottom-located antenna is lower than the top-placed antenna because of the more interspace available between the antenna and the head phantom. If the antenna is located at the top position, the distance between the phantom and mobile housing is exactly 5 mm as per the guidelines of CTIA. For the bottom-positioned antenna, the distance is larger due to the nonplanar structure of the human head phantom. Therefore, SPLSR is lower when the antenna is located at the bottom of PCB. It is also noticed that the SARs of antenna-1 and antenna-2 are not exactly the same due to the nonplanar head phantom and the SAR of each antenna may affect each other. Moreover, the calculated SAR and SPLSR are much below the standard limit because the antenna is packed in the plastic housing, resulting in lesser electromagnetic energy penetration inside human tissues. However, SPLSR meets the criteria of FCC, which is well below 0.3, irrespective of whether the antenna is positioned at the top or bottom of PCB.

TABLE 1.5 Calculated Values of SPLSR

Frequency (GHz)	SAR Distribution over 1 g Tissue				SAR Distribution over 10 g Tissue			
	SAR$_1$ (W/kg)	SAR$_2$ (W/kg)	Distance between Two Peaks of SAR (D) Unit (in cm)	SPLSR (W/kg × cm)	SAR$_1$ (W/kg)	SAR$_2$ (W/kg)	Distance between Two Peaks of SAR (D) Unit (in cm)	SPLSR (W/kg × cm)
PIFAs at the Top Location of PCB								
1.8	0.23	0.21	1.63	**0.27**	0.19	0.13	1.7	0.19
3.5	0.21	0.22	1.65	**0.26**	0.17	0.12	1.7	0.17
PIFAs at the Bottom Location of PCB								
1.8	0.16	0.19	1.9	**0.18**	0.12	0.10	1.6	0.137
3.5	0.17	0.15	2	**0.16**	0.13	0.11	1.57	0.13

1.4 CONCLUSION

In this chapter, thorough investigations of a multi-element antenna system have been carried out. The diversity parameters, MIMO parameters, TRP, SAR, and SPLSR of the designed MIMO are calculated by positioning the multi-element PIFAs at the top and bottom locations of the mobile phone PCB. The diversity parameters fulfilled the criteria of MIMO systems. The diversity parameters, that is, MEG and ECC are close to unity and <0.5, respectively. EDG varies between 3 and 8 in the user proximity. Moreover, MIMO parameters, that is, ME and channel capacity are lower in the user proximity than that in the free space. The loss of power varies between 2 and 11dBm in the user proximity. Furthermore, SAR and SPLSR meet the criteria of both FCC and European standards. It is clearly noticed that the performance of the top-positioned multi-element PIFAs is better than the bottom-located PIFAs, except SAR and SPLSR. Finally, it is concluded that the trade-off between the performance parameters and SPLSR of the top location of the antenna over PCB is a better option than the other location.

KEYWORDS

- **MIMO parameters**
- **PIFA**
- **CTIA**
- **SAR**

REFERENCES

1. Paulraj, A.; Gore, D.; Nabar, R.; Bolcskei, H. An Overview of MIMO Communications—A Key to Gigabit Wireless. *Proc. IEEE* **2004**, *92*, 198–218.
2. Pelosi, M.; Franek, O.; Knudsen, M. B.; Christensen, M.; G. F.; Andersen, J. B. A Grip Study of Talk and Data Modes in Mobile Phones. *IEEE Trans. Antennas Propag.* **2009**, *57*, 856–865.
3. Valkonen, R.; Myllynaki, S.; Huttunen, A.; Holopainen, J.; Ilvonen, J.; Vainikainen, P.; Jantunen, H. Compensation of Finger Effect on Mobile Terminal Antenna by Antenna Selection. *in Proceedings of International Conference on Electromagnetics in Advanced Applications*, Sydney, September 20–24, **2010**, 364–367.

4. Iivonen, J.; Holopainen, J.; Kivekas, O.; Valkonen, R.; Icheln, C.; Vainikainen, P. Balanced Antenna Structure for Mobile Terminals. *Proceedings of the Fourth European Conference on Antennas and Propagation*, Barcelona, Spain, April 12–16, **2010**, 1–5.
5. Zervos1, T.; Alexandridis1, A. A.; Petrovic, V. V.; Dangakis1, K.; Kolundzija, B. M.; Dordevic, A Soras, R. C. Mobile Handset Radiation Efficiency as a Function of the Antenna Position Relative to the Human Head. *WSEAS Trans. Commun.* **2004**, 562–567.
6. Villanen, J.; Ollikainen, J.; Kivekas, O.; Vainikainen, P. Coupling Element Based Mobile Terminal Antenna Structures. *IEEE Trans. Antennas Propag.* **2006**, 54, 2142–2153.
7. Okada, Y.; Yamamoto, M.; Nojima, T. Unbalanced Fed Dipole Antenna Mounted on Ground Plane With L-Shaped Parasitic Elements for Mobile Handsets. *Proc. ISAP*, Taipei, Taiwan, **2008**, 1645395.
8. Huan, L. C.; Ofli, E.; Chavannes, N.; Cherubini, E.; Gerber, H. U.; Kuster, N. Effects of Hand Phantom on Mobile Phone Antenna Performance. *IEEE Trans. Antennas Propag.* **2009**, 57, 2763–2770.
9. Ilvonen, J.; Kivekas, Holopainen, O. J.; Valkonen, R.; Rasilainen, K.; Vainikainen, P. Mobile Terminal Antenna Performance With the User's Hand: Effect of Antenna Dimensioning and Location. *IEEE Antennas Wirel. Propag. Lett.* **2011**, 10, 772–775.
10. Montaser, A. M.; Mahmoud, K. R.; Elmikati, H. A. An Interaction Study between PIFAs Hand-Set Antenna and a Human Hand-Head in Personal Communications. *Prog. Int. Electromagn. Res. B* **2012**, 37, 21–42.
11. Shi, Y.; Sun, H.; Liang,C. -H. SAR Study of Antennas in Wireless Communication Terminals. *Microw. Opt. Tech. Lett.* **2014**, 56, 2361–2365.
12. Plicanic, V.; Lau, B. K.; Ying, Z. Performance of a Multiband Diversity Antenna with Hand Effects. *International Workshop on Antenna Technology: Small Antennas and Novel Metamaterial*, Chiba, Japan, March 4–6, **2008**, 534–537.
13. Plicanic, V.; Lau, B. K.; Derneryard, A.; Ying, Z. Actual Diversity Performance of a Multiband Diversity Antenna with Hand and Head Effects. *IEEE Trans. Antennas Propag.* **2009**, 57, 1547–1556.
14. Buskgaard, E.; Tatomirescu, A.; Barrio, S. C. D.; Franek, O.; Pedersen, G. F. User Effect on the MIMO Performance of a Dual Antenna LTE Handset. *EuCAP 2014: Proceedings of the 8th European Conference on Antennas and Propagation*, The Hague, Netherlands, April 6–11, **2014**, 2006–2009.
15. Zhang, S.; Zhao, K.; Ying, Z.; He, S. Adaptive Quad-Element Multi-Wideband Antenna Array for User-Effective LTE MIMO Mobile Terminals. *IEEE Trans. Antennas Propag.* **2013**, 61, 4275–4283.
16. Singh, H. S.; Pandey, G. K.; Bharti, P. K.; Meshram, M. K. Compact Printed Diversity Antenna for LTE700/ GSM1700/ 1800/ UMTS/ Wi-Fi/ Bluetooth/ LTE2300/ 2500 Applications for Slim Mobile Handsets. *Prog. Electromagn. Res. C.* **2015**, 56, 83–91.
17. Singh, H. S.; Pandey, G. K.; Bharti, P. K.; Meshram, M. K. Design and Performance Investigation of a Low Profile MIMO/Diversity Antenna for WLAN/WiMAX/ HIPERLAN Applications with High Isolation. *Int. J. Radiofreq. Microw. Comput. Aid. Eng.* **2015**, 25, 510–521.
18. Singh, H. S.; Meshram, M. K. Effect of User Proximity on Internal Quad Band Mobile Phone MIMO/Diversity Antenna Performances. *Wirel. Pers. Commun.* **2017**, 95, 1417–1431.

19. Singh, H. S.; Upadhaya, R. Shubair, R. M. Free Space and User Proximity Analysis of Octaband Monopole MIMO/Diversity Antenna for Modern Handset Applications. *Int. J. Radiofreq. Microw. Comput. Aid. Eng.* **2018**, doi:10.1002/mmce.21566.
20. Singh, H. S.; Singh, K.; Vinamrata; Shubair, R. M. A Compact MobileHandsets MIMO/Diversity Antenna for GSM1800 and WiMAX Applications. *International Conference of Electrical and Computing Technologies and Applications (ICECTA2017)*, Ras-Al-Khaimah, Dubai, November 21–23, **2017**, 1–4.
21. Cellular telecommunication association (CTIA). Certification Test Plan for Mobile Station Over the Air Performance. *Method Meas. Radiat. Radiofreq. Power Receiv. Perform.*, **2005**.
22. Gabriel, C. Tissue Equivalent Material for Hand Phantoms. *Phys. Med. Biol.*, **2007**, 52, 4205–4210.
23. Taga, T., Analysis for Mean Effective Gain of Mobile Antennas in Land Mobile Radio Environments. *IEEE Trans. Veh. Technol.* **1990**, 39, 117–131.
24. Dong, L.; Ling, H., Heath, R. W. Multiple-Input Multiple-Output Wireless Communication Systems Using Antenna Pattern Diversity. *IEEE Global Telecommunications Conference*, Taipei, Taiwan, November 17–21, **2002**, 997–1001.
25. Pedersen, K.; Mogensen, P.; Fleury, B. Power Azimuth Spectrum in Outdoor Environments. *Electron. Lett.* **1997**, 33, 583–1584.
26. Karaboikis, M. P.; Papamichael, V. C.; Tsachtsiris, G. F.; Soras, C. F.; Makios, V. T. Integrating Compact Printed Antennas onto Small Diversity/MIMO Terminals, *IEEE Trans. Antennas Propag.* **2008**, 56, 2067–2078.
27. Jusoh, M., Jamlos, M. F.; Kamarudin, M. R.; Malek, F. A MIMO Antenna Design Challenges for UWB Applications. *Prog. Electromagn. Res.* B, **2012**, 36, 357–371.
28. Vaughan, R. G.; Anderson, J. B. Antenna Diversity in Mobile Communications. *IEEE Trans. Veh. Technol.* **1987**, 36, 149–172.
29. Schwartz, M.; Bennett, W. R.; Stein, S. Communication System and Techniques. **1965**, McGraw-Hill, New York, 470–474.
30. Balanis, C. A. Antenna Theory: Analysis and Design (3rd ed.). **2012**, New York: Wiley.
31. Tian, R.; Lau, B. K.; Ying, Z. Multiplexing Efficiency of MIMO Antennas. *IEEE Antennas Wirel. Propag. Lett.* **2011**, 10, 183–186.
32. Geyi. W. Multi-Antenna Information Theory. *Prog. Electromagn. Res.* **2007**, 75, 11–50.
33. Foschini, G. J., Gans. M. J. On Limits of Wireless Communications in a Fading Environment when Using Multiple Antennas. *Wirel. Pers. Commun.* **1998**, 40, 311–335.
34. Durney, C. H.; Massoudi, H.; Iskander, M. F. Radio Frequency Radiation Dosimetry Handbook *USAF School of Aerospace Medicine, Aerospace Medical Division (AFSC)*, Brooks Air Force Base, Armstrong Laboratory.
35. CTIA. Test Plan for Mobile Station Over the Air Performance. *CTIA Revision 3.1*, January **2011**.
36. Federal Communications Commission (FCC), Handsets Multi Xmiter and Ant v01, *648474D04*, **2012**.

CHAPTER 2

Reversible Logic Design Using QCA: Challenges and Future Aspects

RUPALI SINGH and DEVENDRA KUMAR SHARMA

Department of Electronics and Communication Engineering,
SRM Institute of Science and Technology, Ghaziabad, Uttar Pradesh, India

ABSTRACT

Computation using low-power, high-density, and high-speed circuits is the utmost necessity of nanoscale systems. Technology is changing overnight, and the size of the transistor is shrinking day by day. Complementary metal-oxide-semiconductor (CMOS) technology is approaching its limits due to leakage currents, power consumption, difficulties in lithography, etc. Thus, some alternative solution has to be obtained to overcome CMOS limitations and potentially replace CMOS circuits. Reversible logic and quantum-dot cellular automata (QCA) have emerged as promising paradigms which can excel in performance and possible substitute of CMOS in nano-circuits. A reversible logic can be used in the circuits to nullify the energy dissipation during computation. Reversibility is introduced in the circuit by replacing irreversible gates with reversible one. On the other hand, QCA makes use of nanostructures called quantum dots, to build the circuits with compact size, ultra low power, and faster processing capability. This chapter focuses on the major aspects of reversible quantum circuits including basic to the complex structures with their comprehensive analysis. This study targets the design of combinational and sequential circuits using a reversible logic. For that, a unique reversible gate is proposed that can be solely used to design combinational as well as sequential circuits. The reversible gate is implemented in QCA and further subjected to various analyses such as cost analysis, fault characterization, and power analysis. The proposed reversible gate is further utilized to design combinational circuits such as adder, subtractor, and multiplexer, and sequential circuits such as latches and shift register. Moreover, the reversible circuits are analyzed for QCA parameters such as the number of QCA cells, latency, and cost function. Subsequently, this work presents a complete exploration of reversible QCA circuits from basic theory to all-around analysis.

2.1 INTRODUCTION

In recent years, technology in digital computers has improved tremendously in terms of speed, density, and processing power. This progress came mainly due to the development of fabrication technology of small-scale devices and the ability to integrate more devices on a single chip. In 1965, Moore came up with a theory that the number of transistors will double every 18 months. But recent studies indicate that this growth and shrinking of the devices will be restricted by the physical limits of silicon device technology. Complementary metal-oxide-semiconductor (CMOS) is the primary component in integrated circuits. With the advent of nanocomputing, designing of the chips with CMOS has become challenging due to the occurrence of short-channel effects at nanoscale. This motivates researchers to think about the substitute of CMOS transistors. Thus, it is extremely important to find an alternative that can replace CMOS efficiently and subdue its limitations. Quantum-dot cellular automata (QCA) is one of the possible solutions to this problem. QCA is one of the promising future nanotechnologies predicted by Industries Association's International Roadmap for Semiconductors (ITRS). QCA allows operating frequencies of the order of tetrahertz and device density much higher than the current CMOS limits.

QCA makes use of quantum cells to realize QCA circuits. QCA cells consist of four quantum dots placed at four corners of the cell [1]. The quantum dot is either filled with the electron or it is empty. The electron can tunnel through the dots and is bounded within the cell. The flow of information in QCA is current-less, governed by the positioning of electrons in QCA cell; hence, the power dissipation is negligible [2]. Data processing and logical computations in QCA are achieved by the Coulombic interaction between the QCA cells instead of the current flow. The QCA circuits can achieve low power dissipation with a higher device density and very high operating speed. It is challenging to create transistor-less circuits. Moreover, the conventional digital circuits are irreversible in nature. Irreversible circuits lose bits during computation and hence dissipate power. Any bit lost during computation dissipates kT ln2 Joules of heat [3]. To avoid this heat dissipation, reversibility can be introduced in circuits. Ideally, the reversible circuit results in zero power dissipation [4]. Reversible circuits do not lose information during computation. They generate an exclusive output vector for each input vector and vice versa. Thus, designing the circuits using the reversible logic can produce low-power circuits. The reversible circuits are designed using reversible gates. Reversible gates follow the concept of reversibility and have an equal number of input–output terminals. Some of the standard reversible gates are the Feynman gate, Double Feynman gate [5], Fredkin gate [6], Toffoli gate [7], and Peres gate [8]. Many researchers came up with new reversible gates such as the TSG gate [9], new parity preserving gate [10], Sayem gate [11], RM gate [12], RUG gate [13], and many more. These reversible gates emerge with many combinational and sequential circuits. If the implementation of reversible logic circuits is also physically reversible, then the design becomes nondissipative. CMOS cannot be used for implementation as it is not physically reversible. If the reversible circuits are implemented using QCA, then low-power, nanosize, and high-speed circuits can be created.

This chapter focuses on the design of reversible circuits using QCA. First, the reversible logic and QCA concepts are explored and, subsequently, reversible QCA circuits are designed. The work presented here is divided into nine sections. Sections 2.2 and 2.3 describe the elementary concepts and review of work done in the reversible logic and QCA. Section 2.4 gives the design of the proposed reversible gate, design of combinational circuits, sequential circuits, and their simulations. Section 2.5 illustrates the comprehensive analysis of the proposed reversible QCA circuits. Energy dissipation analysis and fault-tolerance characterization are presented in Sections 2.6 and 2.7, respectively. Section 2.8 elaborates future scope and applications. Finally, Section 2.9 concludes the chapter.

2.2 REVERSIBLE LOGIC

As Moore's law suggests, the transistor count in an integrated circuit and, hence, dissipating power doubles every 18 months. The present techniques dissipate more heat as they use irreversible circuits, resulting in the diminished life of circuits. This issue can be handled by introducing a reversible logic in the circuits. The reversible logic computations retain the information, that is, the bits are not erased during reversible operations and, thus, dissipate negligible power. The reversible logic circuit can also be substantially used to regain some part of signal energy that can be reused for successive operations by doing and undoing computation in the forward path and backward path, respectively.

Thus, the reversible logic is likely to be a future paradigm to produce high-speed, power-efficient circuits. The circuits designed using the reversible logic find extensive scope in low-power CMOS design, optical computing, DNA computing, and nanotechnology computing. Major applications of a reversible logic lie in quantum computing.

2.2.1 ELEMENTARY CONCEPTS

A reversible function is the one that has bijective mapping between the input and output vectors. An $n \times n$ reversible gate has $(I_1, I_2, I_3, ..., I_n)$ inputs and $(O_1, O_2, O_3, ..., O_n)$ outputs with a unique mapping between them [6]. Conventional logic gates such as AND and OR are irreversible as in theses gates, it is not possible to determine input states from the output state. Also, in this case, multiple inputs are converted into a single output, which results in information loss and, hence, heat dissipation. The conventional NOT gate is a reversible gate, as it has one input and one output. The customary reversible gate with n inputs and n outputs is shown in Figure 2.1. As shown in Figure 2.1, an $n \times n$ reversible gate must have n input terminals and n output terminals with a unique mapping between them. In any reversible gate, there may exist an additional output vector that is not utilized in the circuit. Such output is referred to as a garbage output. The garbage output is not used as a prime output or it is not useful for successive stages. Sometimes, to generate a valid output, some ancilla input may need to be added to the reversible gate. If additional inputs and outputs, garbage data, are added to an irreversible system, then it is converted to a reversible one by making a one-to-one mapping between the vectors. This is referred to as logical reversibility.

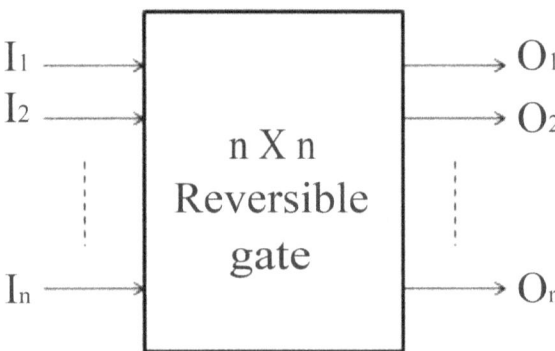

FIGURE 2.1 n x n Reversible gate.

Another way to achieve reversibility is by making circuit physically reversible. In this case, the internal configuration of the circuit should follow the reversibility criterion in a given technology. Thus, introducing either logical or physical reversibility, circuits can be made reversible. Initially, it was reported that fan-outs and feedback are not allowed in reversible logic circuits. Recently, it was established that fan-outs and feedback can be used in a QCA circuit by taking suitable measures [14]. Thus, reversible logic circuits are realized using QCA to resolve the fan-out issue.

2.2.2 RELATED WORK

Reversible circuits are designed using reversible gates. One of the key constraints in the reversible logic is to curtail the number of reversible gates, ancilla inputs, delay, and garbage outputs produced in a circuit. Fredkin, Toffoli, and Peres presented standard reversible gates that can be utilized to implement the number of logic functions [6–8]. Thaplial et al. [9] proposed the TSG gate to design a reversible adder. Then, a new parity preserving gate was reported by Haghparast et al. [10] to detect errors at the output terminal. Gradually, many researchers came up with a number of reversible gates, such as the RM gate, New gate, RUG gate, TQCA gate, RCQCA, PPRG gate, and PRUG gate. Reversible circuits are emerged with different design strategies and optimization methods. Reversible logic circuits such as adders [9, 15, 16], subtractors [17, 18], arithmetic and logic units (ALUs) [12, 13, 19], and counters [20, 21] are reported in the literature. In [22], an efficient reversible adder is proposed using two new reversible gates NRG and MFG. Another reversible gate known as the ANOX gate was presented in [16] to produce a reversible adder. In [17], many combinational circuit designs such as the half-adder, full adder, parallel adder, and multiplier are shown and implemented using CMOS technology. Improved designs of reversible subtractors were proposed by Das and De [18] and Ahmad et al. [22]. Some researchers investigated reversible ALUs and optimized them. Sen et al. [12] investigated the modular design of reversible ALUs using a reversible multiplexer. Sasamal et al. [13] and Nath et al. [19] reported two designs of ALUs. Moreover, application-based reversible circuits such as reversible error-control circuits [23], image stenography circuits [24], and parity-generator circuits for secure nanocommunication [25] were investigated with great detail. After many investigations on combinational circuits, reversible designs of sequential elements emerged. Reversible latches were explored by Thapliyal et al. [26–28]. Sayem et al. [11] reported the Sayem gate to realize different latches, Rad et al. [29] presented the design of reversible flip–flops. But many other sequential elements such as registers, counters, and memory elements are yet to be explored to a greater extent.

This work targets the design of reversible combinational circuits such as adder, subtractor, multiplexer, and some reversible sequential circuits such as D latch, T latch, and register using a single proposed reversible gate.

2.3 QUANTUM-DOT CELLULAR AUTOMATA

This section describes the overview of QCA circuits which covers the elementary concepts and related work reported in the literature. The essential structure of QCA is a QCA cell that has four quantum dots at the corners of a cell and diagonally placed two free electrons [1]. The electrons are bounded in a quantum dot but can quantum-mechanically tunnel from one to another dot and gets final position in either of the two ways of cell polarization as shown in Figure 2.2(a).

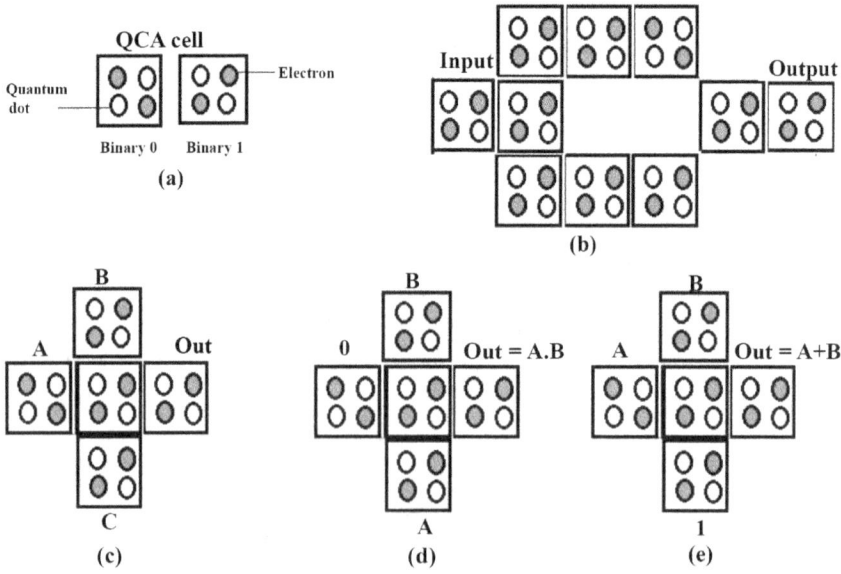

FIGURE 2.2 (a) QCA cell (b) QCA inverter (c) Majority voter (d) Majority voter as AND gate (e) Majority voter as OR gate.

The tunneling of electrons results in the change of cell polarization, which in turn establishes the binary logic 1 and 0 as shown in Figure 2.2. As there exists only the tunneling of electrons and no flow of current or voltage, QCA structures develop an ultra-low-power circuits. The appropriate arrangement of QCA cells forms the QCA wire and other QCA devices, such as the inverter and majority gate as shown in Figure 2.2. The majority gate and inverter are elementary configurations of QCA. The majority gate gives the output 1 or 0 based on the majority of inputs connected. The basic equation for three input majority gates is M(A, B, C) = AB + BC + AC. AND and OR gates can be realized using the majority gate by fixing one of its inputs to logic 0 or 1 [2]. QCA logic gates are interconnected through QCA wires. The wire crossings are either of coplanar or multilayer type. Coplanar wire crossing requires the cell orientation of 90° and 45°.

The flow of information is governed by the clock in QCA. The clocking in QCA circuits gets rid of the metastability problem associated with QCA cells. Initially, Lent and Tougaw [1] came up with the adiabatic switching.

Adiabatic switching is obtained by applying the underlying clocking circuit. In this switching, there are four clock zones: Clock 0, Clock 1, Clock 2, and Clock 3. These clocks are applied to QCA circuits methodically in order to attain the synchronized information flow. Four different phases—switch, hold, release, and relax [30]—are observed in each clock zone as shown in Figure 2.3. Cell polarization occurs in the switch phase followed by the hold phase in which the clock raises to a high level and the cell becomes fully polarized which prevents electron tunneling. The release phase comes with a reduction in barrier and cell polarization with the falling edge of the clock. In the last phase, that is, the relax phase, the cell gets unpolarized with the clock at a low level.

2.3.1 RELATED WORK

As QCA technology emerges with its basic structures, many researchers came up with numerous QCA circuits. Tougaw and Lent [1, 31] introduced the device and concept of logical computation with QCA. The important feature of QCA to ensure the information flow is its clocking scheme that was proposed in [32]. To simulate the logical devices of QCA, a QCA designer tool was proposed, and many arithmetic architectures of QCA were simulated on the tool [33–35]. Then, a method of reduction in majority gates was developed in [36]. Kim et al. [37] proposed a new adder structure with a proper clocking scheme. Later, pipelined structures of adders were proposed in [38]. A new structure of a five-input majority gate of QCA was introduced by Zhang et al. [39]. During this, researchers found that QCA cells are prone to fabrication defects [40]. Thus, the testing of QCA circuits for possible defects was

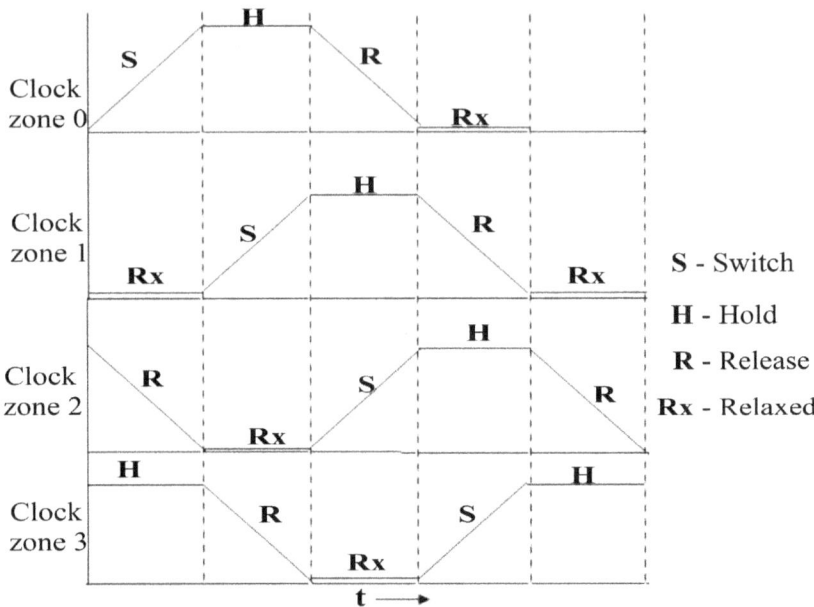

FIGURE 2.3 Clocking zones in QCA circuits.

targeted by many researchers [41], [42]. To improve the fault tolerance of the QCA circuit, new fault-tolerant QCA layout of a majority voter was proposed with its implementation in adder [4345], whereas in [46], the JK latch design was presented based on the fault-tolerant majority gate. The combinational circuits such as adders [44–50], multiplexers [51–53], parity generators [25, 54], encoder and decoder [55, 56], ALU [13, 57, 58] are reported in the literature with the minimum area and latency. The basic sequential element, D flip-flop using QCA, was initially reported by Dehkordi et al. [59]. Dual-edge flip–flop was proposed in [60]. Further, sequential circuits such as flip–flop [61–64], registers [53, 65], counters [66–68], and RAM cell [69, 70] are designed with the QCA analysis of theses circuits. Many reports have been published on the design of QCA circuits, but the design of QCA circuits using the reversible logic needs more attention. Some of the cost-efficient reversible circuits are shown in [29, 71, 72]. Chabi et al. [71] proposed a new reversible gate using which various sequential latches were presented. The memory design was proposed in QCA, but the reversible memory design has not yet been addressed. The optimization of the QCA circuit is important to build low-power and highly dense circuits. There are certain constraints to be followed while reducing the area of the QCA circuit. The minimum distance between neighboring rows and neighboring columns is fixed. Also, the designed circuit should have appropriate cell arrangement without overlapping of adjacent cells. Thus, researchers are now working to curtail the area of the QCA circuit by abiding the standard rules of optimization.

Many researchers mostly put emphasis on the design of QCA circuits without testing the fault tolerance. Moreover, the design of circuits with the improved cost function needs to be addressed more. This motivates us to focus on the design of cost-effective testable circuits.

2.4 REVERSIBLE QCA CIRCUITS

This section targets the design and analysis of the reversible QCA circuits which is the blend of two efficient paradigms: the reversible logic and QCA. First, the design of combinational reversible circuits is explored, and subsequently, sequential reversible circuits are discussed. The reversible circuits are proposed in this section using a novel reversible gate that can be used for designing combinational and sequential circuits. The novel reversible gate is a 3 × 3 gate as shown in Figure 2.4(a), and its QCA layout is proposed in Figure 2.4(b). The QCA layout is designed using the software QCA designer 2.0.3 [35]. The QCA layout proposed here makes use of the XOR structure reported in [73]. The output functions X, Y, Z of reversible gates are realized using the XOR and multiplexer functions.

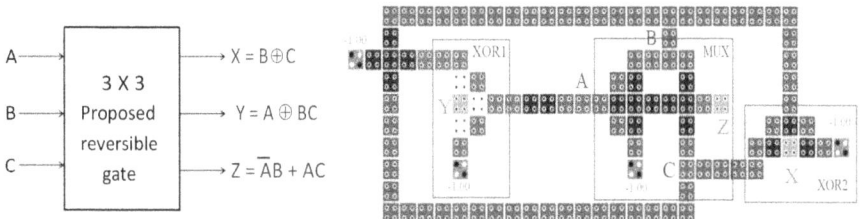

FIGURE 2.4 (a) Proposed reversible 3 x 3 gate (b) QCA layout of proposed reversible gate.

The significance of the proposed gate is that it has a multi-utility property. It can be used in the design of certain crucial combinational circuits as well as sequential circuits. The functionality of the gate can be checked from the simulation waveform, shown in Figure 2.5. The simulation waveform shows that the output X is XOR of inputs B and C, Y is XOR of A and BC, and Z is the multiplexed function of B and C with the selection line being A. The layout is compact utilizing 111 QCA cells with an effective area of 0.12 µm². The latency for the output X is 0.5 clock, that is, 2 clock zones; for output Y, the latency is 1 clock, that is, 4 clock zones; and for the output Z, it is 0.75 clock, that is, 3 clock zones.

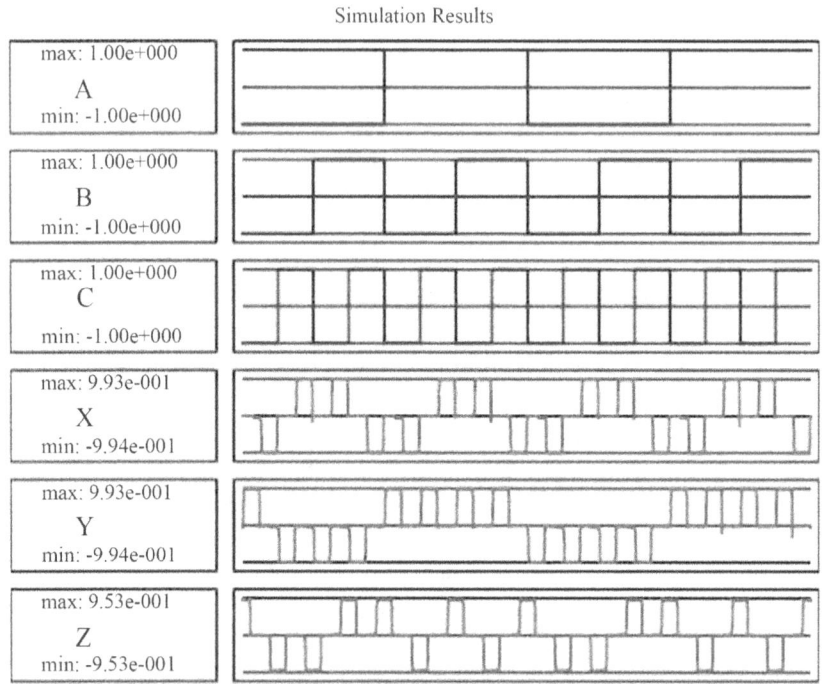

FIGURE 2.5 Simulation waveform of the proposed reversible QCA.

2.4.1 COMBINATIONAL CIRCUITS

There are a number of useful combinational circuits that can be designed using the reversible QCA gate. This section focuses on the design of an adder, a subtractor, and a multiplexer circuits using the proposed reversible gate.

2.4.1.1 ADDER

The most common circuit used in many digital devices is a full adder. The basic unit to design a full adder is a half-adder. The proposed reversible gate can function as a half-adder as shown in Figure 2.6(a). The proposed reversible half-adder is illustrated in Figure 2.6. The output Sum is the XOR function of the inputs In1 and In2, and the output Carry is the logical AND of the inputs In1 and In2. The Sum output is obtained with the latency of 0.5 clock, whereas the Carry output is obtained with the latency of 1 clock, which is clearly observed in the simulation waveform shown in Figure 2.6. Here, 1 clock includes four clocking zones, whereas 0.5 clock indicates two clocking zones.

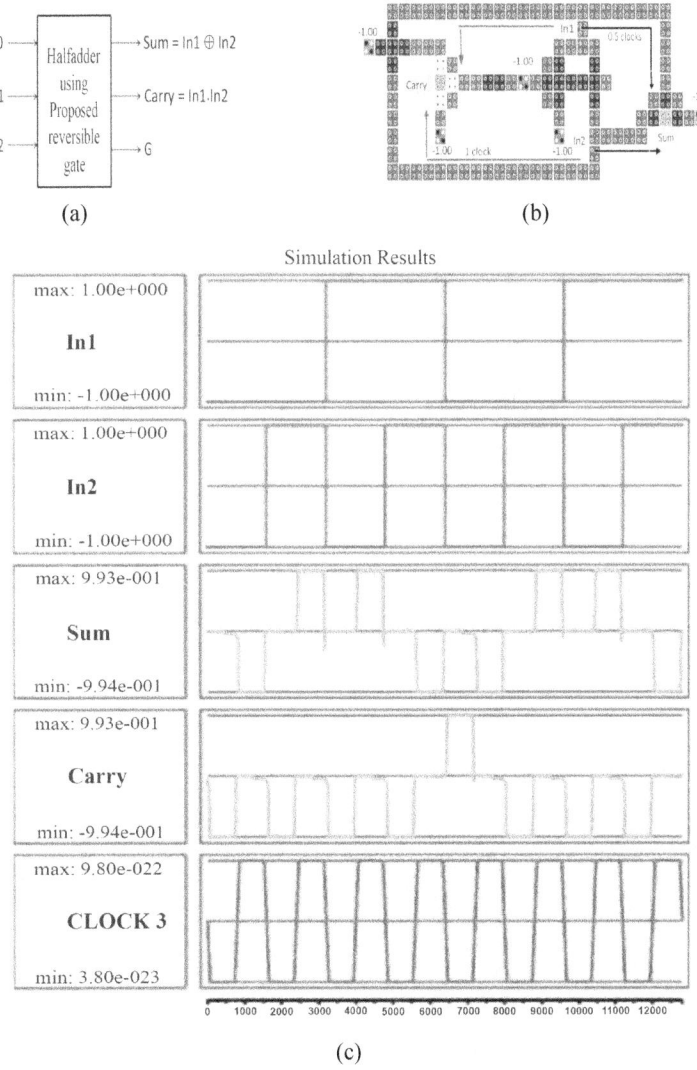

FIGURE 2.6 (a) Half adder using proposed reversible gate (b) Proposed QCA layout of reversible half adder (c) Simulation waveform of proposed half adder.

2.4.1.2 SUBTRACTOR

The proposed reversible gate is further used to design the reversible half-subtractor circuit as shown in Figure 2.7. The outputs Diff and Borrow are obtained as shown in Figure 2.7(a).

The output of the half-subtractor can be verified from the simulation waveform as shown in Figure 2.7(c). It is observed that the Diff output is delayed by 0.5 clock and Borrow is delayed by 1 clock.

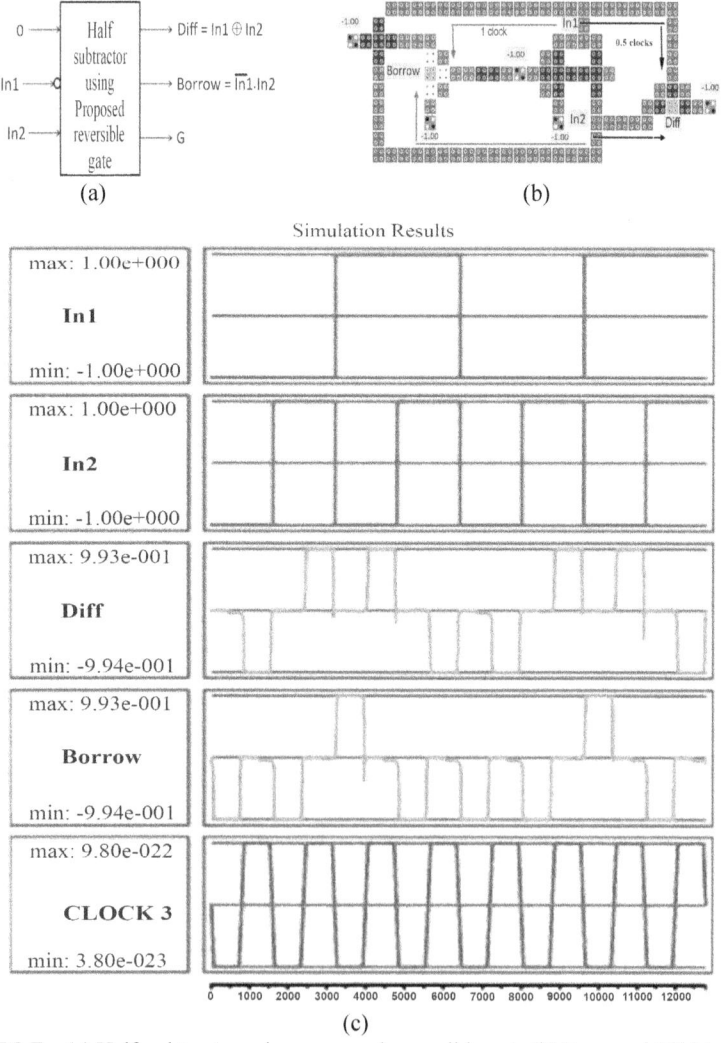

FIGURE 2.7 (a) Half subtractor using proposed reversible gate (b) Proposed QCA layout of reversible half subtractor (c) Simulation waveform of proposed half subtractor.

Reversible Logic Design Using QCA

2.4.1.3 MULTIPLEXER

A multiplexer or a data selector is a necessary circuit in many digital circuits. The characteristic equation for a multiplexer is Out = $\overline{Sel}\ I_{n1}$ + Sel I_{n2}. This section presents the design of a 2:1 multiplexer with the proposed reversible gate.

The reversible gate is operated as a multiplexer; its QCA layout is shown in Figure 2.8. The simulation waveform is given in Figure 2.8(c). The output is delayed by 0.75 clock as shown by the arrow in the proposed QCA layout.

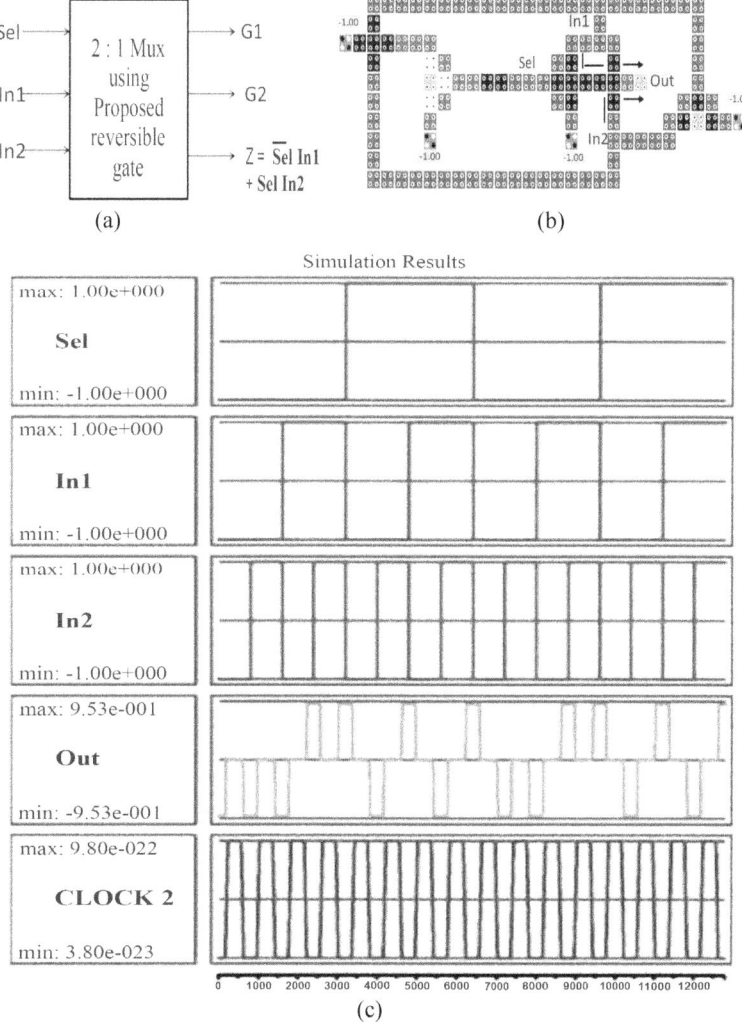

FIGURE 2.8 (a) 2:1 multiplexer using proposed reversible gate (b) Proposed QCA layout of reversible multiplexer (c) Simulation waveform of proposed 2:1 multiplexer.

2.4.2 SEQUENTIAL CIRCUITS

As a sequential circuit is a pivotal part of computing hardware, it is essential to discuss the design of low-power, nanosize reversible sequential circuits. To begin with, the fundamental component of a sequential circuit is a latch. Hence, this section explores the design of reversible latches with their application in a complex sequential circuit such as registers.

2.4.2.1 LATCHES

The operation of a latch is to hold a bit of information. Basically, four types of latches are normally studied. They are SR latch, D latch, T latch, and JK latch. D latch is the most common memory element used to constitute the number of sequential circuits. This section presents the design of a reversible D latch, a T latch, and a shift register using QCA.

2.4.2.1.1 D Latch

This section describes the design of a D latch using the proposed reversible gate. The characteristic equation of a D latch is given by $Q_{n+1} = Q_n E + E\text{¢} D$ [74]. This equation can be easily realized by using the proposed reversible gate as shown in Figure 2.9.

When the output Z of the proposed reversible gate is fed back to the input C, the above equation is obtained and the proposed gate functions as a D latch. The simulation waveform is obtained as shown in Figure 2.9. It is observed from the waveform that the proposed circuit behaves as a D latch. The correctness of the waveform can be verified from Table 2.1. Table 2.1 shows the output Q_{n+1} for different input combinations of Q_n (previous output), E (Enable), and D (input). As the characteristic equation of the D latch suggests, $Q_{n+1} = D$ when $E = 0$, and $Q_{n+1} = Q_n$ when $E = 1$.

TABLE 2.1 Verification of Output for Different Input Combinations

S. No.	Q_n	E	D	Q_{n+1}
1.	x	0	1	1
2.	x	0	0	0
3.	1	1	x	1
4.	0	1	x	0

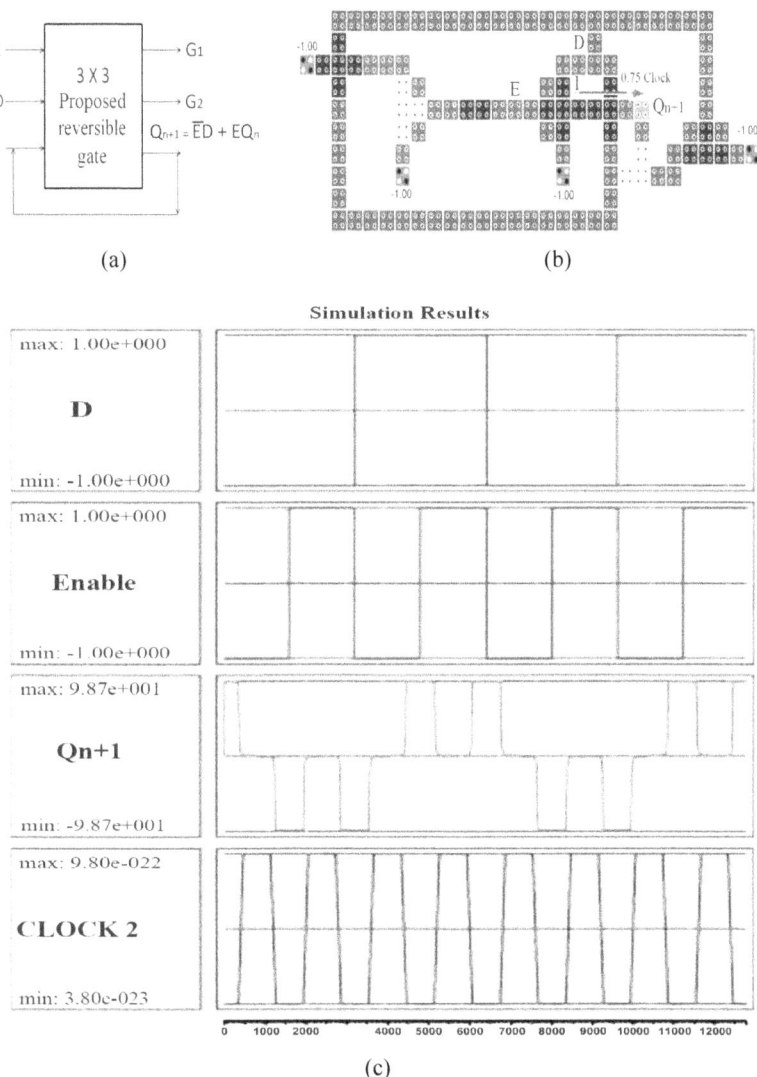

FIGURE 2.9 (a) D latch using proposed reversible gate (b) Proposed QCA layout of reversible D latch (c) Simulation waveform of proposed D latch.

2.4.2.1.2 T Latch

Here, the design and QCA implementation of the T latch are presented using the proposed reversible gate. The proposed reversible gate has three outputs. One of its output equations matches with the characteristic equation of the T latch as depicted in Figure 2.10(a). The latency between input T and output Q_{n+1} is 1 clock and, hence, the output will be delayed by 1 clock. The implementation of the proposed T latch using QCA is illustrated in Figure 2.10(b). The proposed T latch can be simulated on the QCA designer tool. The simulation and verification are shown in Figure 2.10(c). The output can be explained using the marked arrows. The first arrow points to Q_n (previous state) and the next arrow points to Q_{n+1} (current state). "A" corresponds to T = 1, E = 1, Q_n = 1, and the output Q_{n+1} = 0 (toggle). "B" represents T = 0, E = 1, Q_n = 1, and the output Q_{n+1} = 1 (the same as Q_n). "C" shows T = 1, E = 1, Q_n = 1, Q_{n+1} = 0. Thus, the output of the T latch is validated from the simulation waveform.

2.4.2.2 REGISTER

This section describes another crucial circuit of the sequential family that is register. Register can be used either as a data storage register or a shift register. Both the types can be implemented by using the proposed reversible gate. The shift register can be categorized as a serial in serial out (SISO), serial in parallel out, parallel in serial out, and parallel in parallel out. Here, the block diagram of a 3-bit shift register is proposed using the suggested reversible gate. Figure 2.11 displays the proposed SISO shift register and its proposed QCA layout.

The SISO shift register is presented here, using the proposed D latch. As each D latch can store 1 bit of information, three D latches are used here to implement the 3-bit register. The input to the register is provided at D and the output is obtained at Q_n. The enable E represents the clock signal here, which is common to all the latches. The QCA layout of the proposed SISO register is shown here with the latency of 2.75 clock.

In this section, the basic structure of a SISO register is proposed. Based on this methodology, other registers, such as serial in parallel out, parallel in parallel out, parallel in serial out, and universal registers can be designed by the reader as an exercise.

2.5 COMPREHENSIVE ANALYSIS OF REVERSIBLE QCA CIRCUITS

The proposed reversible gate is compared with the existing reversible gates and shown in Table 2.2. The analysis of the proposed gate is carried out based on the cell count, total area, cell area, latency, area usage, and cost

Reversible Logic Design Using QCA

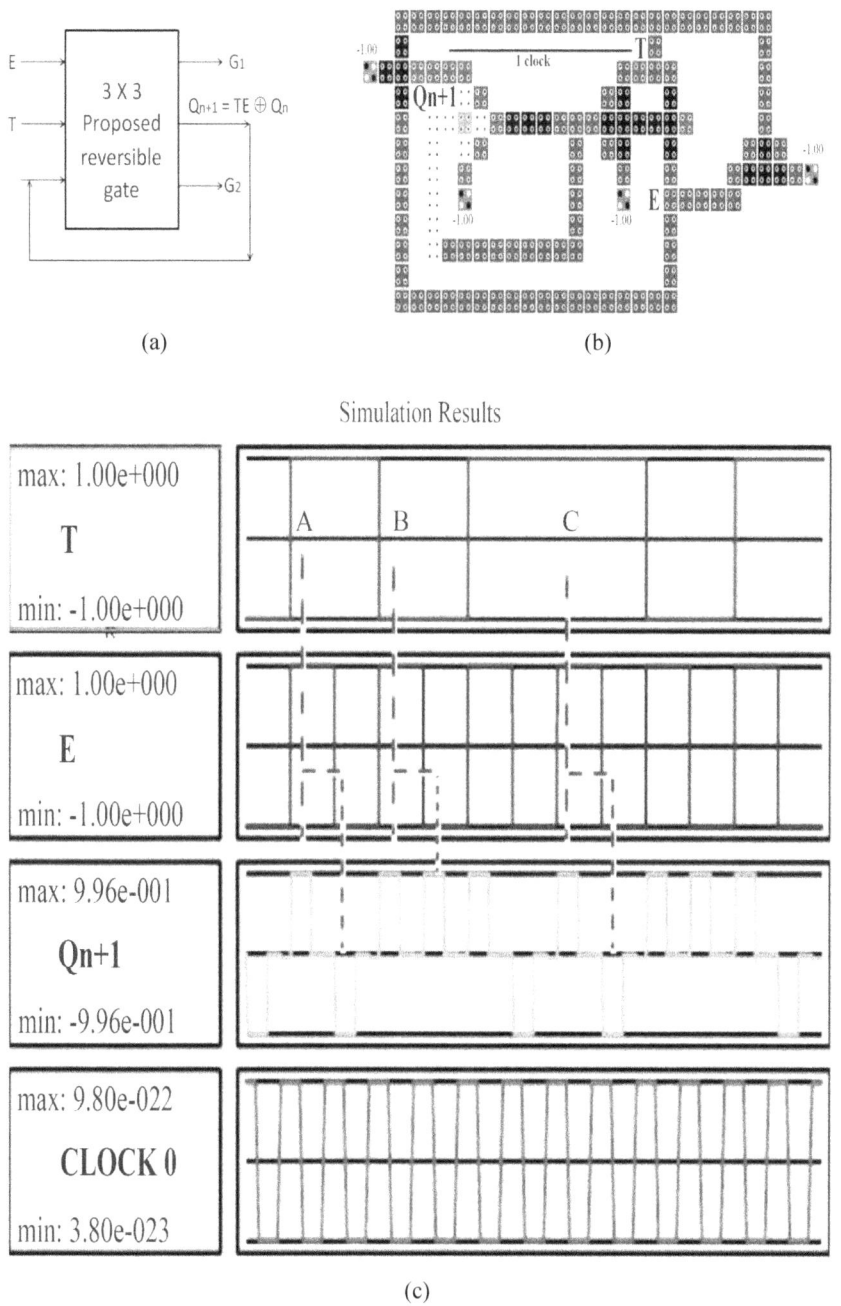

FIGURE 2.10 (a) T latch using proposed reversible gate (b) Proposed QCA layout of reversible T latch (c) Simulation waveform of T latch.

function. The parameters such as the cell area, area usage, and cost function are evaluated using the following equations:

Cell area = Cell count × area of each cell (18 nm 18 nm) (1)

Area usage = Cell area/total area (2)

Cost function = Cell count × cell area × latency (3)

It is apparent from Table 2.2 that the proposed reversible gate has shown improved performance over the previous reversible gates reported in literature. The cost function justifies the efficacy of the circuit in terms of the area and cell count. The reversible gate with the minimum cost function will acquire the maximum efficacy. In turn, the energy dissipation will also be at its minimum value.

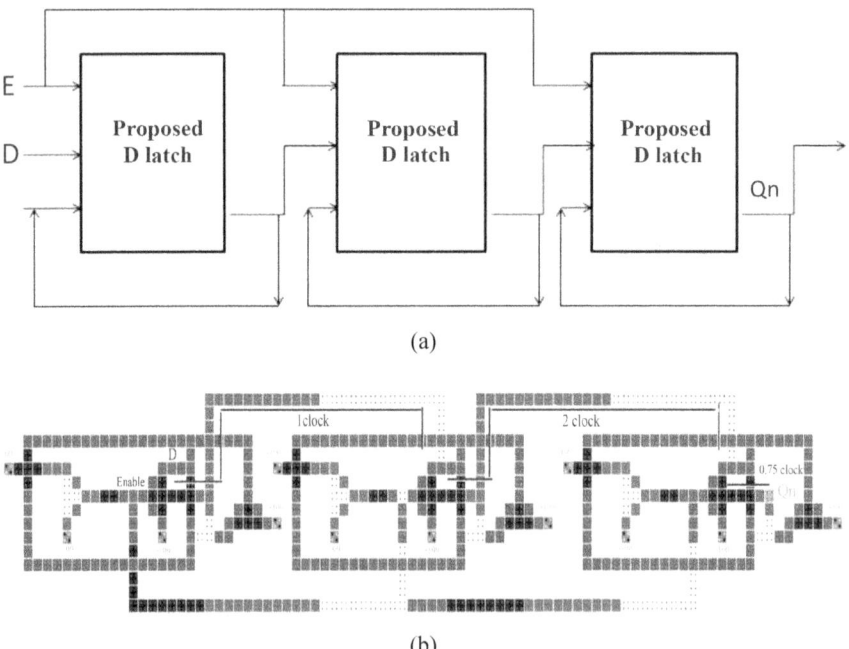

FIGURE 2.11 (a) Proposed serial in serial out shift register using reversible D latch (b) Proposed QCA layout of SISO register.

Further, the proposed reversible circuits are analyzed for parameters such as the number of reversible gates, number of cells, and total area. Table 2.3 depicts the cost parameters of the proposed reversible circuits.

Reversible Logic Design Using QCA 49

TABLE 2.2 Comparative Analysis of the Proposed Reversible Gate with Existing Reversible Gates

S. No.	Reversible Gates	Cell Count	Total Area (in µm²)	Cell Area (in µm²)	Delay	Area Usage (in %)	Cost	Improvement (%)
1.	Fredkin [6]	191	0.37	0.061	1 clock	21.35	11.65	66.60
2.	RUG [13]	211	0.27	0.068	3 clock	25.18	43.04	90.90
3.	RQCA [12]	194	0.21	0.062	3 clock	29.52	36.08	89.24
4.	RCQCA [20]	177	0.24	0.057	1 clock	23.27	10.08	61.50
5.	PRUG [75]	109	0.11	0.035	1 clock	31.81	3.81	NA
6.	Proposed reversible design	111	0.12	0.035	1 clock	29.16	3.88	-

TABLE 2.3 Cost Analysis of the Proposed Reversible Circuits

Reversible Gate	Category	# of Reversible Gates Used	# of Critical Path	Latency (Clock Cycles)	Cell Count	Effective Cell Area (µm²)
Proposed Reversible Circuits	Half-adder	1	1	1 clock	111	0.12
	Half-subtractor	1	1	1 clock	109	0.12
	Multiplexer	1	1	0.75 clock	111	0.12
	D latch	1	1	0.75 clock	113	0.12
	T latch	1	1	1 clock	134	0.15
	3-bit SISO register	3	3	2.75 clock	484	0.56

2.6 ESTIMATION OF ENERGY DISSIPATION

The estimation of power dissipation across QCA circuits is imperative as it can justify the use of QCA in ultra-low-power circuits. Timler and Lent [76] initially came up with the assessment of power dissipation across QCA. Many researchers gave the perspective to calculate energy dissipation across the QCA cell with different mathematical analysis [77, 78]. Srivastava et al. [79] presented an upper bound model to evaluate the QCA power. The model proposed by Srivastava et al. segregates the total energy across QCA cell into two parts which are known as average leakage energy and average switching energy. Average leakage energy is the energy dissipated during clock transition, and average switching energy represents the energy dissipated in the QCA cell during the switching of the clock phase. Based on this power dissipation model, QCA Pro, a simulation tool, was developed to estimate the power dissipated across the QCA cell [80].

Here, the proposed reversible gate is also subjected to energy dissipation analysis using the QCA Pro tool. The energy map of the proposed reversible gate is given in Figure 2.12.

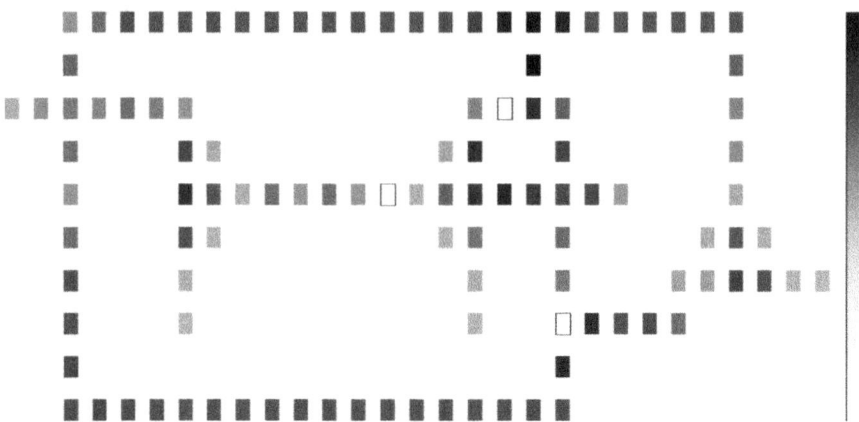

FIGURE 2.12 Energy map of proposed reversible gate.

The energy dissipation is estimated for the proposed reversible gate at three different tunneling energies 0.5Ek, 1.0Ek, and 1.5Ek at 2 K temperature using the QCA Pro tool. The total energy dissipation is calculated by adding average leakage energy and average switching energy. The energy dissipation of the proposed reversible QCA gate is given in Table 2.4.

Table 2.4 shows the comparative study of energy dissipation across the proposed reversible gate and existing reversible gates. It is evident from Table 2.4 that the proposed reversible gate has shown better performance in terms of energy dissipation than the earlier reported reversible gates. The similar analysis can be performed for the other proposed combinational and sequential circuits that can be investigated by the reader.

2.7 TESTING AND FAULT CHARACTERIZATION

QCA circuits are susceptible to various faults or defects that may occur during fabrication or the cell deposition phase of QCA. These defects are mainly cell displacement/cell misalignment and cell omission defects [40]. Cell displacement or cell misalignment fault occurs when a cell is displaced from its original position in any direction during deposition. On the other hand, cell omission defect occurs when a cell or multiple cells are omitted during their placement.

TABLE 2.4 Comparative Study of Energy Dissipation in the Proposed Reversible Gate

Reversible Gates	Average Leakage Energy (eV)			Average Switching Energy (eV)			Total Energy Dissipation (eV)			Improvement in Proposed Reversible QCA Gate (in %)
	0.5Ek	1.0Ek	1.5Ek	0.5Ek	1.0Ek	1.5Ek	0.5Ek	1.0Ek	1.5Ek	1.5Ek (for total energy dissipation)
FRG [6]	0.101	0.283	0.483	0.213	0.175	0.143	0.314	0.458	0.625	48.1%
RCQCA [20]	0.105	0.293	0.506	0.194	0.227	0.191	0.299	0.520	0.697	53.5%
PPRG [81]	0.058	0.168	0.294	0.193	0.166	0.141	0.251	0.334	0.435	25.5%
PRUG [75]	0.052	0.154	0.272	0.109	0.093	0.078	0.161	0.247	0.350	7.42%
Proposed reversible QCA gate	0.0336	0.101	0.181	0.185	0.162	0.139	0.218	0.263	0.324	-

These faults may result in incorrect outputs. Hence, it is imperative to study the fault tolerance of the QCA circuit by inserting such faults during simulation. Here, the proposed QCA layout of the reversible gate is simulated in the presence of cell displacement and cell misalignment faults. Tables 2.5(a) and (b) show the fault characterization of the proposed reversible gate in which FP represents the output fault pattern with 19 different faults.

TABLE 2.5(a) Fault Characterization of the Proposed Reversible QCA Gate

Input Vector	Expected Output Vector	FP1	FP2	FP3	FP4	FP5	FP6	FP7	FP8	FP9
Y0	Y0	Y0	Y0	Y0	Y2	Y2	Y0	Y0	Y0	Y0
Y1	Y4	Y4	Y4	Y4	Y6	Y6	Y5	Y5	Y5	Y4
Y2	Y5	Y5	Y5	Y5	Y7	Y7	Y4	Y5	Y4	Y5
Y3	Y3	Y1	Y3	Y1	Y3	Y3	Y1	Y3	Y1	Y1
Y4	Y2	Y2	Y2	Y2	Y2	Y0	Y2	Y2	Y2	Y3
Y5	Y7	Y7	Y5	Y7	Y7	Y5	Y7	Y7	Y7	Y7
Y6	Y6	Y6	Y6	Y6	Y6	Y4	Y7	Y6	Y6	Y6
Y7	Y1	Y3	Y1	Y3	Y3	Y1	Y1	Y1	Y1	Y2

TABLE 2.5(b) Fault Characterization of the Proposed Reversible QCA Gate

FP10	FP11	FP12	FP13	FP14	FP15	FP16	FP17	FP18	FP19	FT (in %)
Y0	Y4	Y0	Y4	Y0	Y0	Y2	Y0	Y4	Y2	63.15
Y4	Y4	Y4	Y2	Y6	Y4	Y4	Y5	Y0	Y6	47.36
Y5	Y1	Y5	Y1	Y5	Y7	Y7	Y4	Y1	Y7	42.1
Y1	Y1	Y3	Y5	Y1	Y3	Y1	Y3	Y1	Y3	42.1
Y2	Y6	Y2	Y6	Y2	Y2	Y2	Y2	Y6	Y0	68.42
Y6	Y7	Y7	Y1	Y5	Y7	Y7	Y7	Y3	Y5	63.15
Y7	Y5	Y6	Y2	Y6	Y5	Y4	Y6	Y2	Y4	52.63
Y1	Y1	Y1	Y5	Y3	Y1	Y3	Y1	Y1	Y1	63.15

Here, input vectors and expected output vectors are shown in the first two columns of Table 2.5(a) followed by the fault patterns obtained by simulating the proposed gate in the presence of various faults. Highlighted output vectors represent faulty outputs. FT is the fault-tolerant percentage calculated for each output vector. It is evident from Table 2.5 that the proposed reversible gate shows the average fault tolerance of 55.25%. Similarly, the fault tolerance can be obtained for various combinational and sequential circuits proposed in the previous sections.

2.8 APPLICATIONS AND FUTURE ASPECTS

Low-power, high-density, and high-speed circuits are the greatest necessity of nanoscale systems. CMOS technology is approaching its limits due to leakage currents, power consumption, difficulties in lithography, etc. Reversible logic and QCA seem to be the potential paradigms that can excel in performance and can be an alternative of CMOS in nanocircuits. The only necessary but not sufficient condition to obtain reversibility is to have one-to-one mapping between the input and output terminals. The reversible logic is going to be a part of every future computer because it exploits the possibility of negligible power dissipation. Moreover, the implementation of the reversible logic circuit in QCA makes it suitable for nanosize and high-performance computing circuits.

The chapter described the design of QCA-based combinational and sequential circuits using the reversible logic. The work can be extended in future to design larger and complex circuits such as multipliers, dividers, ALUs, counters, and memory cells. Many digital communication-based circuits such as encoders, decoders, pseudo random generators can be configured using the concept of reversible QCA.

While designing these circuits, few constraints can be taken into account. First, new reversible gates should be proposed with minimum hardware complexity and maximum resiliency. Minimum hardware complexity makes the QCA implementation easy and resiliency ensures the multi-utility of the gate, which makes it appropriate for a variety of circuits. Also, hardware complexity can be reduced by minimizing the quantum cost of reversible gates. The quantum cost is the minimum number of 1 × 1 or 2 × 2 gates required to realize the desired gate. Thus, researchers can target the optimization of the quantum cost of reversible gates in turn reversible circuits. Second, the designed reversible gate should have the minimum number of garbage outputs and constant inputs. Further, the reversible circuit must utilize the minimum number of reversible gates, which in turn reduces the area, power, and latency of the circuit. When these circuits are realized using QCA technology, QCA parameters must be considered to enhance the performance. The QCA parameters include the cell count, latency, effective area, etc. Finally, fault tolerance is another significant constraint that should be analyzed before fabricating any QCA circuit. Reliability of any QCA circuit can be enhanced by designing a circuit with a high degree of fault tolerance.

Many issues related to reversible QCA circuits are yet to be addressed. The development of floating-point adders using the reversible logic are not yet targeted. Further, a reversible CPU consisting of reversible ALUs, execution units, pipelines, memory elements, and reversible instruction set needs to be investigated.

The reversible logic finds extensive applications in DNA computing, quantum computing, and optical computing. Due to limitations of CMOS circuits and the supreme performance of reversible QCA circuits, future computers are definitely going to reversible quantum computers.

2.9 CONCLUSION

This chapter described the major aspects of reversible quantum circuits including basic to the complex structures with their comprehensive analysis. This study illustrated the design of combinational and sequential circuits using the reversible logic. A novel reversible gate was proposed, which was used efficiently to design various reversible circuits. These reversible circuits were further implemented using QCA. Moreover, the reversible circuits are analyzed for QCA parameters such as the number of QCA cells, latency, and cost function. The analysis of the circuit is not complete without the estimation of energy dissipation and testing against faults. Thus, the proposed gate was tested for energy dissipation and defects of cell placement. Subsequently, this work presents a complete investigation of reversible QCA circuits from elementary concepts to multifaceted analysis. Further, the study is concluded with applications and future aspects of reversible quantum circuits. A reversible quantum circuit is definitely going to be the foundation of future smart systems and a way toward quantum computing.

KEYWORDS

- **reversible logic**
- **QCA**
- **combinational and sequential circuits**
- **testing**
- **power analysis**

REFERENCES

1. Lent, CS; Tougaw, PD; A device architecture for computing with quantum dots. Proc. IEEE 85 1997, pp. 541–557.
2. Porod, W; Lent, C; Bernstein, G; Orlov, AO; Amlani, I; Snider, GL; Merz, JL; Quantum-dot cellular automata: Computing with coupled quantum dots. Int. J. Electron. 86 1999, pp. 549–590.
3. Landauer, R; Irreversibility and heat generation in the computing process. IBM J. Res. 5 1961, pp. 183–191, doi:10.1147/rd.53.0183.
4. Bennett, CH; Logical reversibility of computation. IBM J. Res. 17 1973, pp. 525–532, doi:10.1147/rd.176.0525.
5. Parhami, B; Fault-tolerant reversible circuits. Proc. 40th Asilomar Conf. Signals, Syst. Comput. Pacific Grove, CA 2006, pp. 3–6.
6. Fredkin, E; Toffoli, T; Conservative logic. Int. J. Theor. Phys. 21 1982, pp. 219–253, doi:10.1007/BF01857727.
7. Toffoli, T; Reversible computing. Int. Colloq. Autom. Lang. Program, 1980, pp. 632–644.
8. Peres, A; Reversible logic and quantum computers. Phys. Rev. A. 32 1985, pp. 3266–3276.
9. Thapliyal, H; Srinivas, MB; A new reversible TSG gate and its application for designing efficient adder circuits. Fifth Int. Conf. Information, Commun. Signal Process 2006, p. 5, http://arxiv.org/abs/cs/0603091.
10. Haghparast, M; Navi, K; A novel fault tolerant reversible gate for nanotechnology based systems. Am. J. Appl. Sci. 5 2008, pp. 519–523.
11. Sayem, ASM; Ueda, M; Optimization of reversible sequential circuits. J. Comput. 2 2010, pp. 208–214, http://arxiv.org/abs/1006.4570.
12. Sen, B; Dutta, M; Goswami, M; Sikdar, BK; Modular design of testable reversible ALU by QCA multiplexer with increase in programmability. Microelectron. J. 45 2014, pp. 1522–1532, doi:10.1016/j.mejo.2014.08.012.
13. Sasamal, TN; Mohan, A; Singh, AK; Efficient design of reversible logic ALU using coplanar quantum-dot cellular automata. J. Circuits Syst. Comput. 27 2018, pp. 85–204, doi:10.1142/S0218126618500214.
14. Yadavalli, KK; Orlov, CSL; Timler, JP; Snider, GL; Fanout gate in quantum-dot cellular. Nanotechnology 18 2007, pp. 7–10, doi:10.1088/0957-4484/18/37/375401.
15. Kumar, R; Ghosh, B; Gupta, S; Adder design using a 5-input majority gate in a novel "multilayer gate design paradigm" for quantum dot cellular automata circuits. J. Semicond. 36 2015, pp. 1–9, doi:10.1088/1674-4926/36/4/045001.
16. Maity, M; Ghosal, P; Das, B; Universal reversible logic gate design for low power computation at nano-scale. Asia Pacific Conf. Postgrad. Res. Microelectron. Electron 2012, pp. 173–177, doi:10.1109/PrimeAsia.2012.6458648.
17. Mahapatro, M;. Panda, SK; Satpathy, J; Saheel, M; Suresh, M; Panda, AK; Sukla, MK; Design of arithmetic circuits using reversible logic gates and power dissipation calculation. Proc. 2010 Int. Symp. Electron Syst. Des. ISED 2010, pp. 85–90, doi:10.1109/ISED.2010.25.
18. Das, JC; De, D; Reversible binary subtractor design using quantum dot-cellular automata. Front. Inf. Technol. Electron. Eng. 18 2016, pp. 1416–1429, doi:10.1631/FITEE.1600999.

19. Nath, T; Kumar, A; Mohan, A; Efficient design of reversible ALU in quantum-dot cellular automata. Opt. Int. J. Light Electron Opt. 127 2016, pp. 6172–6182, doi:10.1016/j.ijleo.2016.04.086.
20. Kumar, N; Wairya, S; Sen, B; Design of conservative, reversible sequential logic for cost efficient emerging nano circuits with enhanced testability. Ain Shams Eng. J. 9 2017, pp. 2027–2037, doi:10.1016/j.asej.2017.02.005.
21. Singh, R; Design and optimization of sequential counters using a novel reversible gate. Int. Conf. Comput. Commun. Autom. Noida 2016, pp. 1–6.
22. Ahmad, F; Ahmed, S; Kakkar, V; Bhat, GM; Newaz, A; Wani, S; Modular design of ultra-efficient reversible full adder-subtractor in QCA with power dissipation analysis. Int. J. Theor. Phys. 57 2018, pp. 2863–2880.
23. Misra, NK; Sen, B; Wairya, S; Novel conservative reversible error control circuits based on molecular QCA. Int. J. Comput. Appl. Technol. 56 2017, doi:10.1504/IJCAT.2017.086558.
24. Debnath, B; Das, JC; De, D; Reversible logic-based image steganography using quantum dot cellular automata for secure nanocommunication. IET Circuits. Devices Syst. 11 2017, pp. 58–67, doi:10.1049/iet-cds.2015.0245.
25. Das, JC; De, D; Quantum-dot cellular automata based reversible low power parity generator and parity checker design for nanocommunication. Front. Inf. Technol. Electron. Eng. 17 2016, pp. 224–236.
26. Thapliyal, H; Vinod, AP; Design of reversible sequential elements with feasibility of transistor implementation. IEEE Int. Symp. Circuits Syst. 2007, pp. 625–628.
27. Thapliyal, H; Ranganathan, N; Kotiyal, S; Design of testable reversible sequential circuits, IEEE Trans. Very Large Scale Integr. Syst. 21 2013, pp. 1201–1209, doi:10.1109/TVLSI.2012.2209688.
28. Thapliyal, H; Ranganathan, N; Reversible logic-based concurrently testable latches for molecular QCA, IEEE Trans. Nanotechnol. 9 2010, pp. 62–69. doi:10.1109/TNANO.2009.2025038.
29. Rad, SK; Heikalabad, SR; Reversible flip-flops in quantum-dot cellular automata. Int. J. Theor. Phys. 56 2017, pp. 2990–3004, doi:10.1007/s10773-017-3466-8.
30. Lent, CS; Liu, M; Lu, Y; Bennett clocking of quantum-dot cellular automata and the limits to binary logic scaling. Nanotechnology 17 2006, pp. 4240–4251, doi:10.1088/0957-4484/17/16/040.
31. Tougaw, PD; Lent, CS; Logical devices implemented using quantum cellular automata. J. Appl. Phys. 75 1994, pp. 1818–1825.
32. Hennessy, K; Lent, CS; Clocking of molecular quantum-dot cellular automata. J. Vac. Sci. Technol., B: Microelectron. Nanom. Struct. 19 2001, pp. 1752, doi:10.1116/1.1394729.
33. Vetteth, A; Walus, K; Dimitrov, VS; Jullien, GA; Quantum-dot cellular automata carry-look-ahead adder and barrel shifter. IEEE Emerg. Telecommun. Technol. Conf. 2002, pp. 2–4.
34. Walus, K; Jullien, GA; Dimitrov, VS; Computer arithmetic structures for quantum cellular automata. Thrity-Seventh Asilomar Conf. Signals, Syst. Comput. 2003, pp. 1435–1439, doi:10.1109/ACSSC.2003.1292223.
35. Walus, K; Jullien, GA; Design tools for an emerging SoC technology : Quantum-dot cellular automata. Proc. IEEE. 94 2006, pp. 1225–1244.
36. Zhang, R; Walus, K; Wang, W; Jullien, GA; A method of majority logic reduction for quantum cellular automata. IEEE Trans. Nanotechnol. 3 2004, pp. 443–450, doi:10.1109/TNANO.2004.834177.

37. Kim, K; Wu, K; Karri, R; The robust QCA adder designs using composable QCA building blocks Kyosun. IEEE Trans. Comput. Aided Des. Integr. Circuits Syst. 26 2007, pp. 176–183.
38. Hänninen, I; Takala, J; Binary adders on quantum-dot cellular automata. J. Signal Process. Syst. 58 2010, pp. 87–103, doi:10.1007/s11265-008-0284-5.
39. Zhang, Y; Lv, H; Liu, S; Xiang, Y; Xie, G; Design of quantum-dot cellular automata circuits using five-input majority gate. J. Comput. Theor. Nanosci. 12 2015, pp. 3675–3681, doi:10.1166/jctn.2015.4259.
40. Tahoori, MB; Huang, J; Momenzadeh, M; Lombardi, F; Testing of quantum cellular automata. IEEE Trans. Nanotechnol. 3 2004, pp. 432–442, doi:10.1109/TNANO.2004.834169.
41. Ma, X; Huang, J; Metra, C; Lombardi, F; Reversible gates and testability of one dimensional arrays of molecular QCA. J. Electron. Test. 24 2008, pp. 297–311, doi:10.1007/s10836-007-5042-2.
42. Thapliyal, H; Ranganathan, N; Conservative QCA gate (CQCA) for designing concurrently testable molecular QCA circuits. Proc. 22nd Int. Conf. VLSI Des. Held Jointly with 7th Int. Conf. Embed. Syst., IEEE, New Delhi. 2009, pp. 511–516, doi:10.1109/VLSI.Design.2009.75.
43. Singh, G; Raj, B; Sarin, RK; Fault-tolerant design and analysis of QCA-based circuits. IET Circuits Devices Syst. 12 2018, pp. 1–7, doi:10.1049/iet-cds.2017.0505.
44. Kumar, D; Mitra, D; Design of a practical fault-tolerant adder in QCA. Microelectron. J. 53 2016, pp. 90–104, doi:10.1016/j.mejo.2016.04.004.
45. Kumar, D; Mitra, D; Bhattacharya, BB; On fault-tolerant design of exclusive-OR gates in QCA. J. Comput. Electron. 16 2017, pp. 896–906, doi:10.1007/s10825-017-1022-7.
46. Khademolhosseini, H; Angizi, S; Nemati, Y; A fault-tolerant design for 3-input majority gate in quantum-dot cellular automata. J. Nanoelectron. Optoelectron. 12 2017, pp. 1–10, doi:10.1166/jno.2017.2175.
47. Ahmadpour, S; Mosleh, M; Nano communication networks new designs of fault-tolerant adders in quantum-dot cellular automata. Nano Commun. Netw. 19 2019, pp. 10–25, doi:10.1016/j.nancom.2018.11.001.
48. Danehdaran, F; Khosroshahy, MB; Navi, K; Bagherzadeh, N; Design and power analysis of new coplanar one-bit full-adder cell in design and power analysis of new coplanar one-bit full-adder cell in quantum-dot cellular automata. J. Low Power Electron. 14 2018, pp. 1–11, doi:10.1166/jolpe.2018.1529.
49. Seyedi, S; Navimipour, NJ; Design and evaluation of a new structure for fault-tolerance full-adder based on quantum-dot cellular automata. Nano Commun. Netw. 16 2018, pp.1–9, doi:10.1016/j.nancom.2018.02.002.
50. Farazkish, R; Khodaparast, F; Design and characterization of a new fault-tolerant full-adder for quantum-dot cellular automata. Microprocess. Microsyst. 39 2015, pp. 426–433, doi:10.1016/j.micpro.2015.04.004.
51. Asfestani, MN; Heikalabad, SR; A unique structure for the multiplexer in quantum-dot cellular automata to create a revolution in design of nanostructures. Phys. B Phys. Condens. Matter. 512 2017, pp. 91–99, doi:10.1016/j.physb.2017.02.028.
52. Kandasamy, N; Ahmad, F; Telagam, N; Shannon logic based novel QCA full adder design with energy dissipation analysis. Int. J. Theor. Phys. 57 2018, pp. 3702–3715, doi:10.1007/s10773-018-3883-3.

53. Sabbaghi-Nadooshan, R; Kianpour, M; A novel QCA implementation of MUX-based universal shift register. J. Comput. Electron. 13 2014, pp. 198–210, doi:10.1007/s10825-013-0500-9.
54. Sheikhfaal, S; Angizi, S; Sarmadi, S; Moaiyeri, MH; Designing efficient QCA logical circuits with power dissipation analysis, Microelectron. J. 46 2015, pp. 462–471, doi:10.1016/j.mejo.2015.03.016.
55. Newaz, A; Billah, M; Maksudur, M; Bhuiyan, R; Ultra-efficient convolution encoder design in quantum-dot cellular automata with power dissipation analysis, Alexandria Eng. J. 57 2018, pp. 3881–3888, doi:10.1016/j.aej.2018.02.007.
56. Bahar, AN; Ahmad, F; Ahmed, K; Performance evaluation of efficient combinational logic design using nanomaterial electronics. Cogent Eng. 9 2017, pp. 1–15, doi:10.1080/23311916.2017.1349539.
57. Bahar, AN, Optimized design and performance analysis of novel comparator and full adder in nanoscale. Cogent. Eng. 4 2016, pp. 1–14, doi:10.1080/23311916.2016.1237864.
58. Babaie, S; Sadoghifar, A; Bahar, AN; Design of an efficient multilayer arithmetic logic unit in quantum-dot cellular automata (QCA). IEEE Trans. Circuits Syst. II Express Briefs. 2018, doi:10.1109/TCSII.2018.2873797.
59. Dehkordi, MA; Shamsabadi, AS; Ghahfarokhi, BS; Vafaei, A; Novel RAM cell designs based on inherent capabilities of quantum-dot cellular automata, Microelectron. J. 42 2011, pp. 701–708, doi:10.1016/j.mejo.2011.02.006.
60. Xiao, L; Chen, X; Ying, S; Design of dual-edge triggered flip-flops based on quantum-dot cellular automata. J. Zhejiang Univ. Sci. C. 13 2012, pp. 385–392, doi:10.1631/jzus.C1100287.
61. Hashemi, S; Navi, K; New robust QCA D flip flop and memory structures. Microelectron. J. 43 2012, pp. 929–940, doi:10.1016/j.mejo.2012.10.007.
62. Singh, R; Pandey, MK; Analysis and implementation of reversible dual edge triggered flip flop using quantum dot cellular automata. Int. J. Innov. Comput. Inf. Control. 14 2018, pp. 147–159.
63. Bahar, AN; Laajimi, R; Ahmed, AK; Toward efficient design of flip-flops in quantum-dot cellular automata with power dissipation analysis. Int. J. Theor. Phys. 57 2018, pp. 3419–3428.
64. Al Shafi, A; Bahar, AN; Ultra-efficient design of robust RS flip-flop in nanoscale with energy dissipation study. Cogent. Eng. 9 2017, doi:10.1080/23311916.2017.1391060.
65. Purkayastha, T; De, D; Chattopadhyay, T; Universal shift register implementation using quantum dot cellular automata. AIN SHAMS Eng. J. 2016, pp. 1–20, doi:10.1016/j.asej.2016.01.011.
66. Sangsefidi, M; Abedi, D; Yoosefi, E; Karimpour, M; High speed and low cost synchronous counter design in quantum-dot cellular automata. Microelectron. J. 73 2018, pp. 1–11, doi:10.1016/j.mejo.2017.12.011.
67. Newaz, A; Habib, A; Maksudur, M; Bhuiyan, R; Ahmad, F; Zahoor, P; Ahmed, K; Designing single layer counter in quantum-dot cellular automata with energy dissipation analysis. Ain Shams Eng. J. 2017, doi:10.1016/j.asej.2017.05.010.
68. Angizi, S; Sayedsalehi, S; Roohi, A; Bagherzadeh, N; Navi, K; Design and verification of new n-bit quantum-dot synchronous counters using majority function-based JK flip-flops. J. Circuits Syst. Comput. 24 2015, pp. 1–16, doi:10.1142/S0218126615501534.
69. Angizi, S; Sarmadi, S; Sayedsalehi, S; Navi, K; Design and evaluation of new majority gate-based RAM cell in quantum-dot cellular automata. Microelectron. J. 46 2015, pp. 43–51, doi:10.1016/j.mejo.2014.10.003.

70. Sasamal, TN; Singh, AK; Ghanekar, U; Design and implementation of QCA D-flip-flops and RAM cell using majority gates. J. Circuits Syst. Comput. 2018, doi:10.1142/S0218126619500798.
71. Chabi, AM; Roohi, A; Khademolhosseini, H; Sheikhfaal, S; Angizi, S; Navi, K; Demara, RF; Towards ultra-efficient QCA reversible circuits. Microprocess. Microsyst. 49 2017, pp. 127–138, doi:10.1016/j.micpro.2016.09.015.
72. Chaves, JF; Ribeiro, MA; Silva, LM; de Assis, LMBC; Torres, MS; Vilela Neto, OP; Energy efficient QCA circuits design: Simulating and analyzing partially reversible pipelines. J. Comput. Electron. 17 2018, pp. 479–489, doi:10.1007/s10825-017-1120-6.
73. Bahar, AN; Waheed, S; Hossain, N; Asaduzzaman, M; A novel 3-input XOR function implementation in quantum dot-cellular automata with energy dissipation analysis. Alexandria Eng. J. 57 2018, pp. 729–738, doi:10.1016/j.aej.2017.01.022.
74. Thapliyal, H; Ranganathan, N; Design of reversible latches optimized for quantum cost, delay and garbage outputs. Proc. IEEE Int. Conf. VLSI 2010, pp. 235–240, doi:10.1109/VLSI.Design.2010.74.
75. Boi, B; Misra, NK; Pradhan, M; Design and evaluation of an efficient parity-preserving reversible QCA gate with online testability. Cogent. Eng. 4 2017, pp. 1–18, doi:10.1080/23311916.2017.1416888.
76. Timler, J; Lent, CS; Power gain and dissipation in quantum-dot cellular automata. J. Appl. Phys. 91 2002, pp. 823–831, doi:10.1063/1.1421217.
77. Huang, J; Ma, X; Lombardi, F; Energy analysis of QCA circuits for reversible computing. Nanotechnology 2006, pp. 3–6, doi:10.1109/NANO.2006.1717011.
78. Liu, M; Robustness and power dissipation in quantum-dot cellular automata. http://www.nd.edu/~qcahome/pdf/nd/Robustness_and_Power_Dissipation_in_Quantum-Dot_Cellular_Automata.pdf. 2006.
79. Srivastava, S; Sarkar, S; Bhanja, S; Estimation of upper bound of power dissipation in QCA circuits. IEEE Trans. Nanotechnol. 8 2009, pp. 116–127, doi:10.1109/TNANO.2008.2005408.
80. Srivastava, S; Asthana, A; Bhanja, S; Sarkar, S; QCAPro: An error-power estimation tool for QCA circuit design. Proc. IEEE Int. Symp. Circuits Syst. 2011, pp. 2377–2380, doi:10.1109/ISCAS.2011.5938081.
81. Roohi, A; Zand, R; Angizi, S; Demara, RF; A parity-preserving reversible QCA gate with self-checking cascadable resiliency. IEEE Trans. Emerg. Top. Comput. 6 2018, pp. 450–459, doi:10.1109/TETC.2016.2593634.

CHAPTER 3

An Introduction to a New Era of Microelectronics Devices and Interconnects

VANGMAYEE SHARDA

Amity University, Uttar Pradesh, India
E-mail vsharma3@amity.edu.

ABSTRACT

The performance of submicron very large scale integrated (VLSI) circuits is growing exponentially day by day. Due to this miniaturization in technology, the quantity of transistors in a VLSI circuit has been increasing (by twofold per 1.8 years, according to Moore's law). As a result of this continuous downscaling, the efficiency requirements of wires (providing connectivity between miniaturized devices) have boosted enormously. Numerous interconnects created from carbon are substituting the Cu/low-k interconnects because of their improved execution regarding power dissipation, delay, and signal veracity. Due to the scaling limitation of the Si metal–oxide–semiconductor field-effect transistor (MOSFET), new options of nanoelectronics devices based on carbon materials are coming into market to give better performance than conventional complementary metal–oxide–semiconductor (CMOS) device. Till now, CMOS is successful in the VLSI field due to its compatibility with miniaturization. But as the silicon technology is facing continuous scaling challenges, MOSFET will reach its limiting size soon. Any upcoming technology that is advantageous for parameters such as crosstalk, delay, power dissipation, or performance should be coordinated by an interconnect methodology which offers analogous technical bounds for evading the inconsistency matters because of interconnects. Apart from developments in semiconductor technology, there is also an emerging possibility for nanoantennas in future nanoelectronics devices due to materials such as carbon nanotubes, graphene, or superconductors. The electronic properties of these carbon-generated materials will allow the extreme miniaturization of antennas. This chapter deals with the new devices, interconnect technologies, and nanoantennas in microelectronics by the use of carbon-generated materials.

3.1 INTRODUCTION

According to Moore's opinion, the minimum feature size of transistors has reduced from 10 μm to the 28–22 nm in 2011. A fast glimpse at the International Technology Roadmap for Semiconductors (2012) demonstrates that the constant reduction of the transistor feature size of semiconductor ICs is projected to approach 7 nm by 2024 [1].

This replacement in the wiring material is also due to the increasing parasitic inductances, capacitances and resistances of interconnects with increment in operating frequencies of circuits in GHz ranges. Also, the high chip temperatures (due to huge power dissipation) in the nanometer regime with continuously growing current densities are making electromigration in copper wires a hazard for submicron very large scale integrated (VLSI) circuits.

Therefore, the new options for devices are coming out with the efforts of researchers. The device-level novel contenders in the postcomplementary metal–oxide–semiconductor (CMOS) epoch consists of FlexFET, single-electron transistor (SET), carbon nanotube FET (CNTFET), triple-gate FET, subthreshold CMOS, FinFET, and gate-all-around FET (GAAFET), etc. At the device level, there are ample solid contenders in the contemporary situation, but all are confronting boundaries levied by interconnect technology [2].

3.2 INTERCONNECT TECHNOLOGIES

3.2.1 CU/LOW-K INTERCONNECT

To produce high-speed integrated circuits (ICs), it is necessary to use interconnections that would allow the rapid transmission of information. Earlier, aluminum has been used almost entirely to make metallic parts on chip wires. More recently, Al–Cu alloys have been used due to better reliability than pure Al. In terms of electrical resistivity, Cu is advantageous in comparison to Al, with the latter being less resistant to electrical conduction

(~40%), which results in a higher speed advantage of 15%. Unfortunately, Cu is hazardous for silicon circuits because it quickly diffuses into the gate, source, and drain regions of the transistor that are fabricated on silicon. This diffusion negatively affects the functionality of the transistor. To overcome this drawback, a new fabrication technique is used which is expensive.

Cu/low-k interconnects used in submicron (~100 nm) CMOS-ICs is negatively affecting the performance of the whole system via enlarged crosstalk, transmission delay of propagating signals, and power dissipation. Cu/low-k interconnects confronted material issues as well as electrical issues at the nanometer scale. Due to the existence of a high-resistive barrier, there will be increment in the resistivity of the material, which is an important issue. Also, the scattering of electrons increases with scaling on the surface and grain boundaries [9]. The second issue related to the material is the lower conductivity of low-k dielectric materials than that of SiO_2. The higher current density demand from interconnects increases with the technology scaling. All these three reasons are resulting in the rise of interconnect temperatures at global wiring [10]. Global interconnect delay also increases with technology scaling. The insertion of a repeater is the solution for minimizing the delay, but the repeaters further increase the overall power dissipation of the chip.

At the global interconnect level, due to high frequencies, the inductive effect plays its role. Also, the skin depth effect for copper at higher frequencies increases the effective resistance of wires. This is generally known as the "skin effect." At high frequencies, the proximity effect also contributes to conductors [10]. Interconnect impedance is affected by the skin effect and proximity effects as a function of frequency. These electrical issues limit the accuracy of parasitic extraction in Cu/low-k interconnects. These challenges led the researchers to look upon innovative options for interconnections that can match up with the technology scaling. After years of research, some devices' friendly options are suggested which are as follows.

3.2.1.1 CNT INTERCONNECT

Carbon nanotubes (CNTs) are the lowest molecule of graphite carbon with exceptional characteristics. CNTs are believed to be the convincing molecular arrangement and known for their outstanding electronic features. Due to this, CNTs have ample participation in the engineering and profitable applications. Having metallic properties, CNTs have a long mean free path (of quite a few micrometers), and they can transmit enormously large current densities (10^3 greater than wires of Cu) [13]. CNTs are grown in the form of seamless cylinders with the walls formed by one atomic layer of graphite known as graphene and having diameter measuring on the nanometer scale [8].

Depending upon the chirality (chirality is the rolling direction of CNTs), CNTs validate either semiconducting or metallic characteristics. This chirality is not under the control of the developer, so the bundle of CNTs consists of metallic as well as semiconducting nanotubes.

Current conduction in this bundle is due to metallic nanotubes only and not the semiconducting ones. CNTs are categorized into single- and multiwalled nanotubes (containing several coaxial cylinder-shaped shells). Although multi-walled CNTs (MWCNTs) are principally metallic, but it is challenging for attaining ballistic carriage for elongated lengths in MWCNTs. Alternatively, electron mean free paths of micron ranges affect single-walled CNTs (SWCNTs). Hereafter, for the interconnect's province, SWCNTs fall in the favored contenders' category [11] for the utmost thought-provoking characteristics of CNTs that are the scattering free (ballistic) and spin preserving movement of electrons in the tube, access to the energy gap, and the capability to have semiconducting as well as metallic behavior which is governed by the diameter of tubes [27].

For forthcoming IC technology, CNTs have been projected to be a conceivable candidate for the interconnection purpose. SWCNTs have enormous latent for purposes in electronics due to their metallic as well as semiconducting features and their capability to transfer large currents. CNTs can carry concentration ranging around 10 $\mu A/nm^2$, whereas Cu interconnects have a current transmitting ability ranging around 10 nA/nm^2.

For interconnects, SWCNT is modeled as an equivalent transmission line. A CNT, because of its band structure, has two propagating channels that are labeled as channel A and channel B. Electrons can spin up and spin down in both channels. Hence, there are four channels [7]. Each channel has its quantum capacitance which is denoted by C_Q in the transmission line model. In $4C_Q$ denotes the quantum capacitance of four channels, C_E is the electrostatic capacitance, R_{mc} is the metal nanotube contact resistance, R_Q denotes the quantum resistance, R_{SCAT} is the scattering resistance, and L_{CNT} is the inductance of the nanotube.

SWCNTs have suitable properties for interconnect application, but they give intrinsic ballistic resistance of 6.5 kΩ that is independent of length of the nanotube. Thus, SWCNT is highly resistive, which adds on to the signal transmission delay due to interconnect. The geometric structure of an

SWCNT, where d is the diameter of the SWCNT and y is its distance from the ground.

To remove this, the intrinsic resistance problems associated with MWCNTs were suggested and substantially validated for the probable interconnect option for interconnects at the intermediate, local, and global levels because MWCNTs provide parallel conduction paths that decrease the parasitic resistance. Depicts an ordered structure for an MWCNT existing on a ground plane.

D_{in} and D_{out} in signify the inner shell diameter and the outer shell diameter, respectively, and y indicates the inner shell height starting from the ground plane. The studies for the comparison of MWCNTs with SWCNTs and Cu have been done, and it has been proved that MWCNTs are beneficial for interconnect applications.

Both SECNT and MWCNT interconnects can attain improved functioning than Cu wires for lengthy interconnects. Though the important fact is that we should know how to provide comparison between SWCNTs and MWCNTs because, nowadays, for closely filled ~100% metallic SWCNT bundles, numerous fabrication confronts should be solved. MWCNT interconnects demonstrate noteworthy enhancement in signal delays in comparison to Cu interconnects (15% lower than Cu delay) for the intermediate- and global-level interconnects. It is also projected that with more technology scaling, this enhancement will be increased. The delays provided by MWCNT interconnects are only slightly longer than that of Cu interconnects (1%–6%) in the case of short or local interconnects. Also, because MWCNTs are simpler to fabricate with not much concern for chirality and density constraint, these could be a smart choice in the case of VLSI interconnects [16].

3.2.1.2 GNR INTERCONNECT

Graphene, a material on which research is started only seven years ago, seems to be more promising for integrated VLSI circuits, as well as for large area transparent conducting film applications. Starting from its invention, graphene provided the possibility of getting awareness of several possessions in smaller magnitudes, and because it has a very large charge carrier mobility, it provided vast possibilities in fabrication of electronic devices. Also, it has provided a promising option to replace silicon electronic devices.

Shown in Figure 3.1 is a small bandgap material, graphene, which is the 2D allotrope of sp^2-bonded carbon, arranged in a honeycomb lattice.

A sp^2-hybridized network is formed by the carbon atoms along with three adjoining neighbors (all of them are residing at a separation of ~1.42 Å from the carbon atom) and leaves one un-hybridized half-filled p-type orbital, vertical to the graphene level for each carbon. Two atoms from two different sublattices make a rhombus unit cell and form a bipartite lattice of graphene. Graphene nanoribbons (GNRs) are strips of graphene with dimension less than 10 nm.

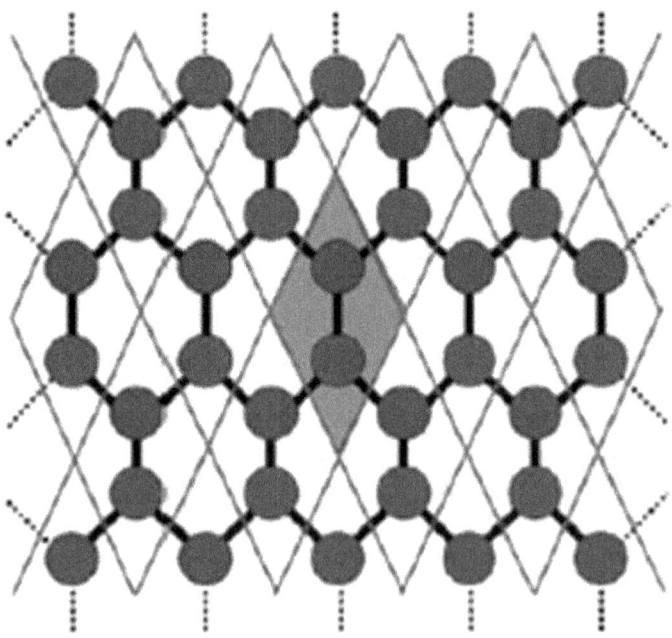

FIGURE 3.1 Graphene honeycomb lattice having two points in the colored area [24].
Source: Reprinted with permission from Ref. [24]. © Royal Society of Chemistry.

GNRs were originally introduced as a theoretical model by Mitsutaka Fujita and co-authors [43] to examine the edge and nanoscale size effect in graphene. Simply put, GNR originated from graphene and hence has inherited similar properties. Graphene comes out in structures like quasi-one-dimensional ribbon due to finite termination. Figure 3.2 represents two diverse conceivable edge arrangements, named as armchair and zigzag.

An Introduction to a New Era of Microelectronics 67

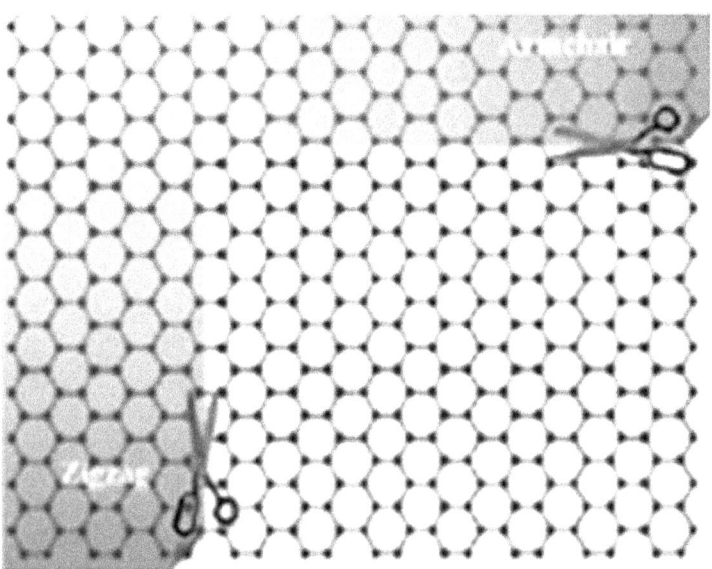

FIGURE 3.2 Representation of carving the 2D graphene pane to attain zigzag armchair and nanoribbons [24].
Source: Reprinted with permission from Ref. [24]. © Royal Society of Chemistry.

They are designated as armchair GNRs and zigzag GNRs, separately and display almost diverse electronic properties ascending on or after their opposing boundary situations. The atoms coming via two different sublattices make bonds alongside the armchair edges, whereas the atoms alongside a zigzag verge originate via the same sublattice.

Compared to CNTs, GNRs are more controllable and cost-effective in terms of fabrication due to the planar nature of graphene [19]. Due to this, GNRs have emerged as an interesting material with affluence of electronic and spin transport properties [23].

3.3 DEVICE TECHNOLOGIES

3.3.1 SINGLE-ELECTRON TRANSISTOR

SET is a nanometer scale device made up of a small island that is conducting (quantum dot) and connected to a source and a drain with tunnels and coupled to the gate junction capacitively (see Figure 3.3). It is based on the tunnel effect that is a quantum phenomenon [25].

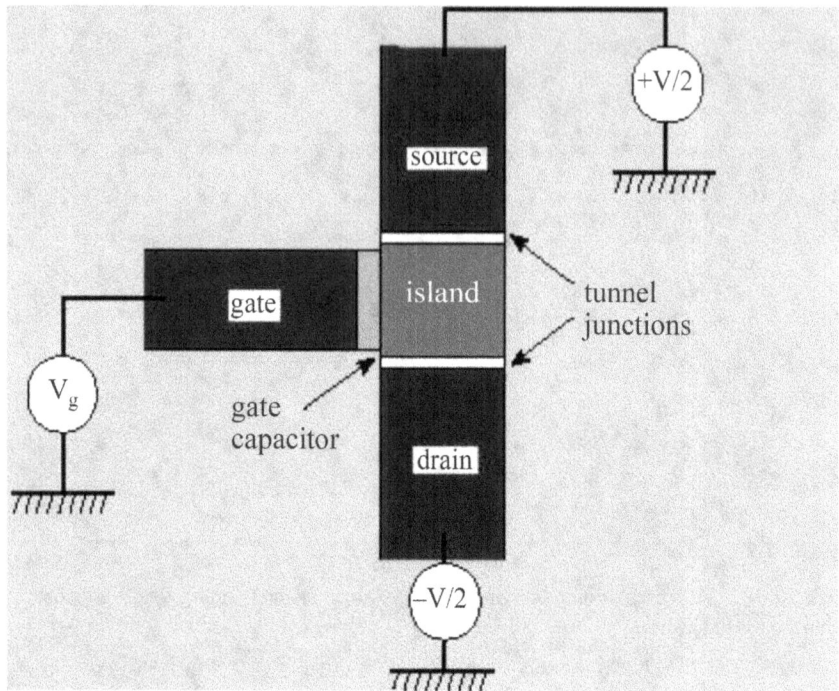

FIGURE 3.3 Structure of the SET [25].
Source: Reprinted with permission from Ref. [24]. Creative Commons license.

It is the key element of the current research area of nanotechnology, which is advantageous in terms of low power consumption and high speed, which are the two main desired factors from any new technology [28].

This transistor turns ON and OFF every time one electron is added in it. This is the reason to call it the "single-electron transistor." These transistors are applied in highly sensitive electrometers, single-electron spectroscopy, infrared radiation detection, voltage stage and charge stage logics, microwave detector, and programmable transistor logic [23, 26].

But there exist some limitations in the implementation of SET. Some of these are their requirement of specific room temperature, randomness in their background charge, co-tunneling, absence of suitable lithography, and unable to link properly to the outside circuit [23, 26]. Researchers in nanotechnology are working on the removal of these problems. Until these problems are removed, it is not a proper technology option.

3.3.2 CARBON NANOTUBE FET

CNTFET first came into existence in 1998 [4]. It uses semiconducting SWCNT for the formation of the channel region field effect transistor. As CNTs are proficient to carry heat (like diamond or sapphire) and due to the small dimension of CNTs, the transistor device made up of CNT, that is, CNTFET can switch using less power than silicon FET [6].

As compared to metal–oxide–semiconductor field-effect transistors (MOSFETs), CNTFETs have good control over the formation of a channel, better threshold voltage, superior electron mobility, current density, and transconductance. The applicable gate capacitance/unit width of CNTFET is almost twofold as compared to p-type metal−oxide semiconductor (PMOS). So, CNTFETs are compatible with high-k gate dielectrics. High electron mobility gives higher current velocity to CNTFETs than MOSFETs [20].

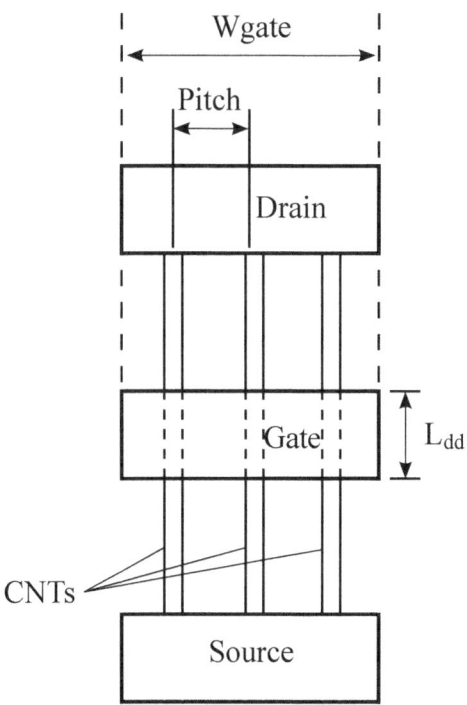

FIGURE 3.4 CNTFET structure.
Source: Modified from Ref. [22].

The CNT region forming channel is undoped, but other regions are heavily doped, thereby acting as a source/drain region. If the extra CNTs are placed, there a linear increment can be attained in the current.

However, because of a small pitch (distance between CNTs) and the diameter of CNT, the screening effect occurs in CNTFET, and the current cannot increase linearly with the number of CNTs [22]. A distinctive assembly of a MOSFET-like CNTFET is demonstrated in Figure 3.4.

Transistor width (W) is changed by determining the ratio of PMOS/NMOS complementary MOS. Similarly, for CNTFET, the count of CNTs are altered as CNTFET practices CNTs for the channel of current conduction amongst the source and the drain of CNTFET. But with exposure to oxygen, CNTs used to degrade. Also, high electric fields and high temperatures make CNTs highly unreliable. Due to this reliability in a single-channel CNTFET, it is observed that the multichannel assembly will be more reliable in the case of CNTFET. Multichannel CNTFET gives stable performance for several months in comparison to the single-channel CNTFET, which works for only some weeks [21]. Another disadvantage of CNTFET is difficulty in mass production and high production cost.

3.3.3 GRAPHENE NANORIBBON FET

In comparison to CNTFET, GNR-FET unveils analogous performance, lesser sensitive for the inconsistent chirality of the channel, and analogous problems of leakage because of inter-band tunneling. For the proper performance of the transistor, the actual width of 1–2 nm with atomic precision is required for nanoribbon. It could be attained with stress patterns or periodic etch patterns [14].

GNR MOSFET shows better performance than GNR Schottky barrier FET (GNR SBFET). The former has improved saturation behavior, high trans-conductance, 50% higher current in the ON state, and higher attainable ON–OFF ratio accompanied by 60% lesser output conductance. The performance of GNR MOSFET in terms of switching and high frequencies is enhanced compared with conventional MOSFETs, which includes a 30% larger range of cut-off frequencies and 20% more switching speed.

GNR MOSFETs are more robust than GNR SBFETs even when the former comprise defect or an impurity. Due to the existence of a lattice vacancy (single), the Schottky barrier thickness of the tunneling device is relentlessly influenced, which in turn can lessen the I_{on} of the GNR SBFET by 46%, which is considerably higher than the I_{on} of the GNR MOSFET. Due to the edge roughness of GNR, there is a higher OFF current and lesser ON current, in general, and due to the entirely changed atomistic GNR configuration in these devices having a small channel, the fickleness of device performance is very hefty.

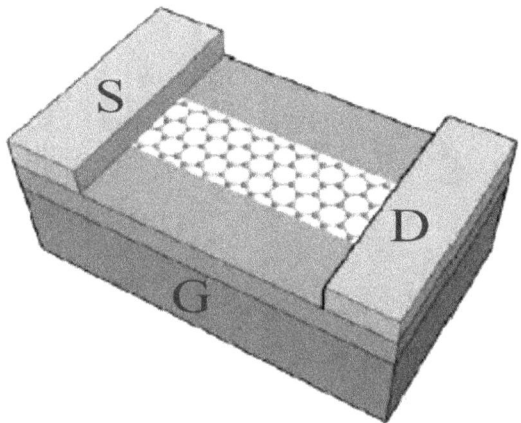

FIGURE 3.5 Schematics of GNRFETs on 10 nm SiO_2 with Pd S/D. P^{++} Si is used as a back gate [16].

Source: Reprinted with permission from Ref [16]. © American Physical Society. https://journals.aps.org/prl/abstract/10.1103/PhysRevLett.100.206803

GNRFETs demonstrated experimentally are achieved by joining the channel to metals with Schottky gates, consequently finding a GNR SBFET. By heavy doping of the source and the drain regions of GNR, the ohmic contacts can principally be attained, which in turn helps in making the operation like that of MOSFET, which is called GNR MOSFET [18].

Due to the positively charged impurity, the ON current (I_{on}) of GNR SBFET could be amplified by 20%. But GNR MOSFET is affected in a very limited manner by this impurity because the top of the barrier of GNR MOSFET is almost invariant to the positively charged impurity. But the carrier transportation of GNRFETs can be disturbed by the negative impurity due to the local increment of electrostatic potential [18].

3.3.4 TRI-GATE TRANSISTOR

These transistors use a single gate stacked on top of two vertical gates, giving three times the surface area for the movement of electrons. According to the reports given by Intel Corporation, these transistors reduce the leakage current and power consumption (less than CMOS transistors). A tri-gate transistor gives 37% higher speed with 50% less power consumption [24, 27]. Intel announced the technology for the very first time in September 2002.

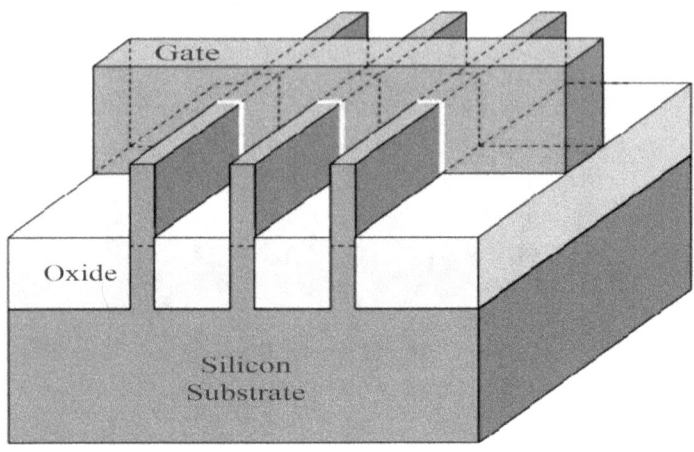

FIGURE 3.6 Tri-gate transistor structure [34].
Source: Image Courtesy Intel Corporation

By 2002, Intel had put efforts on its tri-gate architecture and then the company issued its Ivy Bridge (the new range of CPUs following tri-gate transistor features) in 2011. It shows that it took too long for the mass production of these devices which is the main drawback of these devices.

3.3.5 FLEXFET

This is a double gated transistor having top gate as damascene metal top gate MOSFET and the bottom gate is an implanted JFET (both are self-aligned gates). FlexFET is a planar and have nonepitaxial raised source and drain regions. It is a proper double-gate transistor because its both top and bottom gates provide transistor functioning and are coupled in such a way that single-gate operation affects the operation of other gate also [15].

3.3.6 FinFET

FinFET also comes under the category of a multigate transistor. This term was first used by the University of California, Berkeley (UC Berkeley) researchers. It defines a nonplanar, double-gate transistor having a conduction channel which is enfolded by a thin layer of silicon called "fin."

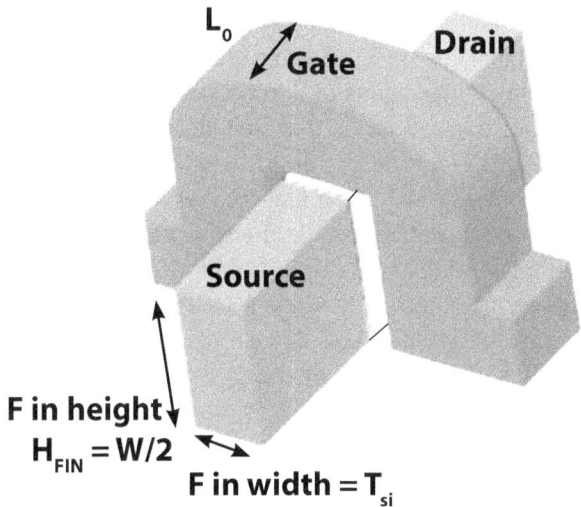

FIGURE 3.7 FinFET structure [33].

Source: Reprinted from Ref. [33]. Courtesy of Synopsys, Inc. https://www.synopsys.com/designware-ip/technical-bulletin/finfet-design.html

Fin generates the physique of the FinFET. In the technical field nowadays, FinFET is generalized as any fin-based multigate transistor, irrespective of the number of gates [5]. The first benchmark model of FinFETs was issued formally by UC Berkeley's Berkeley Short-channel IGFET Model (BSIM) group on March 1, 2012, and is known as BSIM-CMG106.0.0 [30]. It comprises all-important multigate transistor behaviors [31].

FinFETs are analyzed to be 37% faster with less than half dynamic power consumption and reduced static leakage current approximately by 90% than the regular CMOS. So, the circuit's performance can be enhanced in terms of speed by using almost similar or small expanse of power. With this new FinFET device technology, the requirements of nanometer era circuits can be matched and the operation of circuits can be improved [32].

3.3.7 GATE-ALL-AROUND FET

Conceptually, this device is the same as FinFET, but its gate substance encircles the channel area from all sides. GAAFETs could have four or two actual gates. These can be successfully built around a silicon nanowire.

3.3.8 TUNNELING FIELD EFFECT TRANSISTOR

Over the past few years, there has been an expanding requirement of the tunnel field effect transistor (TFET), and scientists are performing extensive research on this transistor. TFET has been established by T. Baba in 1992, as one of the proficient variations to the conservative MOSFET's depending upon several performance aspects that include possibility for subthreshold swing more than 60 mV/decade, extreme low power and extreme low voltage, the consequences of the short channel, reduction in the leakage current, because of the tunneling effect requirement of more speed, competence to operate on subthreshold, and superthreshold voltage region, likeness in the fabrication process as compared with a MOSFET. Considering the above-mentioned aspects, the MOSFET could be replaced by a capable substitute in terms of TFET for the persistence of energy efficient, ultra-low-power, and high-speed applications in the field of ICs.

The structure of TFET is approximately closer to MOSFET, however with a different fundamental switching mechanism. Switching of TFET is done by modulating quantum tunneling through a barrier instead of modulating thermionic emission over a barrier as in traditional MOSFETs. The TFET device is functioned by applying the gate bias so that electron buildup occurs in the intrinsic section. At the ample gate bias, band-to-band tunneling occurs when the conduction band of the intrinsic region brings into line with the valence band of the P-region.

3.4 CNT AND GRAPHENE FOR NANOANTENNA

The on-chip integration of antennas unlocks novel panoramas intended for innovative applications and integrated structures for identification, sensing, wireless communications, and power-garnering applications. The necessities of antenna amalgamation hooked on the IC architecture are diverse from the integration of the circuit. But expertise based on nanoelectronics engraves a compromise among these necessities. Besides, expansion in semiconductor technology, the evolving opportunity for the integration of antennas within future nanoelectronics device platforms based on CNTs, graphene, etc. opens new outlooks. Because of the inherent inductance and capacitance of Nanotubes at extremely high frequencies, nanotubes have been suggested as antennas at infrared (IR) and visible light wavelengths.

Cutting-edge electromagnetic antennas functioning at micro- and millimeter wave frequencies have converted requisite in today's information society [35, 36]. They are enormously used in an extensive variety of applications including mobile or satellite communications, multimedia broadcasting, environmental sensing, radars, or medical systems [37, 38]. This surfeit of applications has unsurprisingly generated massive research and scientific evolution in the field in the past times. However, the exponential progress of the information world is incessantly striking very thought-provoking and sometimes contradictory industrial demands, such as higher communication speed, complex number of functionalities in a single, miniaturized device, future 5G diverse networks, entirely integrated and shrunken sensing solutions, and the competent use of the spectrum and energy resources, to name a few.

The microelectronic features of some constituents will permit an intense shrinking of antennas. There is an involvement of close integration of a rectifying or an active component in the frequencies extending from terahertz ranges up into the optical ranges because of physical reasons. Also, the important factors for antenna action are antenna structures and properties of antenna, which impact their electronic behavior. For this, CNT antennas, plasmonic antennas, and nanowire antennas are in picture nowadays. There is a distinction between nanoelectronics-based integrated antennas and nanoantennas. Nanoelectronics-based antennas are driven by the necessities of monolithic ICs or system-on chip, whereas nanoantennas are nanostructures themselves. Here we will discuss the scope of CNT antennas and graphene antennas.

3.4.1 CNT ANTENNA

CNTs assist an exciting miniaturization because of their slow wave propagation effects. The wavelength of electromagnetic waves promulgating in CNT structures is significantly lesser than the free-space wavelength because of the slow wave propagation of electromagnetic waves. This effect arises due to quantum transport properties in the CNT, granting a kinetic inductance and quantum capacitance along with the geometric inductance and capacitance [39].

Although copper is usually used in applications where high conductivity is essential, it does not preserve its bulk conductivity when scaled down to nanometer magnitudes [40]. Contrary, nanotubes show improved conductivity as compared to Cu when reduced down to the similar diameter.

It is showed [40] that the dc resistance for every unit length of an SWCNT is about 6 kΩ/μm at room temperature. But Cu interconnects having the identical diameter have an even larger resistance for per unit length. This resistance is rather higher than free-space characteristic impedance, and from the conventional radiation resistances in conventional antennas. Thus, this resistance cannot be abandoned. It is also demonstrated that the nanotube up to about 10 GHz has the identical dc and ac resistances [40]. Nevertheless, above-mentioned large impedances can notably be condensed toward the 50 Ω if the capacitive contact is exercised amid the dielectric substrate and CNT instead of resistive contact [40]. This results in the introduction of a thin dielectric in between the CNT and metallic contact. This conformation of the contact, that is, metal/dielectric/nanotube intends 6.5 k resistance in parallel of the capacitor with the global outcome of reduction in the resistance of the CNT.

The distributed electrostatic capacitance and magnetic inductance on a double-interconnect transmission line generate a wave velocity that is archetypally equivalent to the light speed. Though due to the kinetic energy residing in electrons, CNT comprises of an additional inductance. Mathematically, the above-said inductance is almost 10,000 larger than the conventional magnetic inductance, and that is why it leads [40]. CNT act as a quantum transmission line triggered by this hefty inductance for RF range voltages. This CNT line has the characteristic impedance in the ranges of several kiloohms. Also, the wavelength is approximately 50100 times lesser than the free-space wavelength for a specified frequency [40]. By this, the current distribution changes intensely in comparison with a thin-wire macro antenna and must be acknowledged for. As in a metallic wire the charges are rather free of movement, so the conductivities of metallic wires and nanotube are diverse. In nanotubes, the electron movement is because of ballistic transport over the nanotubes through the path length of approximately 100 nm in the tubular structure or thru tunneling among gaps [40] with related high tunneling resistance.

This high inductance in CNT provides a gradual wave proliferation through a CNT broadcast line which is electromagnetic propagation with a phase velocity of the ranges of c0/100–c0/50, where c0 = light speed in free space. CNT nanoantennas which are smaller than the operational wavelength could be used as potential radiation elements and could be carried in the resonance. A CNT nanoantenna is typically tremendously short antenna electrically. It is significantly smaller than free-space wavelength. CNT nanoantennas are considerably smaller than the operating wavelength and can be fetched in the resonance condition and possibly be consumed as radiation components.

The presence of slow wave makes CNT antennas apt for wireless communication among nanocircuits and in the macroscopic situation.

CNT dipoles were discovered to move in a resonance situation at very lesser frequencies as primarily presumed. This can be elucidated from the propagation of electromagnetic waves absorbed by CNTs, thereby creating surface plasmons, having demoted propagation speed, and consequently, smaller wavelengths.

Due to this, CNT dipoles with numerous micrometers in dimension begin resonating in the lowered terahertz section which concentrate along the wavelengths 50100 times elongated in comparison to the CNT dipole length. Due to the enormously high aspect ratio, both metal nanowires and CNTs have AC resistances in ranges of quite a few kΩ per micrometers along with per unit length. High-conduction losses are grounded due to high resistance and which in turn utterly decrements the attainable gain of nanoantenna as well as their proficiency. In [39], the CNT antenna efficacy is valued for the limits of −60 to −90 dB due to the outcomes of prominent conductance losses. A similar condition arises in nanoantennas made up of metal. While there are adequate low power levels in current transmission lines, the integral losses hosted by CNTs or metallic nanoantennas confines their applications substantially. The tactic for evading the resistance problem can be practicing of the arrangement of nanoantenna or a package of nanowires in a parallel manner. This type of arrangement could be helpful in the resistance reduction to a tolerable value though the effect of the slow wave is vanished as conversed in [39]. Hence, making an apt selection of the quantity of nanowires and geometry of antenna, the properties of nanoantenna assemblies must be adjusted.

3.4.2 GRAPHENE NANOANTENNA

There might be a hopeful substitute to CNT antennas in the form of planar structures, for example, 2D graphene layers. Graphene is a 2D material that comprises a monoaural atomic layer made up of carbon atoms well organized as a honeycomb structure, as shown in Figure 3.2. It demonstrates an admirable crystal quality and exceptional electronic properties. Graphene also showcases brilliant slow wave and conductivity properties like CNTs. The attainable slow-wave impact in plasmon modes is of the range of c0/100. In the graphene layer, the population inversion could be attained by forward-biasing or optical pumping for terahertz frequency ranges. Because this produces the magnification of the external (surface) plasmons.

The completion of active circuits and planar structures is allowed by graphene. A patch antenna based on CNTs and GNRs is displayed in Figure 3.8. Estimated investigations have displayed that the antennas having dimensions ranging in few hundred nanometers are appropriate in emitting electromagnetic waves that fall within the terahertz band (0.1–1 THz).

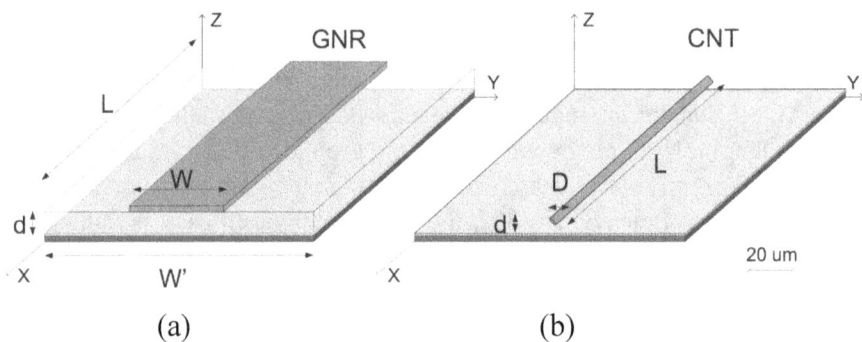

FIGURE 3.8 Antenna (nanopatch) fabricated (a) over a GNR and (b) over a CNT [39].
Source: Reprinted from Ref. [44].

In metallic antennas, graphene is used as a substrate. Researchers [39] have patterned the metallic dipole antenna and array of the dipole antenna onto the layer of graphene. These antennas were designed to function at 120 GHz. Also, the radiation patterns of these kinds of antennas could be organized precisely using the large- and small-resistivity features of graphene.

3.4.3 SUPERCONDUCTING ANTENNA

The use of superconductors allows the accomplishment of superdirectivity antennas of tremendously tiny size. Additionally, superconductors provide abundant exciting purposes for antennas. Superconductors display marvelous properties, for example, low attenuation, low noise level, and low power loss. Superconductors give us an opportunity to frame ultra-small antennas that feature large radiating quality. These antennas are best suited for the amalgamation with Josephson-effect-based radiation detectors [39].

The ultra-sensitive optical detection property is there in superconductors, which is due to the hotspot generation. A photon's occurrence over a superconducting nanoribbon or nanowire produces momentary resistive barrier development in the nanoribbon or the nanowire, and thus affecting a voltage pulse. The interval of decay ranges approximately 30 ps. Due to the short reset time, low noise, and broad wavelength response, superconducting nanowire single-photon detectors are hopefully contenders to substitute other single-photon detectors [39].

3.5 CONCLUSION

Traditional devices as well as interconnects are not accomplishing well in the deep submicron regime of VLSI, for delay, crosstalk, and power dissipation. That is why the novel technologies approaching into market have been examined to work in the applications of submicron VLSI circuits. In recent years, CNT and graphene have engrossed consideration as capable substances for cutting-edge electronic devices together with high-speed transistors that are having a main role in LSI technology. So, there is a rapid increment in the applications of graphene. Nevertheless, the fabrication or processing technologies is still away from the level desired for the authentic construction of devices for hands-on use.

As there is a continuous decrement in the assembly size of devices and components in the circuit, the conditions for antennas and radiating foundations that are used in ICs for chip-to-chip and on-chip communication will be similar. Going along with the common ongoing drift of scaling, antennas residing on-chip will shortly join the micrometer and nanometer regions. The incredible latent for the achievement of innovative devices and schemes (DC to optical ranges) will be stipulated by integrated antennas conceptualized by nanoelectronics.

KEYWORDS

- **carbon nanotube**
- **graphene nanoribbon**
- **FinFET**
- **CNT antenna**
- **GNR antenna**

REFERENCES

1. International Technology Roadmap for Semiconductors (ITRS), 2012 Update, available online: http://www.itrs.net/
2. Ceyhan, A.; Naeemi, A.; Impact of conventional and emerging interconnects on the circuit performance of various post-CMOS devices. Proceedings of the 14th International Symposium on Quality Electronic Design, March 4–6, 2013, 203–209.
3. Pribat, D.; Lee, Y. H.; Carbon nanotubes and graphene for various applications in electronics: competition and synergy. IEEE Technology Time Machine Symposium on Technologies Beyond 2020 (TTM), June 1–3, 2011, 1–2.
4. Tans, S. J.; Verschueren, A. R. M.; Dekker, C.; Room-temperature transistor based on a single carbon nanotube. Nature, 1998, 393, 49–52.
5. Huang, X.; Lee, W. C.; Kuo, C.; Hisamoto, D.; Chang, L.; Kedzierski, J.; Anderson, E.; Takeuchi, H.; Choi, Y. K.; Asano, K.; Subramanian, V.; King, T. J.; Bokor, J.; Hu, C.; Sub-50 nm FinFET: PMOS. IEEE Technical Digest of International Electron Devices Meeting, Washington, DC, USA, December 5–8, 1999, 67–70.
6. Collins, P. G.; Avouris, P.; Nanotubes for electronics. Scientific American, 2000, 283, 62–69.
7. Burke, P. J.; Luttinger liquid theory as a model of the gigahertz electrical properties of carbon nanotubes. IEEE Transactions on Nanotechnology, 2002, 1, 3, 129–144.
8. Hoenlein, W.; Kreupl, F.; Duesberg, G. S.; Graham, A. P.; Liebau, M.; Seidel, R. V.; Unger, E.; Carbon nanotube applications in microelectronics. IEEE Transactions on Components and Packaging Technologies, 2004, 27, 4, 629–634.
9. Steinhogl, W.; Schindler, G.; Steinlesberger, G.; Traving, M.; Engelhardt, M.; Comprehensive study of the resistivity of copper wires with lateral dimensions of 100 nm and smaller. Journal of Applied Physics, 2005, 97, 2, 023706-1-023706-7.
10. Banerjee, K.; Im, S.; Srivastava, N.; Interconnect modeling and analysis in the nanometer era: Cu and beyond. Proceedings of the 22nd Advanced Metallization Conference, Colorado Springs, September 26–29, 2005.
11. Srivastava, N.; Banerjee, K.; Performance analysis of CNT interconnects for VLSI applications. Proceedings of IEEE International Conference on Computer Aided Design, November 6–10, 2005, 383–390.
12. Nieuwoudt, A.; Massoud, Y.; Evaluating the impact of resistance in carbon nanotube bundles for VLSI interconnect using diameter-dependent modeling techniques; IEEE Transactions on Electron Devices, 2006, 53, 10, 2460–2466.
13. Li, H.; Yin W. Y.; Mao, J. F.; Modeling of carbon nanotube interconnects and comparative analysis with Cu interconnects. Proceedings of Asia-Pacific Microwave Conference, Yokohama, December 12–15, 2006, 1361–1364.
14. Fiori, G.; Iannaccone, G.; Simulation of graphene nanoribbon field effect transistors. IEEE Electron Device Letters, 2007, 28, 8, 760–762.
15. Wilson, D.; Hayhurst, R.; Oblea, A.; Parke, S.; Hackler, D.; FlexFet: independently-double-gated SOI transistor with variable V_t and 0.5 V operation achieving near ideal sub-threshold Slope. Proceedings of IEEE International SOI conference, Indian Wells, CA, October 1-4, 2007, 147–148.
16. Wang, X.; Ouyang, Y.; Li, X.; Wang, H.; Guo J.; Dai, H.; Room temperature all semiconducting sub-10-nm Graphene Nanoribbon field-effect transistors. Physics Review Letters, 2008, 100, 20.

17. Li, H.; Yin, W. Y.; Banerjee K.; Mao, J. F.; Circuit modeling and performance analysis of multi-walled carbon nanotube interconnects. IEEE Transactions on Electron Devices, 2008, 55, 6.
18. Yoon, Y.; Fiori, G.; Hong, S.; Iannaccone, G.; Guo, J.; Performance comparison of graphene nanoribbon FETs with Schottky contacts and doped reservoirs. IEEE Transactions on Electron Devices, 2008, 55, 9, 2314–2323.
19. Xu, C.; Li, H.; Banerjee, K.; Graphene nano-ribbon (GNR) interconnects: a genuine contender or a delusive dream? Proceedings of IEEE International Electron Devices Meeting, San Francisco, CA, December 15–17, 2008, 1–4.
20. Sahoo, R.; Mishra, R. R.; Simulations of carbon nanotube field effect transistors. International Journal of Electronic Engineering Research, 2009, 1, 2, 117–125.
21. Cjangxin, C.; Yafei, Z.; Nanowelded carbon nanotubes: from field effect transistor to solar microcells. Nano Science and Technology Series, 2009, 63, ISBN 3-642-01498-4.
22. Cho, G.; Kim, Y. B.; Lombardi, F.; Assessment of CNTFET based circuit performance and robustness to PVT variations. Proceedings of 52nd IEEE International Midwest Symposium on Circuits and Systems, Cancun, August 2–5, 2009, 1106–1109.
23. Jiao, L.; Zhang, L.; Ding, L.; Liu, J.; Dai, H.; Aligned graphene nanoribbons and crossbars from unzipped carbon nanotubes. Nano Res., 2010, 3, 387–394.
24. Duttaa, S.; Pati, S. K.; Novel properties of graphene nanoribbons: a review. Journal of Materials Chemistry, 2010, 38, 8207–8233.
25. Kumar, O.; Kaur, M.; Single electron transistor: applications and problems. International Journal of VLSI Design and Communication Systems, 2010, 1, 4, 24–29.
26. Cartwright, J.; Intel enters the third dimension. Nature, May 6 2011, doi: 10.1038/news.2011.274.
27. Han, C. S.; Assembling, patterning and application of CNT: from research to commercialization. Proceedings of IEEE Nanotechnology Materials and Devices Conference, Jeju, Korea, October 18–21, 2011, 1–4.
28. Kumar, A.; Dubey, D.; Single electron transistor: applications and limitations. Advance in Electronics and Electric Engineering, 2013, 3, 1, 57–62.
29. Lien, J.; Shen, S.; TSMC likely to launch 16 nm FinFET +process at the year-end 2014, and "FinFET turbo" later in 2015-16. DIGITIMES, Retrieved March 31, 2014.
30. BSIM-CMG 107.0.0 models, BSIM Group, University of California, Berkeley. [Online]. Available: www-device.eecs.berkeley.edu/bsim/
31. http://en.wikipedia.org/wiki/Multigate_device
32. Thean, A.; FinFET evolution for the 7 nm and 5 nm CMOS technology nodes. Solid state technology-insights for electronics manufacturing, 2014. Available: http://electroiq.com/blog/2014/01/finfet-evolution-for-the-7nm-and-5nm-cmos-technology-nodes/
33. Kawa, J. FinFET Design, Manufacturability, and Reliability. DesignWare Technical Bulletin. https://www.synopsys.com/designware-ip/technical-bulletin/finfet-design.html
34. http://www.anandtech.com/show/4313/intel-announces-first-22nm-3d-trigate-transistors-shipping-in-2h-2011
35. Balanis, C. A.; Antenna Theory: Analysis and Design. John Wiley & Sons, 2005.
36. Stutzmann, W. L.; Thiele, G. A.; Antenna Theory Design. John Wiley & Sons, 2012.
37. Maral, G.; Bousquet, M.; Satellite Communications Systems: Systems, Techniques and Technology. John Wiley & Sons, 2011.
38. Amundson, M. D.; Von Arx, J. A.; Linder, W. J.; Rawat, P.; Mass, W. R.; Circumferential antenna for an implantable medical device. United States Patent 6456256, 2002.

39. Russer, P.; Fichtner, N.; Lugli, P.; Porod, W.; Russer, J. A.; Yordanov, H.; Nanoelectronics based Integrated Antennas. IEEE Microwave Magazine, December 2010.
40. Carbon Based Smart System for Wireless Application. Nano RF Project. Available: http://project-nanorf.com/
41. Kreupl, F.; Graham, A. P.; Liebau, M.; Duesberg, G. S.; Seidel, R.; Unger, E.; Carbon nanotubes for interconnect applications. Proceedings of IEEE International on Electron Devices Meeting, San Francisco, CA, USA, December 13–15, 2004, 683–686.
42. Srivastava, N.; Banerjee, K.; Performance analysis of CNT interconnects for VLSI applications. Proceedings of IEEE International Conference on Computer Aided Design, November 6–10, 2005, 383–390.
43. Wakabayashi, K.; Fujita, M.; Ajiki, H.; Sigrist, M.; Electronic and magnetic properties of nanographite ribbons. Physical Review B: Condensed Matter and Materials Physics. 1999, 59, 12, 8271–8282. arXiv:cond-mat/9809260. Bibcode:1999PhRvB.59.8271W. doi:10.1103/PhysRevB.59.8271.
44. Broadband Wireless Networking Lab, School of Electrical and Computer Engineering, Georgia Institute of Technology. GRANET: Graphene-enabled Nanonetworks in the Terahertz Band. http://bwn.ece.gatech.edu/granet/projectdescription.html (Accessed Dec. 20, 2020.)

CHAPTER 4

Deep CNN Framework for Classification and Feature Extraction

SHIVKARAN RAVIDAS*, and M. A. ANSARI

Department of Electrical Engineering, School of Engineering, Gautam Buddha University, Greater Noida, Utter Pradesh, India

*Corresponding author. E-mail: mailmekaran@gmail.com

ABSTRACT

The most important task of computer vision is not limited to classification, object detection, alignment, and tracking. Recently, convolutional neural networks (CNNs) have emerged as the most prominent techniques to achieve computer vision tasks. This chapter presents theoretical and practical aspects of CNNs using deep learning. Deep structured CNNs have simply more number of layers. Profound CNNs are utilized for classification as well as for object detection. However, this can be extended for face detection and face recognition. CNNs are similar to the conventional neural network. They both have neurons and learnable weights and biases. Every neuron is given an input, performs dot product, and performs nonlinearity. CNNs have multiple layers. Each layer receives a multidimensional array of inputs and produces the multidimensional output, which becomes input to the next layer. Hence, CNN is a sequence of multiple layers. For acquiring the best execution of such a technique, it needs to exceptionally tune the number of nodes, layers, and rates for learning. Some practical applications are included for image classification and face detection.

4.1 INTRODUCTION

Computer researchers around the globe have been attempting to discover approaches to make machines concentrate more on visual information. Since the last few decades, the deep learning approach has emerged as a new area of research in machine learning [1, 2]. This technique impacts on a wide range of machine learning tasks from face detection to pattern recognition and overcome the traditional artificial intelligence. Deep learning can be defined in many ways. One can define deep learning as, "a class of machine learning technique that utilizes the many layers of nonlinear characteristics of convolutional neural networks (CNNs) with supervised or nonsupervised feature extraction or transformation for pattern classifications."

The early days of computer vision aimed to solve the problem which was difficult for humans but easy for a computer using different algorithms and mathematical rules. Such problems can be explained straightforward through the formal mathematics and set of rules. Now, the real challenge of computer vision is to solve the problem which was hard to explain and describe for humans, for example, recognizing faces, reading handwriting, or object classification. A solution to above problem is to make computers learn and understand the real-world problem with the help of training. The hierarchy of concept is formulated at various abstraction levels and is stack on the basic concept layer, and thus this graph may be very deep. Hence, learning with this approach is called deep learning. The basic learning entity of a deep learning is the neuron. CNNs are used at their highest abstraction level [3].

4.2 ARTIFICIAL NEURAL NETWORKS

Advance computing models to perform operations such as face recognition and object classification are inspired by the structure biological neurons. An artificial neural network (ANN) is replica (up to some extent) of a biological neural network. An ANN is a parallel computational model made up of densely interconnected handling units. These systems are fine-grained execution of nonlinear frameworks. The most significant highlights of these systems are the versatile nature with the capacity of learning.

ANN is a function f of the input $x = (x_1, \ldots, x_d)$ and weights $w_j = (w_{j,1}, \ldots, w_{j,d})$; with a bias b_j and an activation function $\varnothing$, this can be expressed as [4–5]

$$y_j = \varnothing(w_j, x) + b_j \tag{4.1}$$

There are different activation functions that are as follows:

1. The identity function $\varnothing(x) = x$

2. The sigmoidal function $\varnothing(x) = \dfrac{1}{1+\exp(-x)}$

3. The hyperbolic function $\varnothing(x) = \dfrac{\exp(x)-\exp(-x)}{\exp(x)+\exp(-x)} = \dfrac{\exp(2x)-1}{\exp(-x)+1}$

4. The Rectified Linear Unit activation function $\varnothing(x) = \max(0, x)$.

In a neural network, with a large number of layers (in deep learning), this creates problem, especially with back-propagation learning algorithms to estimate parameters. Figure 4.1 shows the different activation function discussed above.

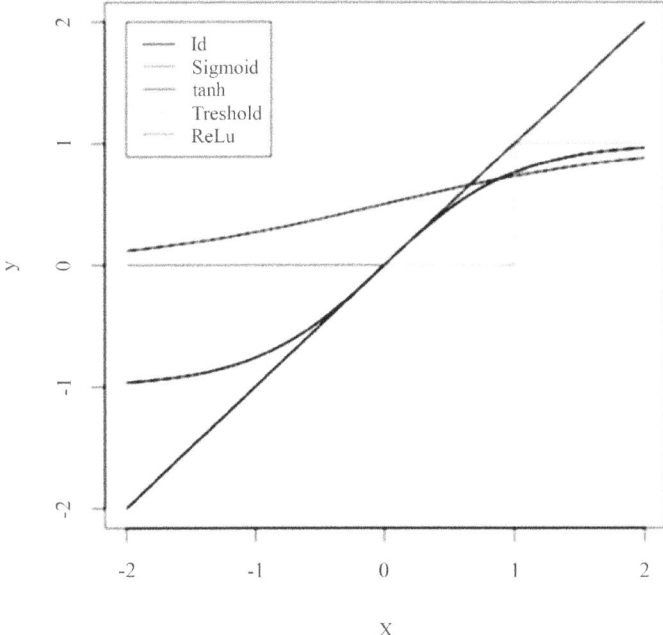

FIGURE 4.1 Different activation functions.

Neurons in ANNs are organized as layers. These layers are partitioned into three principal types: input layer, output layer, and hidden layer as shown in Figure 4.2. The input layer relates to the information that the system gets. The number of neurons in this layer compares to the quantity of contributions to the neuronal system. This layer comprises latent hubs that do not participate in the real signal modification; however, they just transmit the signal to the accompanying layer. The hidden layer has the self-assertive number of layers with the subjective number of neurons. The nodes in this layer partake in the signal adjustment; subsequently, they are dynamic. The last layer is called the output layer that delivers the results of the ANN. The quantity of neurons in the output layer is compared to the quantity of the output estimations of the neural system. The nodes in this layer are dynamic. ANN functions like a human mind. The human mind comprises billions of neurons [6–9].

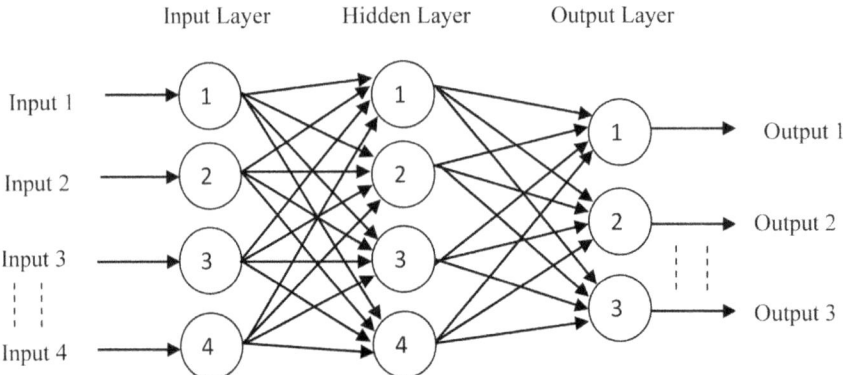

FIGURE 4.2 Artificial neural network structure.

The neurons are interconnected, and their dendrites receive the input signals from environmental stimulations. This signal is processed in the cell body and transmitted by axon to the output terminal. The single artificial neuron works in a similar way. The signal-processing procedure can be expressed mathematically as

$$y(x) = \varnothing \left(\sum_{i=1}^{n} w_i x_i \right) \tag{4.2}$$

where y is the out signal, $\varnothing$ is the activation function, x is the input signal, and w is the weight of every input signal.

4.3 CONVOLUTIONAL NEURAL NETWORKS

Over the past few decades, CNNs have performed extremely well in computer vision tasks [2]. CNNs are widely used by the current state-of-the-art human pose estimation algorithms [3, 4]. They model an image as a composition of functions. The basic idea behind the CNNs is the composition of patterns.

An image can be seen as a composition of higher level parts such as faces and other distinct image patterns. These in turn are again composed of other intermediate visual patterns going up to lower level visual elements such as edges and textures. LeCun et al. [5] proposed a CNN consists of multiple layers of convolutional and subsampling layers starting from low-level to high-level abstractions.

The modern structure of CNNs could be a biologically impressed variant of the multilayer perceptron (MLP). From Huben and Wiesel's early work on the cat's visual area [6], we all know that the visual area contains a fancy arrangement of cells. Every cell is sensitive to tiny subregions of the visual view, referred to as a receptive field. The subregions are covered to hide the whole visual view. These cells act as native filters over the input house and are well suited to use the robust spatially native correlation present in natural pictures. In addition to this, two basic cell types are identified. Easy cells answer specific edge-like patterns inside their several receptive fields. Since the animal visual area is taken into account the foremost powerful visual process system, it looks solely natural to emulate its structure and behavior.

The basic CNN structure is shown in Figure 4.3. It can be visualized from the figure that the CNN structure runs layer by layer in a forward direction. The underlying arrangement of layers reacts to discriminative low-level samples. The following set of layers react to moderate samples that are made up of low-level samples. The motivation for CNN and neural systems, by and large, has been the organic comprehension of the cerebrum. It has been known for a long while that the cerebrum is made up of more than 100 billion neurons, and these neurons are closely associated with each other. CNNs emulate neurons and their associations. A layer in CNN is comprised of $m \times n$ neurons and associated with the neurons of the neighboring layers [10, 11].

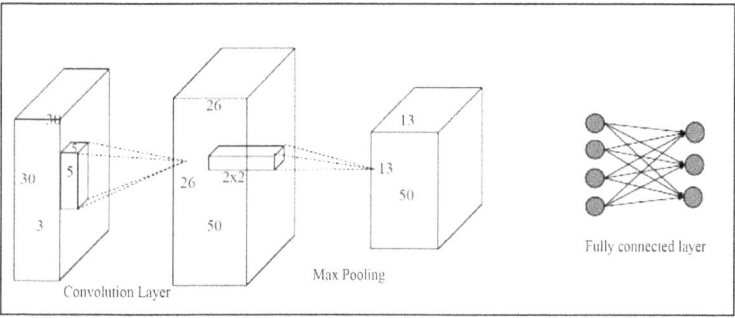

FIGURE 4.3 Various layers in CNN.

For image processing, MLPs are generally not used; instead, CNNs are used. CNNs revolutionized image processing because they have the inherent ability to extract image feature directly [12].

The discreet convolution between two functions f and g can be given as

$$(f*g)(x) = \sum_t f(t)g(x+t). \quad (4.3)$$

Since the image is a two-dimensional (2D) signal, the 2D convolution is given as

$$(K*I)(i,j) = \sum_{m,n} K(m,n)I(i+n, j+m), \quad (4.4)$$

where K is a convolution kernel applied to a 2D signal I (i.e., image).

In 2D convolution, a kernel is scroll on the image. Convolution is computed between the input image and the kernel. The kernel slides in the forward direction by a number s pixel where "s" is called stride. Stride controls the convolution process. A small value of s invites redundancy. Sometimes, we may use zero padding if neurons in the border cannot process the whole receptive field. Convolution between images I with kernel K_t is given as [13]

$$K_t * I(i.i) = \sum_{c=0}^{2} \sum_{n=0}^{4} \sum_{m=0}^{4} K_t(n,m,c) I(i+n-2, i+m-2, c). \quad (4.5)$$

Image is C^i, and the size of the kernel is (k,k,C^i,C^o), where C^o is the number of the output channel.

The pooling layers' segment would lessen the quantity of parameters when the images are excessively enormous. Spatial pooling additionally called subsampling or down-sampling which lessens the dimensionality of each guide, yet holding the significant data. Spatial pooling can be of various kinds such as max pooling, average pooling, and sum pooling. Max pooling is illustrated in Figure 4.4. The subsampling layer acts on small patches of the image. If we take stride larger than 1, then the dimension of the convolutional layer is reduced. One of the biggest advantages of the pooling layer is that it makes the network less sensitive to the changes in the input image. This is the end layer or output layer which is connected to all the neurons from the previous layer. The output stage of a CNN is mostly a number of fully connected layers.

The combination of different layers becomes the architecture of the CNN. There are different types of CNN architectures. Choosing an architecture of CNN depends on the type of application. Therefore, it is important to study the architecture of a CNN. The inventor of CNN, Yann LeCun, proposed a network architecture known as LeNet, shown in Figure 4.5. It was mainly designed for recognizing handwriting.

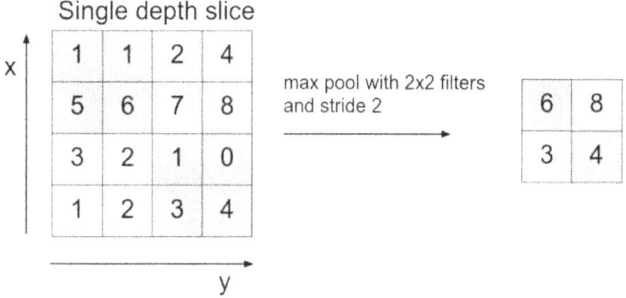

FIGURE 4.4 Effect of dimension after max pooling.

LeNet-5 is an extremely basic network. The LeNet-5 structure comprises of two set of convolutional and normal pooling layers, trailed by a flattening convolutional layer, two fully connected layers, and lastly a softmax classifier. The subsampling layers comprise 2×2 normal pooling layers. The activation function used is the normal $tanh$ sigmoid function. There are a few interesting variations of the LeNet design which are not very popular. One of the major drawbacks of LeNet is that it lacks the measure of processing units which is required to manage such a complex classification problem. Figure 4.6 shows the AlexNet network. It has a similar architecture to LeNet but is much deeper with more number of filters per layers. AlexNet won the ImageNet competition award in 2012 by a large margin [14].

4.4 DEEP LEARNING

The real challenge of computer vision techniques is solving the problems that appear to be simple and instinctive for individuals to perform but are difficult to describe formally. Most of the practical computer vision problems are in an intuitive manner, somewhat automatically, such as reading handwritten text, recognizing spoken words, or inferring objects in images. By letting a computer learn from experience, we avoid the need to formulate all the prior knowledge one would require completing the task at hand [15–17].

If this structure were to be visualized as a graph, each layer of concepts would be stacked on top of a simpler concept layer; the graph can be very

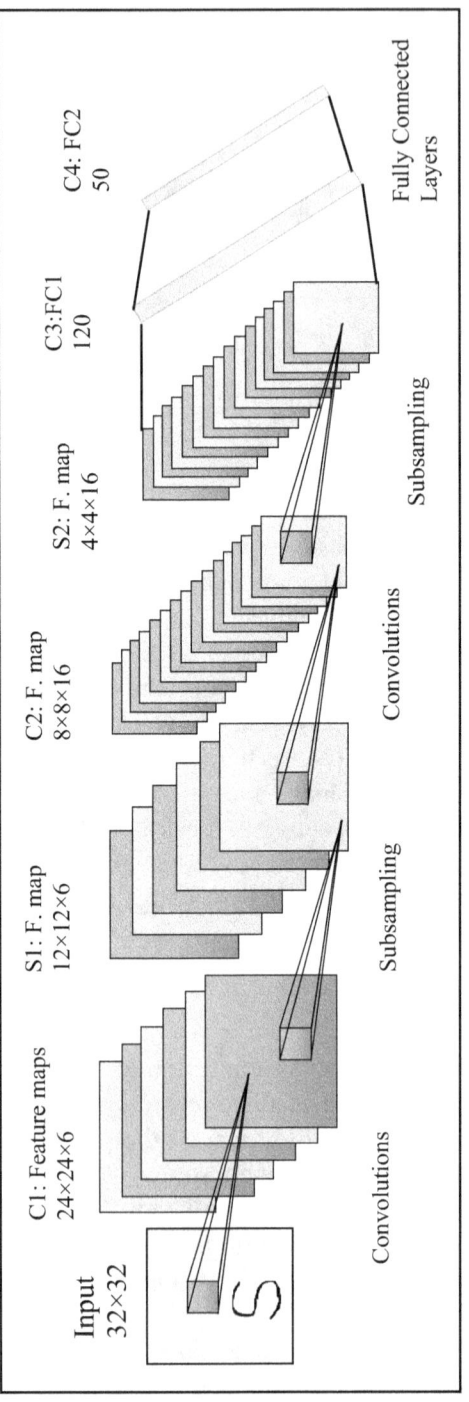

FIGURE 4.5 Modified LeNet Architecture (*Source:* Modified from Ref. [7].

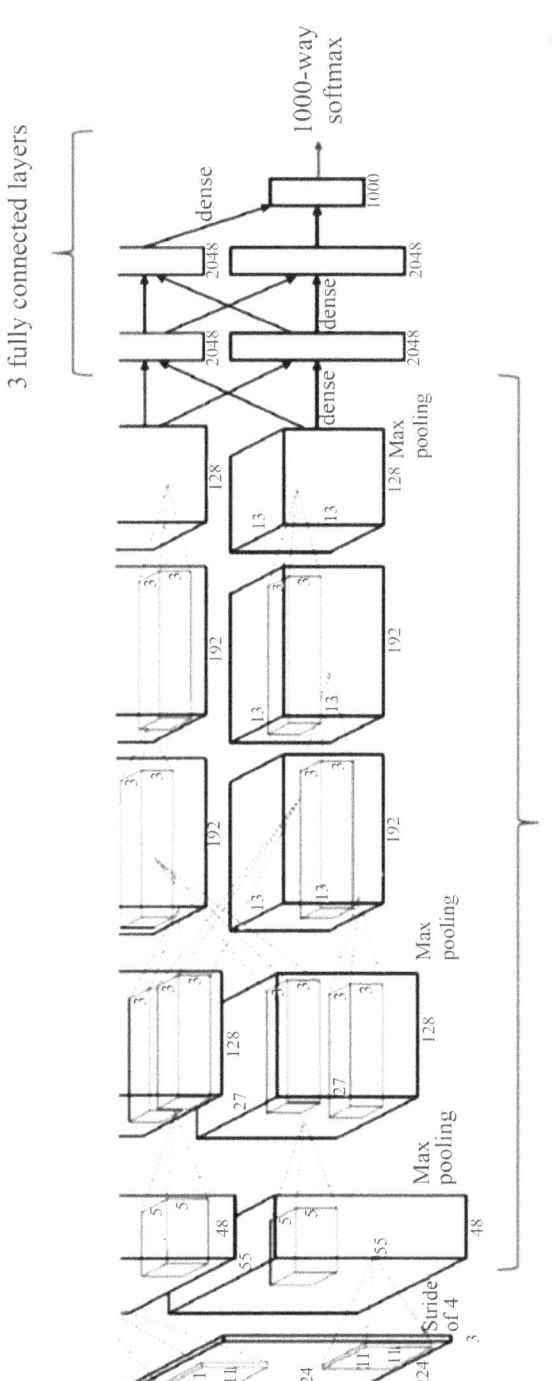

FIGURE 4.6 AlexNet network.

Source: Reprinted from Ref. [21]. https://papers.nips.cc/paper/4824-imagenet-classification-with-deep-convolutional-neural-networks.pdf

deep. The McCulloch-Pitts neuron [17] was an early model of brain function. Rosenblatt [9] proposed a perceptron as the principal model for learning with a teacher, that is, supervised learning. Neurons used today in deep learning are a generalization of the original perception with a few variations. The input and output of a neuron are of a continuous nature, as opposed to the original binary form. Second, replacing the step function, other nonlinear functions are applied over the output. The modern neuron usually takes the following formula [19, 20]:

$$y = \phi (W_x + b), \tag{4.6}$$

where x is the set of externally applied stimuli, that is, input, y is the output, ϕ is the activation function, and W is the weight matrix.

Deep learning is a developing field of computer vision. It involves various hidden layers of neural network systems. The deep learning procedure applies nonlinear transformations and different abstraction levels in the enormous databases. In 2010, deep learning started outperforming other machine learning techniques, which is shown graphically in Figure 4.7.

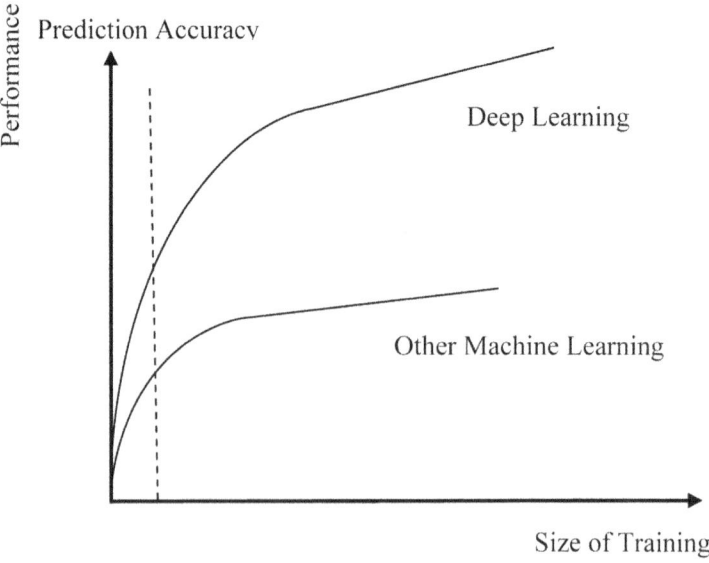

FIGURE 4.7 Comparison of deep learning with other machine learning tools.

Neuroscience has inspired the field of ANNs greatly [10]. The idea of getting several machine units that become intelligent through connections and interactions with one another relies on the neural structure within the brain. The neocognitron [11] presented an incredible model engineering for preparing image greatly impressed by the craniate sensory system visual framework and its structure. This model later turned into the reason for the cutting-edge convolutional network [12, 13].

In addition, the learned features can be extensively abstract as shown in Figure 4.8. The CNNs work intently in the manner in which the biological visual framework works [14, 15].

4.5 RESULTS

A four-class dataset is generated and plotted in different colors. The goal is to train a neural-based classifier that differentiates all the data classes. Here, data is not linearly separable, that is, a straight line cannot separate the dataset into two classes. Figure 4.9 illustrates the four-class data classification using a perceptron network. The network is trained with two inputs and two outputs to classify the input vectors into four categories. The total number of samples taken in each class is $K = 30$. Since the perceptron is known to model the linearly separable functions, therefore, for nonlinearly separable functions, it is required to obtain the separator which is able to minimize the mean squared error. For example, the single-layer perceptron cannot model the eXclusive OR (XOR) Boolean function as it is nonlinearly separable. Hence, it is possible to solve this problem with a two-layer perceptron model. One layer is the hidden layer consisting of neurons directly connected to the input vector with weights, and the other is an output layer consisting of neurons directly connected to the output of the hidden neuron with weights connected to a neuron in the output layer.

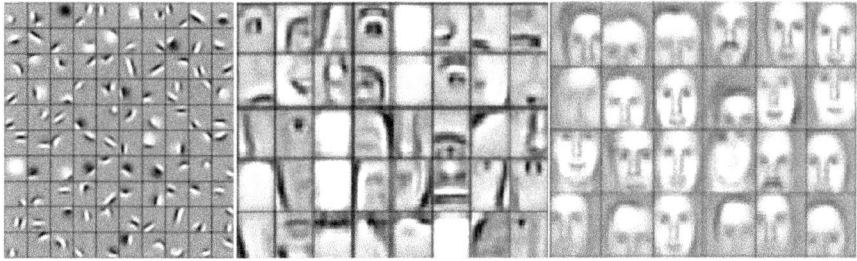

FIGURE 4.8 Facial features extracted by a CNN [4].

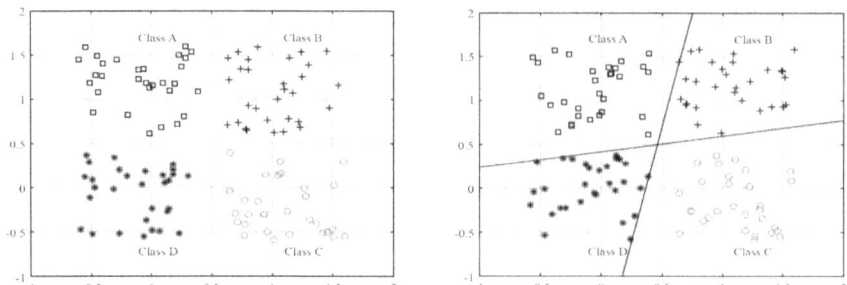

FIGURE 4.9 Classification problem: (a) Four-class data and (b) classification after perceptron training.

Figure 4.9(b) shows that the four classes of samples have been classified successfully. The resulting network structure is given in Figure 4.10.

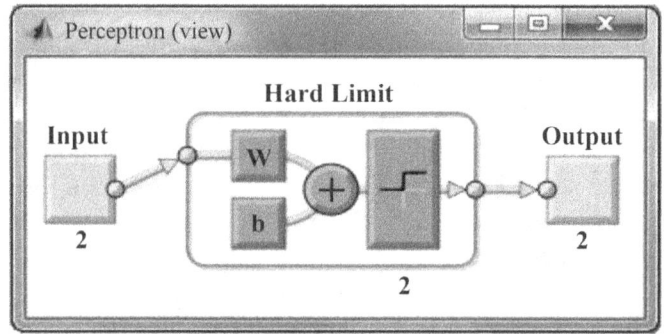

FIGURE 4.10 Network structure.

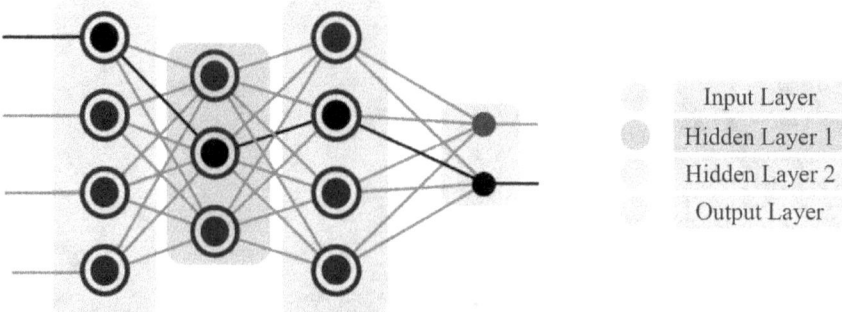

FIGURE 4.11 A typical neural network structure with two hidden layers.

Deep CNN Framework for Classification

Figures 4.11 and 4.12 show the network structures with two hidden layers and an output layer.

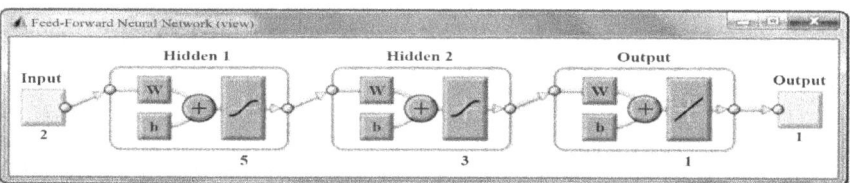

FIGURE 4.12 Feed forward network structure.

The quantity of layers and the quantity of processing elements per layer are imperative choices. To a feedforward, back-engendering topology, these parameters are likewise the most delicate. Figure 4.13 shows the classification result for the complete input space. All the classes are shown with different regions.

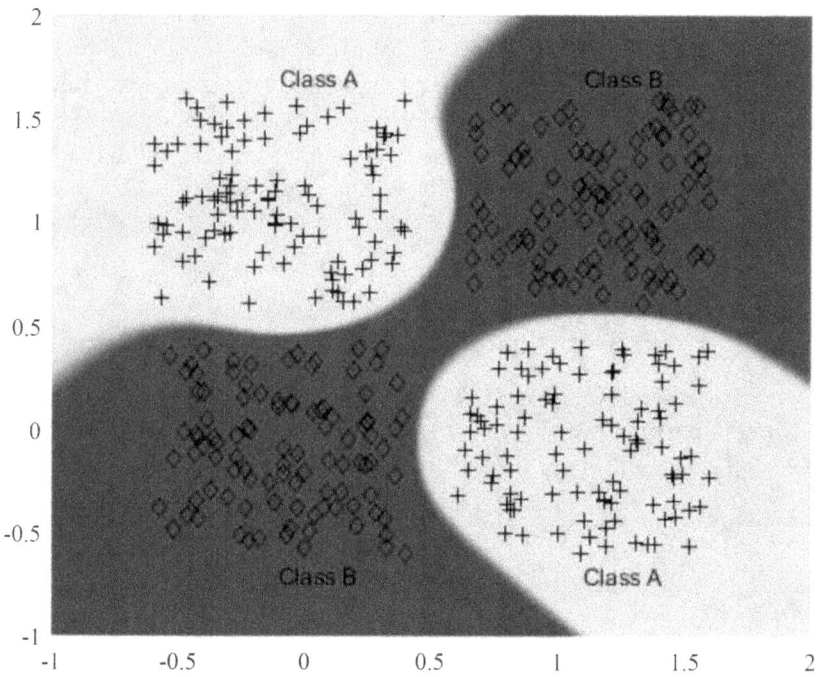

FIGURE 4.13 Classification region.

4.6 CONCLUSION

This chapter describes some core concepts that can help us to understand the workings of deep learning. First, the basic structure of artificial neurons and neural networks is provided. The empirical results of the classification of different classes of data have been shown. The network is trained with a perceptron, and with two hidden layers, also results are shown. The structure of CNN is analyzed. Next, deep neural networks are introduced, and an explanation is given about their primary concepts along with various architectures in use. Finally, a more detailed description of CNNs is provided, which was extensively useful in the experiments of this thesis.

A variation on the original approaches in that weight sharing was used in the neural network with retinal connections, obtaining a fully CNN. It was proved that better generalization is obtained with implication that a smaller training set needed in order to achieve similar results. In order to detect a larger range of face orientation, different training sets were tried. Although good results were obtained with a front-view classifier, the detection of the profile view proved to be a harder problem; the method should be refined in order to obtain better results. Another interesting issue is to examine the capacity of a CNN to gain from a diminished arrangement of preparing training examples while getting equivalent or nearly measure up to outcomes than with a bigger preparing set. Hence, the proposed method is eventually selected from a large set of the most fundamental training models for face detection even when a larger learning set is not available.

KEYWORDS

- **convolutional neural networks**
- **deep learning**
- **computer vision**

REFERENCES

1. Hinton, G., Osindero, S., and Teh, Y. "A fast learning algorithm for deep belief nets," Neural Computation, vol. 18, no. 7, pp. 1527–1554, 2006.

2. Montana, D. J. and Davis, L. "Training feedforward neural networks using genetic algorithms." In: Proceedings of the 11th International Joint Conference on Artificial Intelligence, vol. 1. IJCAI'89. Detroit, MI: Morgan Kaufmann Publishers Inc., pp. 762–767, 1989.
3. Aarts, E. and Korst, J. "Simulated Annealing and Boltzmann Machines: A Stochastic Approach to Combinatorial Optimization and Neural Computing." New York, NY: John Wiley & Sons, Inc., 1989. ISBN: 0-471-92146-7.
4. Yamazaki, A., de Souto, M. C. P., and Ludermir, T. B. "Optimization of neural network weights and architectures for odor recognition using simulated annealing." In: Proceedings of the 2002 International Joint Conference on Neural Networks, Honolulu, HI, USA, May 12–17, 2002.
5. Lecun, Y., Bottou, L., Bengio, Y., and Haffner, P. "Gradient-based learning applied to document recognition." Proceedings of the IEEE, vol. 86, no. 11, pp. 2278–2324, 1998.
6. Goodfellow, I., Bengio, Y., and Courville, A. "Deep Learning." Cambridge, MA: MIT Press, 2016.
7. Zhao, L., Pingali, G., and Carlbom, I. "Real-time head orientation estimation using neural networks. In: Proceedings of the International Conference on Image Processing, Rochester, NY, USA, September 22–25, 2002.
8. The McCulloch-Pitts Model of a Neuron. http://wwwold.ece.utep.edu/research/webfuzzy/docs/kk-thesis/kk-thesis-html/node12.html
9. Rosenblatt, F. "The perceptron: A probabilistic model for information storage and organization in the brain," Psychological Review, vol 65, no. 6, pp. 386–408, 1958.
10. Itti, L. and Koch, C. "Computational modelling of visual attention," Nature Reviews Neuroscience, vol. 2, no. 3, pp. 194–203, 2001.
11. McKenna, S. and Gong, S. "Real time face pose estimation," International Journal on Real Time Imaging [Special Issue on Real-time Visual Monitoring and Inspection], vol. 4, no. 5, pp. 333–347, 1998.
12. Baluja, S. "Probabilistic modeling for face orientation discrimination: Learning from labeled and unlabeled data." Advances in Neural Information Processing Systems, pp. 854–860, 1998.
13. Ba, S. O. and Odobez, J. M. "A probabilistic framework for joint head tracking and pose estimation." In: Proceedings of the 17th International Conference on Pattern Recognition, vol. 4, pp. 264–267, 2004.
14. Kim, J., Kim, S., and Lee, M. "Convolutional Neural Network with Biologically Inspired ON/OFF ReLU." International Conference on Neural Information Processing. New York, NY: Springer, pp. 316–323, 2015.
15. Garcia, C. and Delakis, M. "Convolutional face finder: A neural architecture for fast and robust face detection," IEEE Transactions on Pattern Analysis and Machine Intelligence, vol. 26, no. 11, pp.1408–1423, 2004.
16. Gong, S., McKenna, S., and Collins, J. An investigation into face pose distributions. In: Proceedings of the Second International Conference on Automatic Face and Gesture Recognition, pp. 265–270. IEEE, 16th October 1996, Killington, VT, USA.
17. Ravidas, S. and Ansari, M. A. "An efficient scheme of deep convolution neural network for multi view face detection," I. J. Intelligent Systems and Applications, vol. 3, no. 3, pp. 53–61, 2019.

18. Ravidas, S. and Ansari, M. A. "Analysis of multi-view face detection using deep convolutional neural networks," Indian Journal of Industrial and Applied Mathematics, vol. 9, no. 2, pp. 231–244, 2019.
19. Ravidas, S. and Ansari, M. A. "Deep learning for pose-invariant face detection in unconstrained environment," International Journal of Electrical and Computer Engineering (IJECE), vol. 9, no. 1, pp. 577–584, 2019.
20. Ravidas, S. and Ansari, M. A. "Pose invariant face detection using deep convolutional neural network and calibrated CNN structure," Proceedings of IEEE International Conference NANOfIM, pp. 304–309, 16–17 November 2017, Gautam Buddha University, Greater Noida, India.
21. Krizhevsky, Alex, Ilya Sutskever, and Geoffrey E. Hinton. "Imagenet classification with deep convolutional neural networks." In Advances in neural information processing systems, pp. 1097-1105. 2012.
22. CS321n Convolutional Neural Networks in Visual Recognition. https://cs231n.github.io/convolutional-networks/

CHAPTER 5

Prospects of MMIC Antennas

SATYA SAI SRIKANT[1*], SAPTARSHI GUPTA[1], and ATUL KUMAR PANDEY[2]

[1]*SRM Institute of Science and Technology, Modinagar, Uttar Pradesh, India*

[2]*Scientist G, DRDO-SSPL, Delhi, India*

Corresponding author. E-mail: satya.srikant@gmail.com

ABSTRACT

In this modern digital era, making of small electronics devices with wireless connectivity is the public demand, which put an enormous pressure on the microwave researchers, design engineers as well as scientists, to improve the electromagnetic performance in smaller packages. Wireless communication had already captured the main attention of social life in the present digital era, as it is the fastest growing technology. The medium of wireless communication such as local area networks, wide area networks, and sensor networks is mostly utilized by various industries, automated highways, irrigation fields, houses, education fields, corporate and business areas, and other fields also. The antenna technology plays an important role for any implementation and installation of any wireless communication system. Design of a good antenna design always enhances the system performance and minimizes the system requirements. In the present time, there has been an exponential growth in using terahertz frequencies, that is, millimeter and submillimeter wavelengths for several applications such as security, submarine, satellite, biomedical imaging studies, astronomy, and atmospheric studies. All such applications are now more feasible and possible due to rapid enhancements of microwave-based semiconductor processing technologies. With the help of monolithic microwave integrated circuits (MMIC) techniques, one could design an antenna integrated with high electron mobility transfer/metal semiconductor field effect transistors that resonate more than 100 GHz frequencies. It will open up a new hope for any integrating systems interfaced with the antenna-on-chip technology, which will be very useful for a transreceiver like module. This chapter investigates mostly about the development of various MMIC antennas that interface with the active microwave circuit components for millimeter and submillimeter wave applications.

5.1 INTRODUCTION

As per Constantine A. Balanis, "An Antenna serves to a communication system; the same purpose that eyes and eyeglasses serve to a Human." It means that an antenna plays as one of the most critical components for any communication system. In general, an antenna serves as a perfect transducer between the guided wave and a free space. As per the definition of IEEE standard "Antennas define the aerial as a means for radiating or receiving radio waves" [1]. Basically the antenna operates on the principles of electromagnetic (EM) theory. The word antenna came from the Latin word *antemna* which means, in the Latin language, antenna. The term antenna was first used by Marconi in a lecture in 1909 [2]. Actually, the evolution and concept of antennas began soon after James Clerk Maxwell derived Maxwell's equation for time-varying EM fields and waves [3–5]. In fact, he is remembered as the "Father of Electromagnetic Waves." During the World War II, that is, between the years 1935 and 1940, the antenna technology had initially started based on wire-based radiating elements that operate in frequencies up to a range of an ultrahigh frequency. Hence, one can say that the World War II had launched a new era in the field of antenna technology starting with waveguide, dipole, monopole, horn antennas, reflectors, slots, and apertures [6]. The microwave sources' invention such as magnetron and klystron accelerated and magnified this new era toward the microwave communication. But it was between the middle of the 20th century and the late of the 1970s that antenna technology witnessed drastic changes and improvement in its impedance bandwidth with the bandwidth ratio of more than 50:1. These wideband antennas are rather frequency-independent antennas. These antennas contained the specified geometries with angles rather than linear dimensions. The TV reception, point-to-point and line-of-sight communication, and feed for reflectors are the main applications of these wideband antennas.

Roughly in the early 1980s, a new type of radiating element called the "planar antenna," that is, the microstrip patch antenna was introduced that find many applications with easy fabrication as compared to the earlier antennas. These antennas not only provide easy integration with active components but also provide various antenna characteristics such as gain and radiation pattern in a controlled manner with desired parameters. In the last two decades, all developments were in millimeter-wave antennas that integrated the active and passive circuits with the radiating elements in one compact unit. In recent times, all research work were conducted in the field of the smart antennas, also called as adaptive arrays, where the signal-processing unit along with advanced digital systems is integrated with antennas [7].

5.2 MONOLITHIC MICROWAVE INTEGRATED CIRCUIT

The terahertz (THz) field is almost new, as compared to the conventional microwave engineering. It operates between the 300 GHz and 3 THz frequency span, and now it is characterized as field encompassing techniques (FETs), fabrication approach, and devices. The wavelength for such a frequency span covers between 1 mm and 100 μm which is submillimeter wavelength. Most of the THz components such as cavity resonators, horns, point contact diodes, and polarization filters were invented by Sir Jagdish Chandra Bose in the late 19th century in their elementary form, but it took almost 100 years for the improvement or growth of semiconductor technology in THz frequencies. THz frequencies had found wide applications for astronomy and atmospheric studies that contains various molecular spectral lines along with vital information. No doubt, radio astronomy had played a critical role as a driver for both components development and THz technology [8, 9]. But nowadays, atmospheric studies as well as rapid development in semi-conductor processing capacity enhanced the range of the new utilization of THz not only for wireless communication, broadband communication, and satellite communication but also for biomedical imaging and security [10].

Therefore, the accelerated hike observed with the use of THz frequencies in previous two decades made THz engineering as an emerging field. This chapter is mainly focused on the prospects of MMIC antennas, which means the integration of antennas and active receiver frontends at the THz range with the help of MMIC technology and their wide applications.

The key technology *microwave integrated circuits* (MIC) can be called as one of the major accomplishments of the 20th century. The MIC technology allows the integration of analog and digital circuits both on a single chip with an enhanced performance in addition to smaller sizes of electronic components or devices. The term *monolithic microwave integrated circuits* is identical to and generally associated with *MIC*. It operates in the range of microwave frequency band and consists of monolithic integration with the microwave transistors and other passive ingredients such as capacitors, inductors, resistors, and planar transmission lines. Though previous attempts were taken to have MMIC with silicon technology, but the practical MMIC picked up the pace after the first investigation of the C and X band amplifiers using GaAs technology in the early 1980s of the 20th century [11-13].

5.2.1 ADVANTAGES OF MMIC

The major profit of MMIC technology for application in THz is that the overall transmitter and receiver can be fabricated on an individual chip. It simplifies the interface between radio frequency (RF) and local oscillator frequencies. Also, this technology can be easily integrated in the system because of lower I/O frequencies like IF can be conveyed easily in the transmission line in both the planar (such as microstrip, coplanar waveguide [CPW], and stripline) or in the co-axial line. Parasitic elements can be reduced due to the fabrication of passive and active components on the same substrate. So, this process allows us to design and modeling of complicated circuits, which exhibits the wide bandwidth and works for higher frequencies.

5.2.2 LIMITATIONS OF MMIC

The cost for the initial setup of the lab, research, and development for MMICs is extremely high as it is very difficult to get the required equipment for the fabrication of MMIC. Also, it takes ample time for designing an MMIC process to mature so that it can produce reliable circuits with better yield and high efficiency. But the cost of MMIC fabrication can come down once it goes for mass production, but the gap is still present in order to minimize the dimension and the physical size of circuits. Even though it has some aforementioned limitations, there has been a rapid progress in MMIC research and development provide advanced transistors in near future in the range of GHz to THz.

5.3 ANTENNA CHARACTERIZATION

It is observed in Section 5.2 that the THz bands are widely used for the lower end of the THz spectrum for different kinds of applications and the transistor technology in the present scenario is getting matured day by day. It not only emphasizes the opportunities to integrate passive antenna structures as well as active circuits but also open up the opportunities on a single chip with the help of MMIC antennas and heterojunction transistors. Such a single and miniature chip is very helpful for transmit/receive architecture. With the help of the MMIC technology, the degrees of freedom to design an antenna become less and when the MMIC layer's thicknesses and topology factor increase, this becomes more complex. Hence, during developing and designing the structure of an antenna with MMICs, it is very essential to characterize the structures in terms of voltage standing wave ratio, impedance matching, insertion loss, half-power beamwidth (HPBW), and radiation patterns. So, on the basis of appropriate application, appropriate parameters must be given preference, and the same to be designed. Therefore, for designing the MMIC antennas, one needs to understand the antenna's properties first, and then its characterization definitions considering some examples. To design MMIC antennas for THz applications, one has to develop both quantitative and quantitative understanding toward the challenges in MMIC antenna designs.

5.3.1 DIRECTIVITY

It shows the capability of an antenna to target radiation in a direction provided in space. It is also defined as the ratio of the power radiated by antenna in the inspection direction in the spherical coordinate system (i.e., ɤ, θ°, and ϕ) to power radiated by an isotropic radiator in the same direction. On the basis of antenna size, the directivity has the upper max limit. If D indicates the diameter of the antenna aperture, then one can define the maximum directivity (D_{max}) as [14]

$$D_{max} = 10\log_{10}\left[4\pi\frac{0.785D^2}{\lambda^2}\right]. \qquad (5.1)$$

The directivity occurs when the E-field over the antenna aperture becomes uniform, both in terms of amplitude and phase. With having a diameter of 3λ, the antenna provides the circular aperture D_{max} ~ 19.485 dBi, with the sidelobe label of −17.62 dB, and it is shown in Figure 5.1. This example is to feature the fact that there is also an increase of sidelobe labels whenever the maximum directivity occurs, when the E-field is uniform over the antenna aperture.

It clearly shows that directivity cannot be maximized and sidelobes cannot be minimized simultaneously for a given physical area of the antenna. It also emphasizes to efficiency trade-offs and is more relevant for the MMIC-based antenna design due to an increased cost where the physical size of an antenna is a concerned factor.

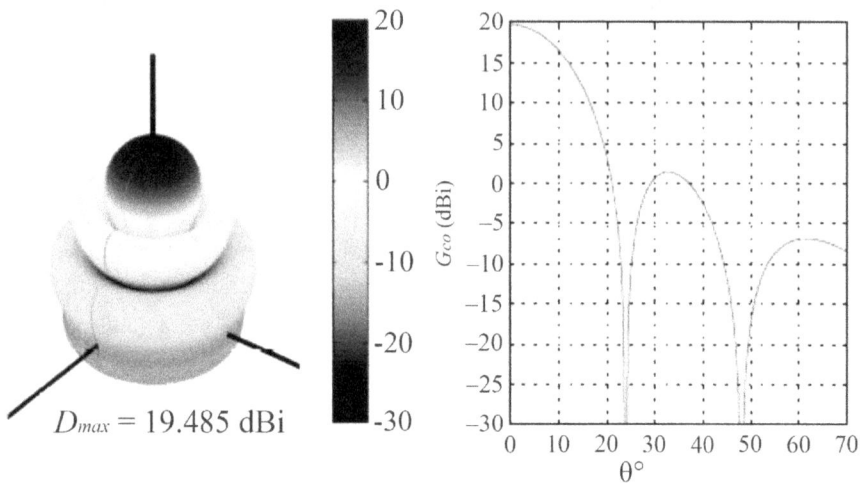

FIGURE 5.1 Radiation patterns: Uniform circular aperture (diameter, $D = 3\lambda$).

5.3.2 OHMIC EFFICIENCY

It is precisely associated with the losses in the antenna structure, and therefore it is defined as the ratio of the total radiated power to the accepted power by the antenna at its input terminal [14]. This is also stated as the ratio between the antenna gain and directivity. The ohmic losses inherent to antenna-building materials indicate the ohmic efficiency value since it is simply the addition of the dielectric and conductor losses in the antenna structure:

$$\eta_{\text{Ohmic}} = \frac{P_{\text{rad}}}{P_{\text{accepted}}} = \frac{\text{Gain}}{\text{Directivity}}. \qquad (5.2)$$

The estimation of the ohmic efficiency can be done using the antenna pattern measurement inside an RF-shielded metallic cavity with an excited mode or in anechoic chambers.

5.3.3 REFLECTION EFFICIENCY

Any type of antenna consists of some input impedance at its I/P port. To transfer the maximum power from a source or generator to the antenna, the impedance of the antenna must match with that of the system characteristics (Z_o). If Γ_A is the reflection coefficient for the antenna impedance Z_A, then the antenna's reflection efficiency is expressed as

$$\eta_{ohmic} = \frac{Z_A - Z_o}{Z_A + Z_o} \qquad (5.3)$$

$$\eta_{refl} = 10 \log_{10}\left[1 - |\Gamma_A|^2\right]. \qquad (5.4)$$

The reflection efficiency is a ratio between the power accepted by antenna terminals with power available from the source or generator.

5.3.4 APERTURE EFFICIENCY

Each antenna has an effective area (A_e) over which it gets the power from the approaching plain wave having certain power flux density (W/m²). The yield power is essentially the duplication of the antenna's effective area with the approaching power flux density [14]. The antenna's effective area is the same as that of the physical area when the aperture field has a uniform or homogeneous distribution of E-field leads to the maximum directivity. The relationship between D and A_e is expressed as

$$D = 4\pi \frac{A_e}{\lambda^2}. \qquad (5.5)$$

This aperture efficiency shows the antenna that couples the power from the approaching plane wave to its O/P terminals. This can also be represented as the ratio of the maximum effective antenna area to its physical area. Mathematically, it is represented as

$$\eta_{ap} = \frac{\max A_e}{A_{physical}}. \qquad (5.6)$$

It is an important characterization parameter that is mostly considered in practical antenna applications to optimize. For aperture efficiency, such types of applications are used to characterize for the offset feed reflector, Cassegrain reflector, and prime focus reflector, which desire the feed antenna along with the reflector. Such types of systems are commonly used for base station microwave links for mobile communication, satellite communication, and radio astronomy. Henceforth, one can say that aperture efficiency in the reflector antenna framework does not only depend on feed antenna radiation patterns but also depends on the term f/D, where f and D are shown in Figure 5.2. Also, the optimization of the aperture efficiency for reflector antennas occurs for the uniform distribution of the E-field over an aperture, and it comes with trade-offs. An ideal radiator is required for the uniform distribution of the E-field over an aperture to ensure that a balanced amplitude of the E-field radiate in every direction. In any case, for all intents and purposes, this type of isotropic antenna is impossible, and therefore the feed pattern with finite directivity, that is, the tapered E-field distribution over an aperture is preferable. It reflects well-known overflow and light efficiency trade-offs, which are shown in Figure 5.2.

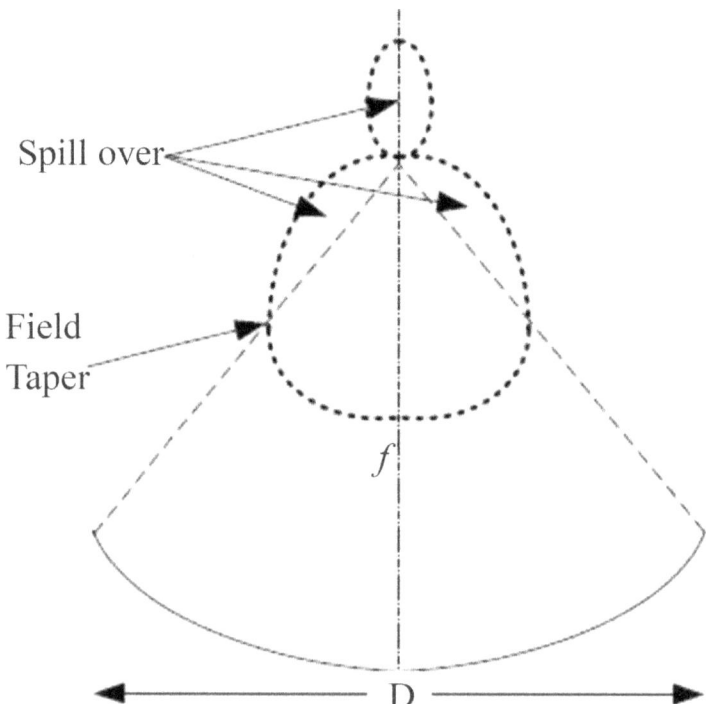

FIGURE 5.2 Feed pattern of the prime focus reflector, influence, and f/D ratio showing max (η_{ap}).

An approximate equation (5.7) is chosen to understand the spillover and illumination efficiency trade-off factor for the rotational symmetrical feed pattern, whose directivities lie between 6 and 14 dBi, with a prime focus reflector ($f/D = 0.433$). It is shown in Figure 5.3 where illumination, spillover, and aperture efficiencies are numerically calculated:

$$G(\theta,\phi) = Cos^n\left(\frac{\theta}{2}\right)[\sin\phi\hat{\theta} + \cos\phi\hat{\phi}]. \tag{5.7}$$

The maximized η_{ap} of approximately 80%, whose feed directivity is 9.25 dBi, can be observed in Figure 5.3. It translates to the E-field taper of 9.26 dB at the reflector edge. Such calculations are also performed for other f/Ds (practical values); the optimum directivity reflector and taper values are listed in Table 5.1. Thus, the planes of equal electric (E) and equal magnetic field (H) planes with the ideal feed pattern, cross-polarization = 0, and excellent rotational symmetry in the maximum efficiency η_{ap} pattern (theoretical values) do not exceed more than 80%.

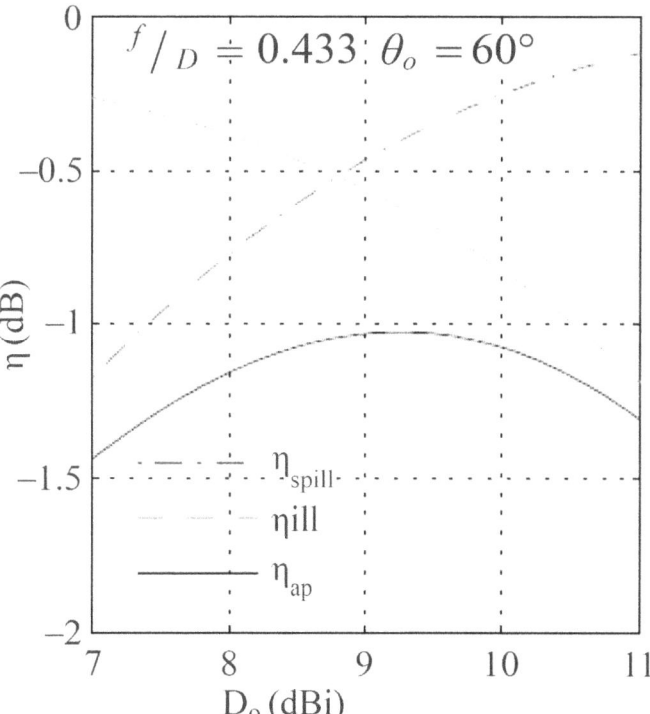

FIGURE 5.3 Spillover and illumination efficiency of the trade-off factor.

So, the maximum efficiency η_{ap} degrades further for any practical feed patterns, which consists of definite levels of cross-polar ingredient and with less rotational beam (symmetric). Likewise, such feed design does not have uniform period of the transmitted E-field. This causes nonuniform stage appropriation on aperture and results in the further deterioration of the η_{ap} value. Thus, in practice, BOR1 (body of revolution) Type 1 efficiency, phase efficiency, and polarization efficiency become supplementary and subefficiency terms in the aperture efficiency estimations [15-17].

TABLE 5.1 Optimized Do and Taper Values (η_{ap} is Maximized)

θ (°)	f/D	D_o(dBi)	Taper (dB)	η_{ap} (dB)
45	0.604	11.92	10.01	−0.96
50	0.536	10.95	9.79	−0.98
55	0.480	10.05	9.54	−1.00
60	0.433	9.26	9.26	−1.02
65	0.392	8.50	8.97	−1.05
70	0.357	7.78	8.64	−1.08
75	0.326	7.10	8.28	−1.12
85	0.298	6.46	7.92	−1.15

BOR1 subefficiency generally defines the amount of power radiated by an antenna in the first-order ϕ-variations in the pattern.

The power transmitted from the antenna in higher order modes does not influence on axis directivity after the reflector [18]. Therefore, there is a loss for the radiation in the higher order ϕ, deviation of pattern, which causes decreases in directivity. On accounting all these factors, the aperture efficiency can be represented as

$$\eta_{ap} = \eta_\phi \eta_{BOR1} \eta_{spill} \eta_{pol} \eta_{ill}. \tag{5.8}$$

Considering the reflector antenna and practical feed systems, the overall efficiency can be represented as the product of aperture efficiency along with ohmic efficiency and reflection efficiency as

$$\eta_{total} = \eta_{ohmic} \eta_{BOR1} \eta_{refl} \eta_{ap}. \tag{5.9}$$

It is extremely valuable to comprehend while planning MMIC-based planar antennas that the area accessible for the structure is exceptionally constrained or it is costly to save huge areas for passive antenna structures.

5.4 ANTENNA TOPOLOGIES

There exist numerous attractive and optimized designs and topologies interfaced with active transistors for millimeter and submillimeter wave antennas.

Hence, it is required to have best solutions for antennas that are fully suitable with the MMIC layer structure. Thus, with the proper MMIC technique, the entire antenna integrated receiver (Rx) can be fabricated.

5.4.1 ANTENNA CLASSIFICATIONS

Many antenna engineers/researchers had designed several ways of design and geometries/structures that convert applied electric current excitation in to radiated EM waves in a free space, after Heinrich Hertz discovered the dipole structure radiator of EM waves in 1886 [19]. The various literatures on these different antenna structures are usually found in [14, 19–22]. As per the literature survey, the antenna structures (radiating) are classified in four distinct ways as shown in Figure 5.4. The simplest kinds of antenna elements are dipoles, circular/square loops, slots that are based on the matching of the input impedance, and single resonance over limited bandwidths. These structures are generally fed by transverse electromagnetic (TEM)/quasi-TEM line methods. The second kind depends on step-by-step tapering out slot lines to such an extent that they begin radiating, which are regular in Vivaldi sorts of antennas. The third kind of structures can be made on joining of single resonance structures and expansion of appropriate phase shift for one component to the following. This sort of methodology helps in accomplishing extremely wide bandwidths and is often utilized in planning log-periodic antennas. The keep going sort depends on transmitting structures obtained from the transverse electric (TE) or transverse magnetic (TM) modes of waveguides. So, the horn kind of antennas falls under this category alongside slots that are normally excited by waveguides.

5.4.2 SELECTION CRITERIA OF AN ANTENNA ELEMENT

It is very important to classify the radiating antenna's elements. The main choice criteria in this process are to choose the antenna (radiating) elements as planar metal layers of MMIC. It is also equally important to select/identify the polarization of antennas and their elements. The chosen antenna along with the elements must have the feed from quasi-TEM lines (because of planar structures such as microstrip, CPW, and striplines), and also these lines are preferable for maximum radiation in the broadside direction, that is, 90° to the plane consisting of MMIC.

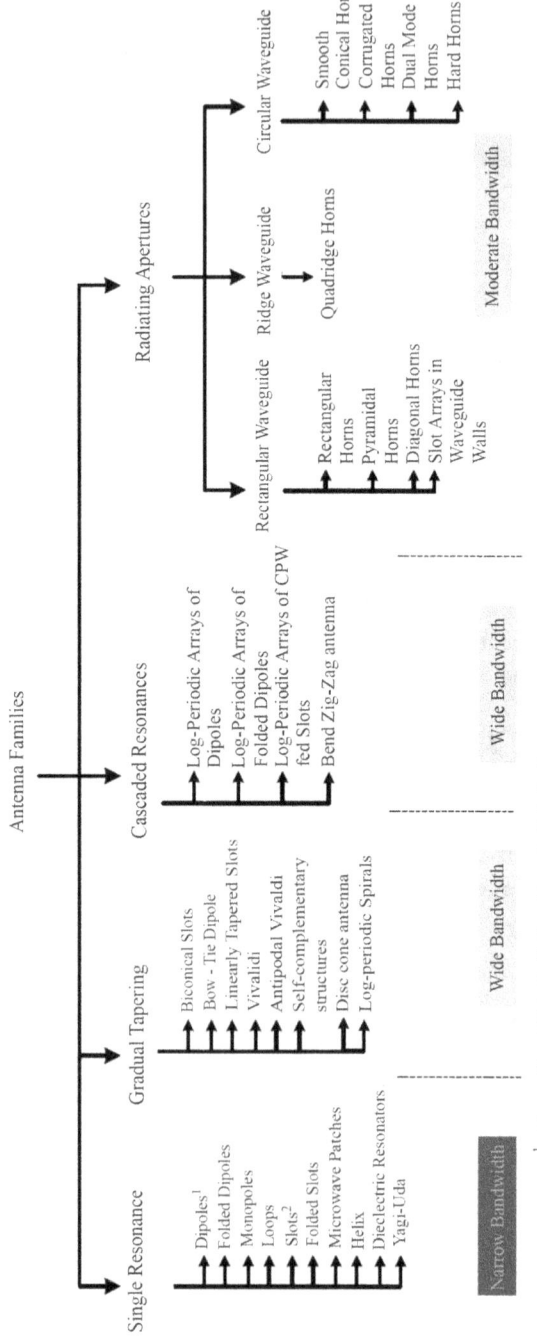

FIGURE 5.4 Classification of Antenna families

In spite of these properties, it should be high-coupling efficiencies (Gaussian in nature) with low ohmic losses and low dielectric losses for the selected antenna elements with proper impedance matching when it is desired to work or use in quasi-optical systems over 5%–10% bandwidth. Technically, it is understood that one cannot able to obtain high Gaussian effect (i.e., flat bandwidth) and with good radiation patterns from basic antenna elements. An antenna array with necessary elements can produce the desired results. One the basis of this discussion, one can summarized the selection criterion in the following ways:

1. Should be designed in the planar geometry
2. Compatible to MMIC processes
3. Linearly or circularly polarized
4. Broad-side radiation
5. Must be microstrip feeding
6. Impedance matching at each point
7. Coupling effects to be considered
8. EM as well as circuit effect to be considered while designing at high frequency
9. Less ohmic loss
10. Always preferred for 10% of bandwidth.

In order to select the radiating structures as shown in Figure 5.4, the aforementioned selection criteria must be followed considerably. No doubt, dipole antennas like folded dipoles and bowtie can be made planar, which can be easily constructed on a single metal layer; yet, they are excluded from the selection because of few crucial reasons, which are as follows:

1. As MMIC processes depend on thin dielectric layers, the dipole framed on the top metal layer remains near the ground plane, making its I/P impedance low (few ohms).
2. The structures like dipole desire the balanced feeding method, which would need a balun on each component.
3. Few antennas such as Vivaldi and Linearly tapered slots etc. cannot be used in MMIC fabrication because their radiation occurs in the same plane of the antenna structure, which is known as the end-fire direction.

Due to the above reasons, the designing and fabrication of the MMICs antenna are limited to microstrip fed patch antennas and slot antennas. The microstrip antennas can be made in single metal layer and also the slots are possible in an MMIC procedure, which offers patterning of the ground plane and a top alloy layer to make a microstrip line to excite them.

The basic radiation patterns as shown in Figure 5.5(a–c) are shown for a microstrip patch on the infinite ground plane, dipole-free space, and $\lambda/2$ slot infinite ground plane.

The slots and microstrip fed patch are also a fair choice in considering simplicity in feeding, fabrication, and input impedance. It is observed from radiation patterns that none of them would couple the emitted power to the fundamental mode. Hence, it is required alteration in the pattern in order to achieve further rotationally symmetric beam, which has smaller beam width and higher directivity. Hence, the microstrip patch antenna and slots are the best and fairer choice considering simplicity in feeding, input impedance, fabrication, and planarity. It is also seen that the inherent radiation pattern with a single microstrip or slot element is unsuitable for high efficiency. Instead of this, the smaller arrays of patches and slots can be built to shape the beam. Additionally, based on the limit of beam direction, the following grouping can be done for antenna topologies, dependent on the arrays of patches and slots:

1. Most of the microstrip patches must have the emitted energy in $\theta = 0°$ (spherical coordinate system) known as the broadside pattern.
2. Inverse broadside radiating where $\theta = 180°$, that is, slot exhibit maximum radiation in the below plane of the chip.

5.4.3 SELECTION OF THE SUBSTRATE FOR ANTENNA CHARACTERIZATIONS

It is very important to extract relevant information about the selection of substrates, their electric properties, and dielectric layers for antenna design, particularly in MMIC antennas. These substrates will play an important role for antenna computations and their performances. The important factor to analyze with the substrates used for designing the MMIC antenna is computing the cut-off frequencies. Since any antenna structure planned at frequencies higher than the cut-off frequency may cause the excitation of undesirable substrate modes and would degrade not only the radiation pattern of the given structure but also its efficiencies. The cut-off frequency for the TE and TM modes [14, 21, 23–25] for a ground dielectric slab is given by

$$f_c = \frac{c}{4h\sqrt{\varepsilon_r - 1}} \qquad (5.10)$$

where h is the thickness of the substrate of microstrip, c is the velocity of light (3×10^8 m/s), and ε_r is the relative permittivity of the substrate.

5.4.4 BROADSIDE MMIC ANTENNAS WITH VARIOUS GEOMETRIES

The designs of planar antennas like microstrip patch are primarily fall under broadside antenna geometries. The topologies with various process using microstrip patches can be designed, compromising the factor between the ohmic loss and impedance bandwidths. As it is observed analytically that the broadband microstrip patch can be designed using a thick substrate and a low dielectric constant [23], the MMIC process does not provide an optimum choice. It may be due to the MMIC process with either microstrip patches having a low dielectric constant suffer from poor ohmic efficiency or microstrip patches having a high dielectric constant suffer from a narrow band. Hence, for the broadband patch antenna, it is defined in terms of the Gaussian coupling efficiency, dielectric loss, ohmic loss, and reflection loss, which is considered to be an important role in wireless and satellite communications.

It is seen in the microstrip patch array (2×1) with an infinite ground plane as shown in Figure 5.5(d), the H-plane of an array shows null along with the ground plane, whereas the E-plane does not dissolve along the ground produces not only the unequal E- and H-planes but also it reduces the coupling to the Gaussian beam. Hence, a combo of two microstrip patches was designed, detached by a half-wavelength (~l/2) in the E-plane helps in reducing the beam width in the E-plane. The two patches can be combined in phase by making the utilization of feed through the Microstrip tee lines, with fitting impedance matching the quarter wavelength transformer (as shown in Figure 5.5(d)). The main disadvantage of such designing with phase feeding of the microstrip patch array take up more space on MMIC and simultaneously, the feed lines causes not only emits the spurious radiations but also it degrades he overall coupling to fundamental Gaussian beam mode. Due to this reason, it not only causes the losses but also produces the unsymmetries in the radiation pattern.

To overcome this limitation, one of the microstrip patches is rotated by 180° as shown in Figure 5.5(e). It means that the plane wave incident from the broadside direction will be in-phase with the E-field in the emanating edges of microstrip patches; however, the out-of-phase current will be on the microstrip feed lines. In this way, an unbalanced antenna array (microstrip) is deliberately built differential or balanced for conservative integration with the mixers.

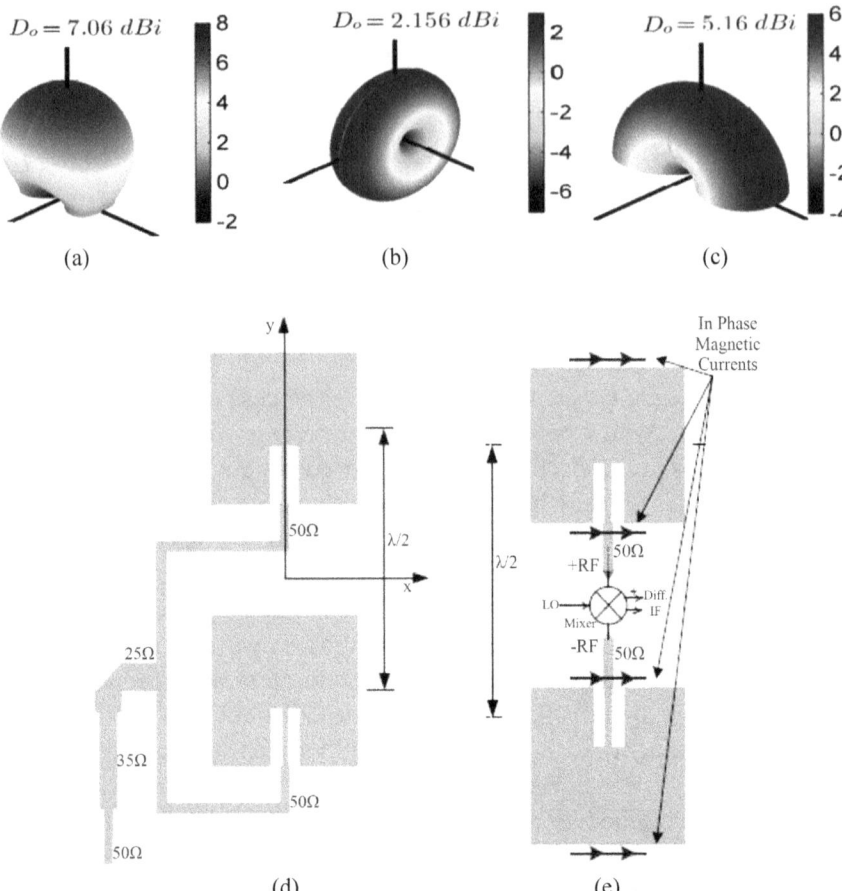

FIGURE 5.5 Radiation patterns for (a) microstrip patch on infinite ground plane (b) dipole-free space (c) $\lambda/2$ slot-infinite ground plane (d) Microstrip array 2×1 (e) microstrip array 2×1 with one of the microstrips rotated by 180 degree

It is observed that the direction of the incident broadside plane wave not only causes in-phase E-field in the radiating edges but it also causes phase shifted current on the microstrip feed lines of the microstrip patches. The main disadvantage of such MMIC design is that it has very less Gaussian beam analysis, that is, the beam waist side is typically 0.25λ. To overcome this, with designing of the microstrip array of 2×2 (as shown in Figure 5.6) which is nothing but the phase addition of microstrip array of 2×1 by an extra array of 2×1. Here in this MMIC design, it is observed that the Gaussian beam analysis of this array not only shows the improved coupling but also provides the size of the beam waist of the order of 0.5λ. Since the area of the beam waist is exceptionally closer to the ground, it may very well be considered as consistent regarding the wavelength. Such a topology is appealing as it offers a high coupling and possesses a little zone on MMIC; yet, at the same time, the beam waist is lower than the practical limit of 0.9 λ. The array element number can be doubled, that is, the microstrip patch arrays with 4 × 4 further increases the beam waist (as shown in Figure 5.7). It is observed that the simulated results of the microstrip patch array with 4 × 4 offer a shorter beam width with the cost of expanded sidelobe levels as all microstrip patches in array are energized with a uniform phase and amplitude.

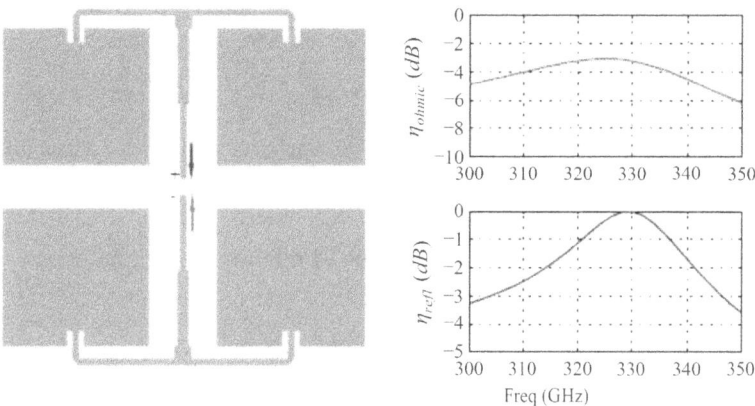

FIGURE 5.6 Design of a microstrip patch array 2 × 2 showing ohmic and reflection efficiencies.

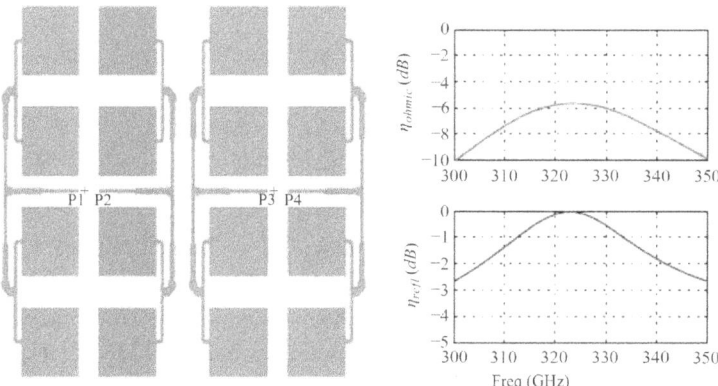

FIGURE 5.7 Design of a microstrip patch array 4 × 4 showing ohmic and reflection efficiencies.

All the microstrip lines consist of four metal layers with three dielectric layers made up of benzocyclobutene (BCB) (ε_r = 2.7) [26]. The BCB layer thickness is 5 µm and top material used here is gold (Au) of 3-µm thick. This substrate is shown in Figure 5.8.

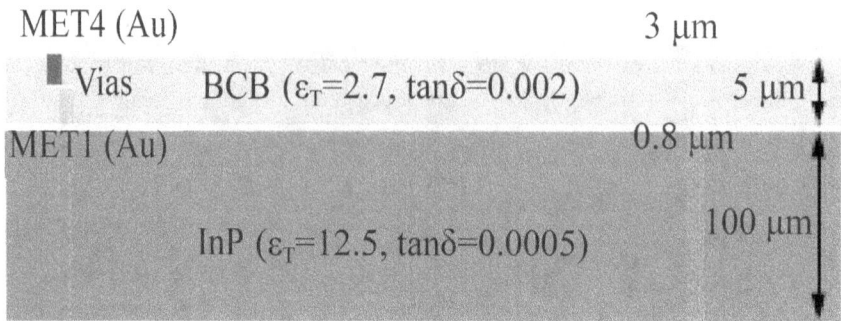

FIGURE 5.8 Microstrip patch antenna designed/simulated on the three-layered dielectric substrate (ε_r = 1 air; ε_r = 2.7 BCB, and ε_r = 12.5 InP).

Hence, as a summary, the advantages of making MMIC antenna topologies are as follows:

a. Spurious radiation from the matched feed lines cancels out producing null cross polarization.
b. Minimizes the complexities of microstrip feed lines with proper impedance matching.
c. Producing the differential RFs out from the multiple pair of microstrip carrying out of phase signals.
d. Spurious harmonics get reduced.
e. Easy to integrate with microwave active devices like balanced mixers.
f. Losses such as ohmic losses and reflection loss get minimized.
g. Compact integration.
h. Minimized the cross-polarizations levels.
i. Side lobes get minimized, causing increase in major lobes.

All the MMIC antenna designs represented in this chapter are evaluated in terms of reflection, ohmic, and Gaussian coupling efficiencies for satellite application (i.e., space wave propagations) whose center frequency is close to 350 GHz. Fair comparisons were made among the MMIC topologies and their simulated results of essential parameters such as efficiencies and bandwidth, and their areas are presented in Table 5.2.

TABLE 5.2 Comparison of MMIC Planar Antenna

Microstrip Patch Topology	Z_c (Ω)	BW (%)	η_{ohmic} (dB)	η_G (%)	Area (μm²)
Patch array 2 × 1	50	2.148	-3	91.65	350 × 750
Patch array 2 × 2	50	3.012	-3.48	94.86	875 × 875
Patch array 4 × 4	50	3.998	-6.47	77.32	1550 × 1550

5.5 CONCLUSIONS

This chapter deals with the detail characterization of MMIC antennas for various applications, especially for wireless communications and space wave propagations. It also shows the brief applications of active devices using MMIC technology for various applications. It is seen in this chapter that out of various antenna characterization parameters, both the reflection and ohmic efficiencies are the important factors for every application of antennas. So, one should design the MMIC antenna, considering the minimization of antenna losses and enhancement of impedance BW, which is ever be a big design issue. It is also seen in this chapter that the main characteristic parameters for MMIC antennas are aperture and Gaussian coupling efficiencies that affect the performance. The aperture efficiency is mainly used when the MMIC antenna is used as a feed for reflectors. Hence, for a given size of the aperture, there will be a maximum directivity.

It is observed from this chapter that the Gaussian efficiency is responsible for reflection on the coupling of emission/radiation from the antenna when considered to MMIC applications. For submillimeter wave operations, the characterization of the planar antenna (MMIC type) in terms of Gaussian efficiency is more significant along with reflection and ohmic efficiencies. The joining of antennas with MMIC is plausible at submillimeter wavelengths and viable decision is to coordinate antenna with active devices, for example, mixer. Considering the goal of reducing Gaussian efficiency values, a single antenna element is generally not desired and therefore one can use the combinations of small arrays of the planar antenna to provide the radiation pattern with a higher Gaussian efficiency with less ohmic and reflection losses.

This MMIC antenna technology plays an important role for any implementation and installation of any wireless and space wave communication system. In the present time, there has been exponential growth and a great demand in using THz frequencies, that is, millimeter and submillimeter wavelengths for several applications such as defense, security, submarine, satellite, biomedical imaging studies, astronomy, and atmospheric studies. All such applications are now more feasible and possible due to rapid enhancements of microwave-based semiconductor processing technologies. With the help of submillimeter wave techniques, designing an antenna integrated with active devices resonates more than THz frequency. This chapter investigates mostly about the development of various MMIC antennas which interface with the active devices for millimeter and submillimeter wave applications.

KEYWORDS

- **wireless communication**
- **MMIC**
- **planar antennas**
- **terahertz**
- **millimeter and submillimeter wave**

REFERENCES

1. IEEE. "IEEE standard definitions of terms for antennas," IEEE Std. 145-1983, June 1983.
2. Garratt, G.R.M. "The Early History of Radio from Faraday to Marconi" (London: Institution of Electrical Engineers, 1994).
3. Maxwell, J.C. "A dynamic theory of the electromagnetic field," Philosophical Transactions of the Royal Society of London, 1865, 155, pp. 459-512.
4. Maxwell, J.C. "A Treatise on Electricity and Magnetism (1873, 1881, 1891) Bde 1 u. 2" [Unabridged reprint of the last edition 1891] (Mineola, NY: Dover, 1954). ISBN 0-486-60636-8 and 0-486-60637-6.
5. Carmeli, M. "Group Analysis of Maxwell's Equations," Journal of Mathematical Physics, 1969, 10, p. 1699.
6. Christopher, H.S.; Shiers, G. "History of Telecommunications Technology: An Annotated Bibliography" (Lanham, MD: Scarecrow, 2000).
7. Sarkar, T.K. History of Wireless (New York, NY: Wiley-IEEE Press, 2006).
8. Siegel, P.H. "Terahertz technology," Microwave Theory and Techniques, IEEE Transactions, 2002, 50 (3), pp. 910–928.
9. Dragoman, D.; Dragoman M. "Terahertz fields and applications," Progress in Quantum Electronics, 2004, 28 (1), pp 1–66.
10. Yang, Y., Mandehgar, M., Grischkowsky, D. "Broadband THz pulse transmission through the atmosphere," Terahertz Science and Technology, IEEE Transactions, 2011, 1 (1), pp. 264–273.
11. Marsh, S. Practical MMIC Design (Norwood, MA: Artech House, 2006).

12. Robertson, I. D.; Lucyszyn, S. RFIC and MMIC Design and Technology, 1st edition, The Institution of Engineering and Technology, London, United Kingdom, 2001, pp. 429–463.
13. Pengelly, R.; Turner, J. "Monolithic broadband GaAs FET amplifiers," Electronics Letters, 1976, 12 (10), pp. 251–252.
14. Balanis, C. Antenna Theory: Analysis and Design (New York, NY: Wiley Publications, 2005).
15. Kildal, P.S. Foundations of Antenna Engineering: A Unified Approach for Line-of-Sight and Multipath, Kildal, Sweden, 2015.
16. Rosengren, K.; Kildal, P.S. "Study of distributions of modes and plane waves in reverberation chambers for the characterization of antennas in a multipath environment," Microwave and Optical Technology Letters, 2001, 30 (6), pp. 386-391. http://dx.doi.org/10.1002/mop.1323.
17. Kildal, P.S. "Factorization of the feed efficiency of paraboloids and Cassegrain antennas." Antennas and Propagation IEEE, 33 (8), pp. 903-908, 1985.
18. Kildal, P.; Sipus, Z. "Classification of rotationally symmetric antennas as types BOR 0 and BOR 1," IEEE Antennas and Propagation Magazine, 1995, 37 (6), p. 114.
19. Kraus, J.D.; Marhefka, R. Antennas: For All applications (Boston, MA: McGraw-Hill, 2002).
20. Liu, D.; Ulrich, P.; Janusz G.; Brian, G. Advanced Millimeter-wave Technologies: Antennas, Packaging and Circuits (New York, NY: Wiley, 2009).
21. Rebeiz, G. "Millimeter-wave and terahertz integrated circuit antennas," Proceedings of the IEEE, 1992, 80 (11), pp. 1748-1770.
22. Gupta, K.C.; Hall, P.S. Analysis and Design of Integrated Circuit Antenna Modules (New York, NY: John Wiley, 2000).
23. Kumar, G.; Ray, K. "Broadband Microstrip Antennas." (London: Artech House, 2003).
24. Pozar, D. Microwave Engineering. (New York, NY: John Wiley & Sons, 2004).
25. Srikant, S.S. "An overview on monolithic microwave integrated circuits," Turkish Journal of Engineering, Science and Technology, 2014, 3, pp. 123-126.
26. Heiliger, H.M.; Nagel, M.; Roskos, H.G.; Kurz, H.; Schnieder, F.; Heinrich, W.; Hey, R.; Ploog, K. "Low-dispersion thin film microstrip lines with cyclotene (benzocyclobutene) as dielectric medium," Applied Physics Letters, 1997, 70 (17), pp. 2233.

CHAPTER 6

A 3D Analytic Modeling of Threshold Voltages of FD SOI MOSFET

KRISHNA MEEL[1*], RAM GOPAL[2], and DEEPAK BHATNAGAR[3]

[1]*Department of Science and Humanities, BK Birla Institute of Engineering and Technology, Pilani, Rajasthan, India*

[2]*CSIR—Central Electronics Engineering Research Institute, Pilani, Rajasthan, India*

[3]*Department of Physics, University of Rajasthan, Jaipur, Rajasthan, India*

Corresponding author. E-mail: krishna.meel@bkbiet.ac.in

ABSTRACT

This chapter presents a new approach for deriving analytical models for front- and back-gate threshold voltages by solving Laplace and Poisson's equation in multilayer structure of small geometry fully depleted-silicon-on-insulator (SOI) *metal–oxide–semiconductor field-effect transistor*s. A three-dimensional Poisson's equation is solved analytically by applying Green's function technique not only within SOI film but also within the front- and back-oxide regions. By utilizing these expressions, formulae of front- and back-threshold voltages comprising inversion effect of side-wall interfaces have been formulated. The influence of back-gate bias and drain voltage have also been included. A new subthreshold model can be developed with the help of potential expression obtained in this chapter as well.

6.1 INTRODUCTION

For the last two decades, enhancement-mode *metal–oxide–semiconductor field-effect transistor*s (MOSFETs) fabricated on a silicon-on-insulator (SOI) film have received much attention in very large-scale integration (VLSI) application. There are several advantages of SOI over bulk MOSFETs like reduced short channel effects [1, 2], punch through suppression [3], increased subthreshold slope [4], mobility enhancement [5], increased radiation hardness, and saturation current enhancement [6, 7]. As the size of device is shrinking to compensate the packaging density, which results the gate length and width of SOI MOSFET is narrowed down considerably so to overcome inter-device interactions in bias case. Each device is isolated by forming separate islands or trench/mesa isolation structure [8] of SOI film prior to device fabrication. Analytical modeling of electrical behavior of semiconductor devices is playing an important role in their development. CMOS circuits fabricated on SOI wafers are gaining high importance in present day VLSI and ultra large-scale integration (ULSI) technology. As we have already mentioned that SOI technology shows better performance over its bulk counterpart in many different ways like lower leakage current, latch up free, high radiation tolerance, fast switching due to lower capacitance, less power dissipation due to steeper subthreshold characteristics that allow the transistor to be operated at lower voltages and so on. Although SOI CMOS technology is now being widely used, there still exist the need to develop an accurate analytical device models for SOI-based MOSFETs suitable for circuit simulation. In order to achieve high integration in ULSI, the geometry of SOI MOSFETs is very small by reducing channel length as well as channel width that give rise to a strong coupling of potential in front-, back- and side-wall oxide regions. It is becoming more difficult to use one-dimensional (1D) or even two-dimensional (2D) models to describe the behavior of many small device structures. Therefore, the three-dimensional (3D) analytical device model is necessary to address these geometric dependencies and for accurate electrical characterization of small geometry devices. Especially short channel and narrow width effect have a combined effect on threshold voltage, which is a very crucial parameter to estimate various features of the device.

In this chapter, a new approach is considered for deriving front- and back-threshold voltage models by solving 3D Poisson's equation not only within the SOI film [9] but also within the oxides, that is, front-oxide and back-oxide regions. In this way, there are three different zones, that is, front oxide, SOI film, and back oxide are defined in which Poisson's equation is solved as it is shown by a rectangle ABCD (active portion) in Figure 6.1. The surface potential expression for SOI MOSFET can also be obtained from the solution of 3D Poisson's equation and thereby other important subthreshold characteristics can be derived [10]. The schematic 3D cross-sectional view of SOI MOSFET is given in Figure 6.1(A).

A 3D Analytic Modeling of Threshold Voltages

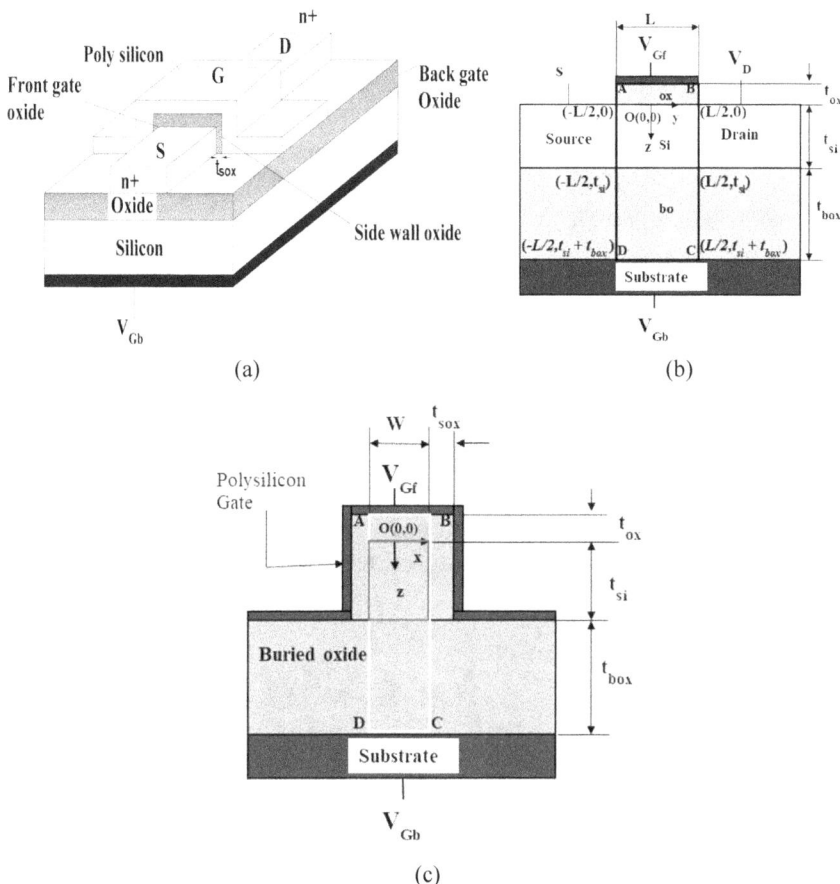

FIGURE 6.1 (A) Schematic 3D view, cross-sectional view along, (B) the channel length, and (C) width of active portion of SOI MOSFET.

6.2 THEORETICAL MODEL

Figure 6.1 shows 3D and the cross-sectional view of the fully depleted (FD) SOI MOSFET along the channel length and width, respectively. A solid box enclosed by four planes passing through four sides of the rectangle (ABCD) along the channel length and width from $z = -t_{ox}$ to $t_{Si} + t_{box}$ is the active portion of the device as shown in Figure 6.1. The plane ABCD in Figure 6.1(a) shows the plane passing through center of active portion of the device along the channel length, L ($y = -L/2$ to $+L/2$) and in Figure 6.1(b) the plane ABCD is along the channel width, $W(x = -W/2$ to $+W/2)$.

The origin O ($x=0$, $y=0$, $z=0$) is assumed at the center point of the front-oxide and silicon interface plane. The thicknesses of front-gate oxide, buried oxide, and SOI film are t_{ox}, t_{box}, and t_{si}, respectively. In order to account for the coupling effect of all the four interfaces for fully depleted SOI film having uniform doping, a 3D Poisson's equation under the electrostatic condition for n-channel MOSFET in front oxide, depleted silicon film, and back oxide, respectively can be given as

$$\nabla^2 \phi_{ox} = 0 \tag{6.1}$$

$$\nabla^2 \phi_{si} = \frac{qN_A}{\varepsilon_0 \varepsilon_{si}}, \tag{6.2}$$

$$\nabla^2 \phi_{bo} = 0 \tag{6.3}$$

where ε_0 is the vacuum dielectric constant, ε_{Si} is the relative permittivity of silicon, and N_A is the acceptor impurity concentration. At the front gate and source end; the boundary conditions assumed to solve (6.1)–(6.3) are written as

$$\phi_{ox}(x, y, z = -t_{ox}) = V'_{Gf}, \tag{6.4}$$

$$\phi_{ox}(x, -L/2, z) = \frac{\phi^f_{ss} - V'_{Gf}}{t_{ox}} z + \phi^f_{ss}, \tag{6.5}$$

$$\phi_{si}(x, -L/2, z) = V_{bi}, \tag{6.6}$$

$$\phi_{bo}(x, -L/2, z) = \frac{V'_{Gb} - \phi^b_{ss}}{t_{box}}(z - t_{si}) + \phi^b_{ss}, \tag{6.7}$$

$$V'_{Gf} = V_{Gf} - V^f_{FB},$$

While those at the drain end and at back gate are

$$\phi_{ox}(x, L/2, z) = \frac{\phi^f_{ss} + V_D - V'_{Gf}}{t_{ox}} z + \phi^f_{ss} + V_D, \tag{6.8}$$

$$\phi_{si}(x, L/2, z) = V_{bi} + V_D, \tag{6.9}$$

$$\phi_{bo}(x, L/2, z) = \frac{V'_{Gb} - \phi^b_{ss} - V_D}{t_{box}}(Z - t_{si}) + \phi^b_{ss} + V_D, \tag{6.10}$$

$$\phi_{bo}(x, y, z = t_{Si} + t_{box}) = V'_{Gb} \tag{6.11}$$

$$V'_{Gb} = V_{Gb} - V^b_{FB}.$$

Now, the boundary conditions for front-oxide–silicon interface and back-oxide–silicon interface can be written as

$$\phi_{ox}(x, y, z = 0) = \phi_{Si}(x, y, z = 0), \quad (6.12)$$

$$\frac{\partial \phi_{ox}}{\partial z}(x, y, z = 0) = \eta \frac{\partial \phi_{Si}}{\partial z}(x, y, z = 0), \quad (6.13)$$

$$\phi_{si}(x, y, z = t_{si}) = \phi_{bo}(x, y, z = t_{si}), \quad (6.14)$$

$$\eta \frac{\partial \phi_{si}}{\partial z}(x, y, z = t_{si}) = \frac{\partial \phi_{bo}}{\partial z}(x, y, z = t_{si}), \quad (6.15)$$

Here V_{Gf} is the front-gate voltage, V_{Gb} is the back-gate bias, and $V_{FB}^{f,b}$ are the front- and back-gate flat-band voltages, respectively. For n$^+$–p source and drain junctions, the built-in potential is $V_{bi} = E_{g/2} + (kT/q)\ln\{N_A/n_i\}$ where n_i—intrinsic concentration, E_g—energy band gap, and V_D—source-to-drain applied voltage. The front- and back-interface source end potential are $\phi_{SS}^f = V_{bi}(z = 0)$ and $\phi_{SS}^b = V_{bi}(z = t_{si})$, respectively. Since the front-gate voltage also appears along the side-wall interface. Finally the boundary conditions at the side-wall interface are modified from those used in previously derived 3D SOI MOSFET model. Here the potential appearing across the side interface, $\phi'_{Gs}(z)$ is a function which varies with the thickness of SOI film. The boundary conditions are

$$\frac{\partial \phi}{\partial x}(x = \pm W/2, y, z) = \mp \frac{\phi(x = \pm W/2, y, z) - \phi'_{Gs}(z)}{t_s}, \quad (6.16)$$

where,

$$\phi'_{Gs}(z) = -\frac{(V'_{Gs} - V'_{Gs})}{t_{box}} z + V'_{Gs}\left(1 + \frac{t_{Si}}{t_{box}}\right) - V'_{Gs}\left(\frac{t_{Si}}{t_{box}}\right),$$

$$t_s = (\epsilon_{Si}/\epsilon_{ox}) t_{sox}$$

$$V'_{Gs} = V_{Gf} - V_{FB}^s$$

having t_{sox}—side-wall oxide thickness and V_{FB}^s—flat-band voltage at side interfaces. As the crystallography of side oxide-silicon and front oxide-silicon interfaces is different therefore their flat-band voltages are also different. The flat-band voltages of different oxide interfaces are inclusive of the respective fixed charge densities, Q_f besides work function difference ϕ_{ms}. The flat band voltage is $V_{FB} = \phi_{ms} - Q_f/C_o$, where C_o is the capacitance associated with different oxide layers [11]. In order to solve 3D Poisson's equations (6.1)–(6.3), we have used Green's function which has been derived considering the homogeneous boudary conditions given in Eqs. (6.4)–(6.16) associated with Eqs. (6.1)–(6.3). The new multizone Green's function has been derived to obtain the explicit solution of the aforesaid differential equations. The procedure in detail is explained in the next section.

6.2.1 GREEN'S FUNCTIONS AND SOLUTIONS

The Laplace equations together with Poisson's equation are needed to be solved in multizone structure with three media joined on two oxide/silicon interfaces as shown in Figure 6.1. Appropriately for three-zone structure, we have derived new Green's functions considering their basic definitions associated with Eqs. (6.1)–(6.3) subject to homogeneous conditions of boundary values equations (6.4)–(6.16) at the outer as well as real boundary conditions. In this chapter, we show that we can find out Green's function $G(x, y, z; x', y', z')$ for all three zones joined on interfaces. Let us assume the source point (x', y', z') fixed at silicon film [see Figure 6.1(a)] and consider $G(x, y, z; x', y', z')$ as a function of x, y, and z, which vary throughout the three-zone system including interfaces. Thus Green's function set, representing silicon combined with the effects of adjoining layers, that is, front- and buried-oxide, is defined as

$$\left. \begin{array}{l} \nabla^2 G_{ox}^{Si}(x, y, z; x', y', z') = 0, \\ \nabla^2 G_{ox}^{Si}(x, y, z; x', y', z') = \delta(x-x')\delta(y-y')\delta(z-z'), \\ \nabla^2 G_{bo}^{Si}(x, y, z; x', y', z') = 0. \end{array} \right\} \quad (6.17)$$

Similarly, if the source point (x', y', z') is assumed to be located in front oxide, Green's functions consisting of the effects of other layers are represented by the differential equations, written as

$$\left. \begin{array}{l} \nabla^2 G_{ox}^{ox}(x, y, z; x', y', z') = \delta(x-x')\delta(y-y')\delta(z-z'), \\ \nabla^2 G_{Si}^{ox}(x, y, z; x', y', z') = 0, \\ \nabla^2 G_{bo}^{ox}(x, y, z; x', y', z') = 0. \end{array} \right\} \quad (6.18)$$

and those in case when point (x', y', z') is kept fixed in buried oxide, are governed by the following equations:

$$\left. \begin{array}{l} \nabla^2 G_{ox}^{bo}(x, y, z; x', y', z') = 0, \\ \nabla^2 G_{si}^{bo}(x, y, z; x', y', z') = 0 \\ \nabla^2 G_{bo}^{bo}(x, y, z; x', y', z') = \delta(x-x')\delta(y-y')\delta(z-z'). \end{array} \right\} \quad (6.19)$$

A 3D Analytic Modeling of Threshold Voltages

Here, subscripts in Green's functions is indicating three different layers, as such it is single function $G(x, y, z; x', y', z')$ appeared in Eqs. (6.17)–(6.19). Each set of differential equations pertains to the individual layer having combined effects of other two layers owing to location of source points at the particular layer indicated by superscripts. Now we multiply Eqs. (6.1)–(6.3) by $G(x, y, z; x', y', z')$ and Eqs. (6.17)–(6.19) by ϕ and then subtract the latter from the former ones and then by applying Green's theorem to yield

$$\begin{aligned}\phi_{Si} = &\frac{1}{\eta}\oint\left[\phi_{ox}\nabla G^{Si}_{ox} - G^{Si}_{ox}\nabla\phi_{ox}\right]\cdot dS \\ &+ \frac{1}{\eta}\oint\left[\phi_{bo}\nabla G^{Si}_{bo} - G^{Si}_{bo}\nabla\phi_{bo}\right]\cdot dS \\ &+ \oint\left[\phi_{Si}\nabla G^{Si}_{Si} - G_{Si}\nabla\phi_{Si}\right]\cdot dS \\ &+ \iiint\frac{qN_A(z)}{\varepsilon_0\varepsilon_{Si}}G^{Si}_{Si}(x', y', z'; x, y, z)\,dx'\,dy'\,dz'. \end{aligned} \quad (6.20)$$

that is, the potential for silicon layer and for front/buried oxide layers the same are given as

$$\begin{aligned}\phi_{ox} = &\oint\left[\phi_{ox}\nabla G^{ox}_{ox} - G^{ox}_{ox}\nabla\phi_{ox}\right]\cdot dS \\ &+ \oint\left[\phi_{bo}\nabla G^{ox}_{bo} - G^{ox}_{bo}\nabla\phi_{bo}\right]\cdot dS \\ &+ \eta\oint\left[\phi_{Si}\nabla G^{ox}_{Si} - G^{ox}_{Si}\nabla\phi_{Si}\right]\cdot dS \\ &+ \eta\iiint\frac{qN_A(z)}{\varepsilon_0\varepsilon_{Si}}G^{ox}_{Si}(x', y', z'; x, y, z)\,dx'\,dy'\,dz'. \end{aligned} \quad (6.21)$$

and

$$\begin{aligned}\phi_{bo} = &\oint\left[\phi_{ox}\nabla G^{bo}_{ox} - G^{bo}_{ox}\nabla\phi_{ox}\right]\cdot dS \\ &+ \oint\left[\phi_{bo}\nabla G^{bo}_{bo} - G^{bo}_{bo}\nabla\phi_{bo}\right]\cdot dS \\ &+ \eta\oint\left[\phi_{Si}\nabla G^{bo}_{Si} - G_{Si}\nabla\phi_{Si}\right]\cdot dS \\ &+ \eta\iiint\frac{qN_A(z)}{\varepsilon_0\varepsilon_{Si}}G^{bo}_{Si}(x', y', z'; x, y, z)\,dx'\,dy'\,dz'. \end{aligned} \quad (6.22)$$

respectively. The present formalism can be extended up to any number of media joined at the interfaces. Green's functions obtained by solving Eqs. (6.17)–(6.19) include the combined effects of all the three layers and also the consideration of Eqs. (6.12)–(6.15) at the interface include the material properties in Green's functions. The first to third integral of Eqs. (6.20)–(6.22) at the interfaces also cancel out each other therefore only external boundary integral in these equations are evaluated. Green's functions are still valid if the interface trap densities are included in boundary values given through Eqs. (6.12)–(6.15), but for this condition the evaluation of integrals at the interfaces becomes mandatory. Green's functions appeared in the above integral equations, as per Appendix 6A, are written as

$$G_{ox}^{Si} = -\frac{2\eta}{LT_{sc}} \sum_{m,n=1}^{\infty} g_{mn} \frac{f_{Si}^{(n)}(z') f_{ox}^{(n)}(z)}{\lambda_{mn}\Delta_n} \sin \beta_m (y'+L/2) \sin \beta_m (y+L/2), \quad (6.23a)$$

$$G_{Si}^{Si} = -\frac{2}{LT_{sc}} \sum_{m,n=1}^{\infty} g_{mn} \frac{f_{Si}^{(n)}(z') f_{Si}^{(n)}(z)}{\lambda_{mn}\Delta_n} \sin \beta_m (y'+L/2) \sin \beta_m (y+L/2), \quad (6.23b)$$

$$G_{bo}^{Si} = -\frac{2\eta}{LT_{sc}} \sum_{m,n=1}^{\infty} g_{mn} \frac{f_{Si}^{(n)}(z') f_{bo}^{(n)}(z)}{\lambda_{mn}\Delta_n} \sin \beta_m (y'+L/2) \sin \beta_m (y+L/2), \quad (6.23c)$$

for the silicon layer derived from set (6.17), and those corresponding to set (6.18) can be obtained by replacing the common eigenfunction $f_{Si}^{(n)}(z')$ of Eq. (6.23) by $f_{ox}^{(n)}(z')$ related to oxide zone as

$$G_{ox}^{ox} = -\frac{2\eta}{LT_{sc}} \sum_{m,n=1}^{\infty} g_{mn} \frac{f_{ox}^{(n)}(z') f_{ox}^{(n)}(z)}{\lambda_{mn}\Delta_n} \sin \beta_m (y'+L/2) \sin \beta_m (y+L/2), \quad (6.24a)$$

$$G_{Si}^{ox} = -\frac{2}{LT_{sc}} \sum_{m,n=1}^{\infty} g_{mn} \frac{f_{ox}^{(n)}(z') f_{Si}^{(n)}(z)}{\lambda_{mn}\Delta_n} \sin \beta_m (y'+L/2) \sin \beta_m (y+L/2), \quad (6.24b)$$

$$G_{bo}^{ox} = -\frac{2\eta}{LT_{sc}} \sum_{m,n=1}^{\infty} g_{mn} \frac{f_{ox}^{(n)}(z') f_{bo}^{(n)}(z)}{\lambda_{mn}\Delta_n} \sin \beta_m (y'+L/2) \sin \beta_m (y+L/2), \quad (6.24c)$$

Similarly, the replacement of $f_{Si}^{(n)}(z')$ of Eq. (6.23) by eigenfunction, $f_{bo}^{(n)}(z')$ for buried oxide gives the set of Green's functions representing the solutions of Eq. (6.19), written as

$$G_{ox}^{bo} = -\frac{2\eta}{LT_{sc}} \sum_{m,n=1}^{\infty} g_{mn} \frac{f_{bo}^{(n)}(z') f_{ox}^{(n)}(z)}{\lambda_{mn}\Delta_n} \sin \beta_m (y'+L/2) \sin \beta_m (y+L/2), \quad (6.25a)$$

$$G_{Si}^{bo} = -\frac{2}{LT_{sc}} \sum_{m,n=1}^{\infty} g_{mn} \frac{f_{bo}^{(n)}(z') f_{Si}^{(n)}(z)}{\lambda_{mn} \Delta_n} \sin \beta_m (y'+L/2) \sin \beta_m (y+L/2), \quad (6.25b)$$

$$G_{bo}^{bo} = -\frac{2\eta}{LT_{sc}} \sum_{m,n=1}^{\infty} g_{mn} \frac{f_{bo}^{(n)}(z') f_{bo}^{(n)}(z)}{\lambda_{mn} \Delta_n} \sin \beta_m (y'+L/2) \sin \beta_m (y+L/2), \quad (6.25c)$$

where

$$g_{mn}^{-}(x,x') = \frac{\left(\sinh \lambda_{mn}(W/2-x') + \lambda_{mn} t_s \cosh \lambda_{mn}(W/2-x')\right)}{\left(\sinh \lambda_{mn}(W/2) + \lambda_{mn} t_s \cosh \lambda_{mn}(W/2)\right)}$$

$$\times \frac{\left(\sinh \lambda_{mn}(W/2+x) + \lambda_{mn} t_s \cosh \lambda_{mn}(W/2+x)\right)}{\left(\cosh \lambda_{mn}(W/2) + \lambda_{mn} t_s \sinh \lambda_{mn}(W/2)\right)}; x < x'$$

$$g_{mn}^{+}(x,x') = \frac{\left(\sinh \lambda_{mn}(W/2+x') + \lambda_{mn} t_s \cosh \lambda_{mn}(W/2+x')\right)}{\left(\sinh \lambda_{mn}(W/2) + \lambda_{mn} t_s \cosh \lambda_{mn}(W/2)\right)}$$

$$\times \frac{\left(\sinh \lambda_{mn}(W/2-x) + \lambda_{mn} t_s \cosh \lambda_{mn}(W/2-x)\right)}{\left(\cosh \lambda_{mn}(W/2) + \lambda_{mn} t_s \sinh \lambda_{mn}(W/2)\right)}; x < x'$$

The use of Green's functions given through Eq. (6.23) in evaluating integral equation (6.20) results in the potential distribution within silicon film only as the common eigenfunction $f_{Si}^{(n)}(z')$ belongs to silicon film only. The second set of Green's functions given through Eq. (6.24) having common eigenfunction, $f_{ox}^{(n)}(z')$, as a result, the integral equation (6.21) yields the solution that corresponds to the front oxide. On the other hand, by using third set of Green's function given by Eq. (6.25) on Eq. (6.22), would give rise to the potential relation for buried oxide. Now by using these aforesaid Green's functions and integral equations (6.20)–(6.22) by applying boundary conditions given through Eqs. (6.4)–(6.16). The solutions of Eqs. (6.1)–(6.3) in, respectively, SOI film, front oxide, and buried oxide layers can be expressed as

$$\phi_{Si} = \phi_{Si}^0 + \frac{2}{t_{Si}} \sum_{n=1}^{\infty} \frac{R_n f_{Si}^{(n)}(z)}{\alpha_n \Delta_n} \left[\phi_{SD}^{(n)}(U,V) \frac{\cosh(\alpha_n y)}{\cosh(\alpha_n L/2)} \right.$$

$$+ \frac{1}{2} V_D \zeta_n \frac{\sinh(\alpha_n y)}{\sinh(\alpha_n L/2)}$$

$$\left. + \frac{2}{L} \sum_{m=1}^{\infty} P_{mn}(V'_{Gf}, V'_{Gb}) \frac{\cosh(\lambda_{mn} x) \sin \beta_m (y+L/2)}{\beta_m S_{mn}(t_s) \cosh(\lambda_{mn} W/2)} \right] \quad (6.26)$$

$$\phi_{ox} = \phi_{ox}^0 + \frac{2}{t_{Si}}\eta \sum_{n=1}^{\infty} \frac{R_n f_{ox}^{(n)}(z)}{\alpha_n \Delta_n} \left[\phi_{SD}^{(n)}(U,V) \frac{\cosh(\alpha_n y)}{\cosh(\alpha_n L/2)} \right.$$
$$+ \frac{1}{2}V_D \zeta_n \frac{\sinh(\alpha_n y)}{\sinh(\alpha_n L/2)}$$
$$\left. + \frac{2}{L}\sum_{m=1}^{\infty} P_{mn}(V'_{Gf}, V'_{Gb}) \frac{\cosh(\lambda_{mn} x)\sin \beta_m (y+L/2)}{\beta_m S_{mn}(t_s)\cosh(\lambda_{mn} W/2)} \right] \qquad (6.27)$$

$$\phi_{bo} = \phi_{bo}^0 + \frac{2}{t_{Si}}\eta \sum_{n=1}^{\infty} \frac{R_n f_{bo}^{(n)}(z)}{\alpha_n \Delta_n} \left[\phi_{SD}^{(n)}(U,V) \frac{\cosh(\alpha_n y)}{\cosh(\alpha_n L/2)} \right.$$
$$+ \frac{1}{2}V_D \zeta_n \frac{\sinh(\alpha_n y)}{\sinh(\alpha_n L/2)}$$
$$\left. + \frac{2}{L}\sum_{m=1}^{\infty} P_{mn}(V'_{Gf}, V'_{Gb}) \frac{\cosh(\lambda_{mn} x)\sin \beta_m (y+L/2)}{\beta_m S_{mn}(t_s)\cosh(\lambda_{mn} W/2)} \right]. \qquad (6.28)$$

where

$$\phi_{Si}^0 = \frac{1}{2}Kz^2 - \left(\frac{1}{2}Kt_{Si}^2 + Kt_{Si}t_b - V'_{Gb}\right)\left(\frac{z+t_g}{T_{sc}}\right) + \left(\frac{t_{Si}+t_b-z}{T_{sc}}\right)V'_{Gf}$$

$$\phi_{ox}^0 = V'_{Gf} - \eta\left[\left(\frac{1}{2}Kt_{Si}^2 + Kt_{Si}t_b - V'_{Gb} + V'_{Gf}\right)\left(\frac{z+t_{ox}}{T_{sc}}\right)\right]$$

$$\phi_{bo}^0 = V'_{Gb} - \eta\left[\left(\frac{1}{2}Kt_{Si}^2 + Kt_{Si}t_g - V'_{Gf} + V'_{Gb}\right)\left(\frac{t_{Si}+t_{box}-z}{T_{sc}}\right)\right]$$

$$\phi_{SD}^{(n)}(U,V) = \frac{K}{\alpha_n^2} - \frac{1}{R_n}\left(U\chi_n^f + V\chi_n^b\right) + \left(V_{bi} + \frac{1}{2}V_D\right)\zeta_n,$$

$$P_{mn}(U,V) = \left\{1-(-1)^m\right\}\Omega_n(U,V)$$
$$-\frac{\beta_m^2}{\lambda_{mn}^2}\left\{\phi_{SD}^{(n)}(U,V) - \frac{1}{2}V_D\zeta_n - (-1)^m\left(\phi_{SD}^{(n)}(U,V) + \frac{1}{2}V_D\zeta_n\right)\right\}$$

followed by

$$\Omega_n(U,V) = \frac{K}{\alpha_n^2} + \frac{\chi_n^b}{R_n}(U-V) + \frac{\left(V_{FB}^f - V_{FB}^s\right)}{R_n}\left(\sec(\alpha_n t_{ox}) + \chi_n^b\right).$$

Other series parameters are defined as

$$\zeta_n = \chi_n^f + \chi_n^b, \qquad R_n = 1 + Q_n,$$

$$\chi_n^f = \frac{\tan(\alpha_n t_{ox})}{\alpha_n t_{ox}}, \qquad \chi_n^b = Q_n \frac{\tan(\alpha_n t_{box})}{\alpha_n t_{box}}$$

$$S_{mn}(t_s) = 1 + \lambda_{mn} t_s \tanh(\lambda_{mn} W/2),$$

Here U and V corresponding to V'_{Gf} and V'_{Gb}, respectively, are the dummy parameters used in Eqs. (6.26)–(6.28). These parameters can be modified accordingly in the other expressions.

If we analyze explicit potential expressions (6.26)–(6.28) corresponding to their respective layers, it consist of basically two components: the first represent the long channel behavior whereas the second terms in series forms shows the short channel effects. The series over α_n in these expressions converges fast and therefore only four terms of the series are sufficient to be summed up for accurate results. Hence, we retain the series summation throughout the formalism of threshold voltages, which are described in the following sections.

In expression (6.26), since the series over α_n is highly convergent therefore the first two terms are sufficient to be summed up but the series over m is not convergent so as to truncate up to fundamental mode. Therefore, it needs minimum of 10 terms to be summed up to achieve considerable results. So to use this expression to derive threshold voltage formulae is not advisable. Therefore it is worthwhile to impose some simplifying assumptions to make the expression (6.26) compact and easy to manage. For this, we restrict [cosh $(\lambda_{mn} x)/S_{mn}(t_s)\cosh(\lambda_{mn} W/2)$] to [cosh $(\lambda_{1,n} x)/S_{1,n}(t_s)\cosh(\lambda_{1,n} W/2)$] in series over m and latter independent of m. Now the series over m can be easily summed up. The series over m converges slowly as compared to the series over α_n. Moreover, the functions of x and y coordinates are strongly coupled with each other; therefore, the summation of series cannot be done and hence Eq. (6.26) with these assumptions can be approximated as

$$\phi_{Si} = \phi_{Si}^0 + \frac{2}{t_{Si}} \sum_{n=1}^{\infty} \frac{R_n f_{Si}^{(n)}(z)}{\alpha_n \Delta_n} \left[\phi_{SD}^{(n)}(U,V) \frac{\cosh(\alpha_n y)}{\cosh(\alpha_n L/2)} \right.$$

$$\left. + \frac{1}{2} V_D \zeta_n \frac{\sinh(\alpha_n y)}{\sinh(\alpha_n L/2)} + \frac{\cosh(\lambda_{1n} x)}{S_{1n}(t_s)\cosh(\lambda_{1n} W/2)} E_{1n}(y) \right] \quad (6.29)$$

$$E_{1n}(y) = \frac{2}{L} \sum_{m=1}^{\infty} P_{mn}(V'_{Gf}, V'_{Gb}) \frac{\sin \beta_m(y + L/2)}{\beta_m} \quad (6.30)$$

The term $E_{1n}(y)$ is an infinite series and summation of same is obligatory in order to have compact formulation; therefore, we will further simplify this by substituting $P_{mn}(V'_{Gf}, V'_{Gb})$ from Eq. (6.28b) in Eq. (6.30) which consist of three terms given as

$$E_{1n}(y) = \sum_{n=1}^{\infty}\left[\frac{2}{L}\Omega_n(V'_{Gf}, V'_{Gb})\sum_{m=1}^{\infty}\{1-(-1)^m\}\frac{\sin\beta_m(y+L/2)}{\beta_m}\right.$$

$$-\left(\phi_{SD}^{(n)}(U,V) - \frac{1}{2}V_D\zeta_n\right)\frac{2}{L}\sum_{m=1}^{\infty}\frac{\beta_m}{\lambda_{mn}^2}\sin\beta_m\left(y+\frac{L}{2}\right)$$

$$\left.+\left(\phi_{SD}^{(n)}(U,V) + \frac{1}{2}V_D\zeta_n\right)\frac{2}{L}\sum_{m=1}^{\infty}\frac{\beta_m(-1)^m}{\lambda_{mn}^2}\sin\beta_m\left(y+\frac{L}{2}\right)\right] \quad (6.31)$$

Here we have put $\lambda_{1n}^2 = \beta_1^2 + \alpha_n^2$

In order to solve Eq. (6.31), we will adopt the same procedure as it was done in reference [9]. The solution of three infinite series associated with each term is taken from there and by substituting these series solution in Eq. (6.31) we obtain

$$E_{1n}(y) = \sum_{n=1}^{\infty}\left[\Omega_n(V'_{Gf}, V'_{Gb})\right.$$

$$\left.-\left[\phi_{SD}^{(n)}(U,V)\frac{\cosh(\alpha_n y)}{\cosh(\alpha_n L/2)} + \frac{1}{2}V_D\zeta_n\frac{\sinh(\alpha_n y)}{\sinh(\alpha_n L/2)}\right]\right]. \quad (6.32)$$

Finally, we will achieve simplified expression (6.33) by substituting Eq. (6.32) in Eq. (6.29). Thus, leading an approximate form of Eq. (6.26) is expressed by

$$\phi_{Si} = \phi_{Si}^0 + \frac{2}{t_{Si}}\sum_{n=1}^{\infty}\frac{R_n f_{Si}^{(n)}(z)}{\alpha_n \Delta_n}\left[\phi_{SD}^{(n)}(U,V)\frac{\cosh(\alpha_n y)}{\cosh(\alpha_n L/2)}\right.$$

$$+\frac{1}{2}V_D\zeta_n\frac{\sinh(\alpha_n y)}{\sinh(\alpha_n L/2)}\left(1 - \frac{\cosh(\lambda_{1n}x)}{S_{1n}(t_s)\cosh(\lambda_{1n}W/2)}\right)$$

$$\left.+\frac{\dot{U}_n(V'_{Gf}, V'_{Gb})\cosh(\lambda_{1n}x)}{S_{1n}(t_s)\cosh(\lambda_{1n}W/2)}\right] \quad (6.33)$$

The threshold voltage result obtained from Eq. (6.26) and simplified Eq. (6.33) have been compared and found in a good agreement to each other. Now we will derive the threshold voltages at different conditions.

6.2.2 THRESHOLD VOLTAGES

To derive the formulae of threshold voltages V_T, under different conditions, we have followed the procedure given in reference [9]. So in order to include the coupling effects of front- and back-surface potentials, two virtual electrodes at minima positions of both the surface potentials are represented by Eqs. (6.9) and (6.10) from reference [9], respectively. The electrode positions y_m and y'_m can be found by using Eq. (6.11) by replacing ϕ with ϕ_{si} in Eqs. (9) and (11).

The electrode positions y_m and y'_m cannot be the same unless otherwise $\phi_s^f = \phi_s^b$ or $V_D = 0$. These cannot be formulated explicitly therefore we have calculated these values numerically by using Newton–Raphson method. Nearly, about three to four iterations in this method give fairly accurate results without consuming much time.

In SOI MOSFET, the silicon film is assumed to be very thin as the depletion reaches within the entire film. As a result, both front- and back-gates are coupled and condition of one gate depends on the condition of another. In order to analyse these dependences, we formulate front- and back-gate biases that incorporate the charge coupling effects in terms of surface potentials. To derive the expressions of threshold voltages for different cases, we can use the simplified relation (6.33). By using Eqs. (6.9) and (6.10) for the front-gate voltage and back-gate voltage, repectively [9], in Eq. (6.33) results in these two equations

$$\frac{2t_g}{t_{Si}} \sum_{n=1}^{\infty} \frac{R_n \chi_n^f}{\Delta_n} \Lambda_n \left[\phi_{SD}^{(n)}(V'_{Gf}, V'_{Gb}) \frac{\cosh(\alpha_n y_m)}{\cosh(\alpha_n L/2)} + \frac{1}{2} V_D \zeta_n \frac{\sinh(\alpha_n y_m)}{\sinh(\alpha_n L/2)} \right] = H_f \quad (6.34)$$

and

$$\frac{2t_b}{t_{Si}} \sum_{n=1}^{\infty} \frac{R_n \chi_n^b}{\Delta_n} \Lambda_n \left[\phi_{SD}^{(n)}(V'_{Gf}, V'_{Gb}) \frac{\cosh(\alpha_n y'_m)}{\cosh(\alpha_n L/2)} + \frac{1}{2} V_D \zeta_n \frac{\sinh(\alpha_n y'_m)}{\sinh(\alpha_n L/2)} \right] = H_b \quad (6.35)$$

respectively. Where

$$H_f = \phi_s^f + \left(\frac{1}{2} Kt_{Si}^2 + Kt_{Si}t_b \right) \frac{t_g}{t_{Si} + t_b + t_g}$$

$$- \frac{2t_g}{t_{Si}} \sum_{n=1}^{\infty} \frac{R_n \chi_n^f}{\Delta_n} \frac{\Omega_n(V'_{Gf}, V'_{Gb})}{S_{1,n}(t_s)\cosh(\lambda_{1,n}W/2)}$$

$$- \frac{t_g}{t_{Si} + t_b + t_g} V'_{Gb} - \frac{t_{Si} + t_b}{t_{Si} + t_b + t_g} V'_{Gf}, \quad (6.36)$$

$$H_b = \phi_s^b + \left(\frac{1}{2}Kt_{Si}^2 + Kt_{Si}t_g\right)\frac{t_b}{t_{Si}+t_b+t_g}$$
$$-\frac{2t_b}{t_{Si}}\sum_{n=1}^{\infty}\frac{R_n\chi_n^b}{\Delta_n}\frac{\Omega_n(V_{Gf}',V_{Gb}')}{S_{1,n}(t_s)\cosh(\lambda_{1,n}W/2)}$$
$$-\frac{t_g+t_{Si}}{t_{Si}+t_b+t_g}V_{Gb}' - \frac{t_b}{t_{Si}+t_b+t_g}V_{Gf}', \tag{6.37}$$

and

$$\Lambda_n = 1 - \frac{1}{S_{1,n}(t_s)\cosh(\lambda_{1,n}W/2)}.$$

Here we can easily observe the difference between the solutions obtained in [9] and in this chapter when the solutions are done within the front/back/side oxides also. By comparing equations obtained from earlier model [9] with Eqs. (6.34) and (6.35) of present model, we found that here the solution is a series summation over n where as in our earlier solution $n = 1$ gives fair results. Once Eqs. (6.34) and (6.35) are solved to get solution for front-threshold voltages which is given as

$$V_{Gf} = V_{Gf}^0 + \Delta V_{Gf}. \tag{6.38}$$

Here V_{Gf}^0 is the front-gate voltage, which is unaffected by short channel length expressed by

$$V_{Gf}^0 = V_{FB}^f + V_{Gf}^{0'},$$

having

$$V_{Gf}^{0'} = \left(1+\frac{t_g}{t_{si}}\right)\phi_s^f - \frac{t_g}{t_{si}}\phi_s^b + \frac{1}{2}Kt_{si}t_g. \tag{6.38a}$$

ΔV_{Gf} is the front-gate voltage shift which is because of short channel effect expressed as

$$\Delta V_{Gf} = \frac{\left(\frac{t_g}{t_{si}}\right)\Gamma_b(V_{Gf}^{0'},V_{Gb}^{0'}) - \left(1+\frac{t_g}{t_{si}}\right)\Gamma_f(V_{Gf}^{0'},V_{Gb}^{0'})}{1-\left[\Upsilon_f+\Upsilon_b\right]}, \tag{6.38b}$$

which includes

$$\Gamma_f(V_{Gf}^{0'},V_{Gb}^{0'}) = \frac{2t_g}{T_{sc}}\sum_{n=1}^{\infty}\left(\frac{\chi_n^f}{\Delta_n}\right)F_n(V_{Gf}^{0'},V_{Gb}^{0'};y_m), \tag{6.38c}$$

$$\Gamma_b\left(V_{Gf}^{0'}, V_{Gb}^{0'}\right) = \frac{2t_b}{T_{sc}} \sum_{n=1}^{\infty} \left(\frac{\chi_n^b}{\Delta_n}\right) F_n\left(V_{Gf}^{0'}, V_{Gb}^{0'}; y_m'\right), \qquad (6.38d)$$

$$\Upsilon_f = \frac{2t_g}{T_{sc}} \sum_{n=1}^{\infty} \frac{\chi_n^f}{\Delta_n} \left[\Lambda_n \left\{\left(1 + \frac{t_g}{t_{si}}\right)\chi_n^f - \frac{t_b}{t_{si}}\chi_n^b\right\} \frac{\cosh(\alpha_n y_m)}{\cosh(\alpha_n L/2)} \right.$$
$$\left. -\frac{T_{sc}}{t_{si}} \frac{\chi_n^b}{S_{1n}(t_s)\cosh(\lambda_{1n} W/2)} \right] \qquad (6.38e)$$

$$\Upsilon_b = \frac{2t_b}{T_{sc}} \sum_{n=1}^{\infty} \frac{\chi_n^b}{\Delta_n} \left[\Lambda_n \left\{\left(1 + \frac{t_b}{t_{Si}}\right)\chi_n^b - \frac{t_g}{t_{Si}}\chi_n^f a\right\} \frac{\cosh(\alpha_n y_m')}{\cosh(\alpha_n L/2)} \right.$$
$$\left. +\frac{T_{sc}}{t_{Si}} \frac{\chi_n^b}{S_{1n}(t_s)\cosh(\lambda_{1n} W/2)} \right] \qquad (6.38f)$$

$$F_n(U,V;y) = \left(\phi_{SD}^{(n)}(U,V) \frac{\cosh(\alpha_n y)}{\cosh(\alpha_n L/2)} + \frac{1}{2} V_D \zeta_n \frac{\sinh(\alpha_n y)}{\sinh(\alpha_n L/2)}\right) \Lambda_n$$
$$+ \frac{\Omega_n(U,V)}{S_{1n}(t_s)\cosh(\lambda_{1n} W/2)} \qquad (6.38g)$$

As we can observe in Eq. (6.38b), the front-gate bias shift ΔV_{Gf} comprises the short-channel effect. The scaling down of channel length induces ΔV_{Gf} to increase in negative direction, whereby the front-gate bias V_{Gf} degrades. This can be understood by analyzing the numerator and denominator of Eq. (6.38b). Besides, ΔV_{Gf} also depends on drain voltage V_D which introduces drain-induced barrier lowering (DIBL) effects that degrades V_{Gf}. Now it is evident that the front interface of short channel device can be switched on by lower value of V_{Gf} as compared with long channel device.

Likewise, the back-gate bias can be derived as

$$V_{Gb} = V_{Gb}^o + \Delta V_{Gb} \qquad (6.39)$$

where

$$V_{Gb}^o = V_{FB}^b + V_{Gb}^{0'},$$

with

$$V_{Gb}^{0'} = \left(1 + \frac{t_b}{t_{Si}}\right)\phi_s^b - \frac{t_b}{t_{Si}}\phi_s^f + \frac{1}{2}Kt_{Si}t_b. \qquad (6.39a)$$

Expressions (6.38a) and (6.39a) are the same as obtained in reference [12] for large active area devices. The expression for change in back-gate bias is

$$\Delta V_{Gb} = \frac{\left(\frac{t_b}{t_{Si}}\right)\Gamma_f\left(V_{Gf}^{0'}, V_{Gb}^{0'}\right) - \left(1+\frac{t_b}{t_{Si}}\right)\Gamma_b\left(V_{Gf}^{0'}, V_{Gb}^{0'}\right)}{1-\left[\Upsilon_f + \Upsilon_b\right]}. \tag{6.39b}$$

From Eqs. (6.39b) and (6.38b), it is observed that back-gate bias shift ΔV_{Gb} is apparently different from ΔV_{Gf}. By using Eq. (6.39) along with Eqs. (6.39a) and (6.39b), one can decide back-gate bias for accumulation or inversion mode of back-gate interface for analyzing front-gate threshold voltage. Also in a similar way Eq. (6.38) along with Eqs. (6.38a) and (6.38b) are useful to decide operation mode of front-gate interface while analyzing back-gate threshold voltage. Therefore, Eqs. (6.38) and (6.39) describe the front- and back-interface coupling of SOI MOSFET in terms of their respective surface potential at the virtual electrodes. By combining these relations, we can describe both front-gate and back-gate threshold voltages.

6.2.2.1 FRONT THRESHOLD VOLTAGE

Here the threshold condition of front interface, that is, $\phi_s^f = 2\psi_B^f$, if back interface of SOI MOSFET is at accumulation ϕ_s^b is reduced to zero for fully depleted transistor or substrate bias V_B for partially depleted one [9]. Equations (6.38), (6.38a), and (6.38b) the front-gate biasing parameters are assumed to $V_{Gf} \equiv V_{Tf}^A$, $V_{Gf}^{0'} \equiv V_{Tf}^{A0'}$ and $\Delta V_{Gf} \equiv \Delta V_{Tf}^A$, that is, the front-threshold voltages at back-interface accumulation. In the same way, the corresponding back-gate biases under the similar condition can be found out with the help of Eqs. (6.39), (6.39a), and (6.39b), which are $V_{Gb} \equiv V_{Gb}^A$, $V_{Gb}^{0'} \equiv V_{Gb}^{A0'}$ and $\Delta V_{Gb} \equiv \Delta V_{Gb}^A$. In this situation, the threshold voltage V_{Tf}^A becomes independent of back-gate bias V_{Gb}.

Now if the back interface is at inversion, that is, $\phi_s^b = 2\psi_B^b$, ψ_B^b is the Fermi potential at back interface, then Eqs. (6.38), (6.38a), and (6.38b) become $V_{Gf} \equiv V_{Tf}^I$, $V_{Gf}^{0'} \equiv V_{Tf}^{I0'}$ and $\Delta V_{Gf} \equiv \Delta V_{Tf}^I$, respectively, that is, threshold voltages at back-interface inversion. Also the back-gate biasing parameters gets modified versions of Eqs. (6.39), (6.39a), and (6.39b) as $V_{Gb} \equiv V_{Gb}^I$, $V_{Gb}^{0'} \equiv V_{Gb}^{I0'}$ and $\Delta V_{Gb} \equiv \Delta V_{Gb}^I$, respectively, if we put $\phi_s^f = 2\psi_B^f$ and $\phi_s^b = 2\psi_B^b$. For this case, V_{Tf}^I reaches a considerably low value and that is independent of back-gate bias. Thus, one can decide the back-gate bias V_{Gb} range by knowing the onsets of back-interface accumulation ($\phi_s^b = 0$) and inversion ($\phi_s^b = 2\psi_B^b$).

If back interface is in the depletion mode, depletion threshold voltage V_{Tf}^D varies with V_{Gb} as ϕ_s^b strongly depends on back-gate bias; its value ranges about zero to $2\psi_B^b$. Accordingly, the back-gate bias lies within the range between V_{Gb}^A and V_{Gb}^I. Beyond this, ϕ_s^b is invariant and shield the effect of back-gate voltage in the real devices. Therefore to derive the formula for depletion threshold voltage, we consider Eq. (6.34) and apply the strong inversion criterion ($\phi_s^f = 2\psi_B^f$) at the front interface. After arranging it gives the expression of front-gate voltage V_{Gf} and then we replace V_{Gf} by V_{Tf}^D to yield

$$V_{Tf}^D = V_{Tf}^{D0} + \Delta V_{Tf}^D, \qquad (6.40)$$

$$V_{Tf}^{D0} = V_{Tf}^{D0'} + V_{FB}^f,$$

$$V_{Tf}^{D0'} = 2\psi_B + \left\{ 2\psi_B - V_{Gb}' + \frac{1}{2}Kt_{Si}^2 + Kt_{Si}t_b \right\} \left(\frac{t_g}{t_{Si} + t_b} \right). \qquad (6.40a)$$

The threshold voltage shift for front gate due to short channel effects is

$$\Delta V_{Tf}^D = -\frac{\Gamma_f\left(V_{Tf}^{D0'}, V_{Gb}'\right)}{\varrho_f - \xi_f}, \qquad (6.40b)$$

where

$$\varrho_f = \frac{t_{Si} + t_b}{T_{sc}},$$

$$\xi_f = \frac{2t_g}{T_{sc}} \sum_{n=1}^{\infty} \frac{\chi_n^f}{\Lambda_n} \left[\frac{\cosh(\alpha_n y_m)}{\cosh(\alpha_n L/2)} \chi_n^f \Lambda_n - \frac{\chi_n^b}{S_{1n}(t_s)\cosh(\lambda_{1n} W/2)} \right].$$

The depletion threshold voltage represented by Eq. (6.40) along with Eqs. (6.40a) and (6.40b) pertains the combined effects of V_{Gb}, V_D and short channel length.

6.2.2.2 BACK THRESHOLD VOLTAGE

If the back-interface switch on first as compared to front interface, then strong inversion criterion ($\phi_s^b = 2\psi_B^b$) is applicable at the back interface.

For this case, V_{Gf} is a controller for back depletion threshold voltage V_{Tb}^D. The threshold voltages V_{Tb}^A and V_{Tb}^I corresponding to their onsets of front-interface accumulation ($\phi_s^f = 0$) and inversion ($\phi_s^f = 2\psi_B^f$) can be obtained from Eq. (6.39). Similarly, the respective front-gate voltages for accumulation and inversion cases, that is, V_{Gf}^A and V_{Gf}^I pertaining to their onsets can be obtained by using Eq. (6.38). Accordingly, the range $V_{Gf}^A < V_{Gf} < V_{Gf}^I$ of V_{Gf} about these onsets can be decided. Now, if the strong inversion criterion is applied at back interface and by solving Eq. (6.35) for back-gate voltage and then by replacing it by V_{Tb}^D results

$$V_{Tb}^D = V_{Tb}^{D0} + \Delta V_{Tb}^D, \tag{6.41}$$

where V_{Tb}^{D0} is the long channel threshold voltage which can be given as

$$V_{Tb}^{D0} = V_{Tb}^{D0'} + V_{FB}^b,$$

$$V_{Tb}^{D0'} = 2\psi_B + \left\{ 2\psi_B - V_{Gf}' + \frac{1}{2} K t_{Si}^2 + K t_{Si} t_g \right\} \left(\frac{t_b}{t_{Si} + t_g} \right), \tag{6.41a}$$

and the short channel threshold voltage shift, ΔV_{Tb}^D, is expressed as

$$\Delta V_{Tb}^D = -\frac{\Gamma_b \left(V_{Gf}', V_{Tb}^{D0'} \right)}{\varrho_b - \xi_b}, \tag{6.41b}$$

$$\varrho_b = \frac{t_{Si} + t_g}{T_{sc}},$$

$$\xi_b = \frac{2t_b}{T_{sc}} \sum_{n=1}^{\infty} \left(\frac{\chi_n^b}{\Delta_n} \right) \chi_n^b \left[\frac{\cosh(\alpha_n y_m)}{\cosh(\alpha_n L/2)} \Lambda_n - \frac{1}{S_{1n}(t_s) \cosh(\lambda_{1n} W/2)} \right].$$

The back-gate threshold voltage expression (6.41) along with Eqs. (6.41a) and (6.41b) comprises the effects of V_{Gf}, V_D and channel length. The formalism is based on the assumption of no mobile charges in depleted SOI film of the transistor.

6.3 RESULTS AND DISCUSSION

The surface potential distribution versus channel length ($x = 0$) using simplified expression (6.33) and general equation (6.26) to validate the simplification imposed on Eq. (6.26) is presented in Figure 6.2(a) and (b). The upper and the lower curves represent the potential distribution at front interface ($z = 0$) and back interface ($z = t_{si}$), repectively, for different values of channel lengths. Results obtained from Eq. (6.33) matche with Eq. (6.26) at both the interfaces for all the values of L for the entire range of y values. Since we have calculated the threshold voltages at minima position, a little deviation at the source and drain end of front-surface potential ($z = 0$) does not affect the threshold voltage much. On the other hand, potential distributions along the width at $y = 0$ are plotted in Figure 6.2(b). The results of Eq. (6.33) also matches very well with those of Eq. (6.26) for different values of W. An insignificant deviation has been calculated at the side interfaces ($x = \pm W/2$) even for the width up to $W = 0.3$ μm. As all the calculations for threshold voltages are done at the minima positions, the results are not affected due to little deviation at side interface. From these results, the simplifying assumptions on Eq. (6.33) are justified. The summation of series over α_n in Eq. (6.26) up to first three to four terms and summation of series over m is sufficient for the calculations.

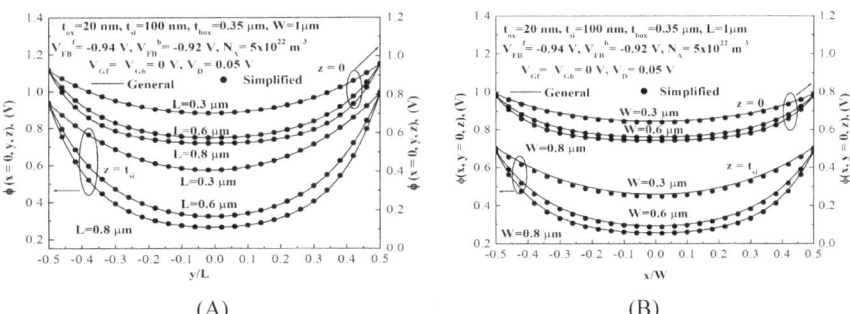

FIGURE 6.2 (A) Surface potential distribution considering expressions (6.26) and (6.33). Potential distribution along the channel length of the device for different values of L. (B) Surface potential distribution considering expressions (6.26) and (6.33). Potential distribution along the channel width at different values of W.

The result of front-threshold voltage calculated from the expressions (6.40) and (6.40b) is shown in Figure 6.3. Narrow width effects can be easily observed here as the channel length is sufficiently high and the results are associated if the device is operated when the back interface is in depletion mode. The results are in a good matching with that of model with PISCES [13]. Figure 6.4 has been plotted by utilizing Eq. (6.39) and Eq. (6.39b) for V_{Gb}, considering the threshold condition of front interface at onsets of back gate interface in inversion ($\phi_s^b = 2\psi_B$) and accumulation

($\phi_s^b = 0$). This shows that negative values of V_{Gb} can change the operational modes of the device from depletion-to-accumulation.

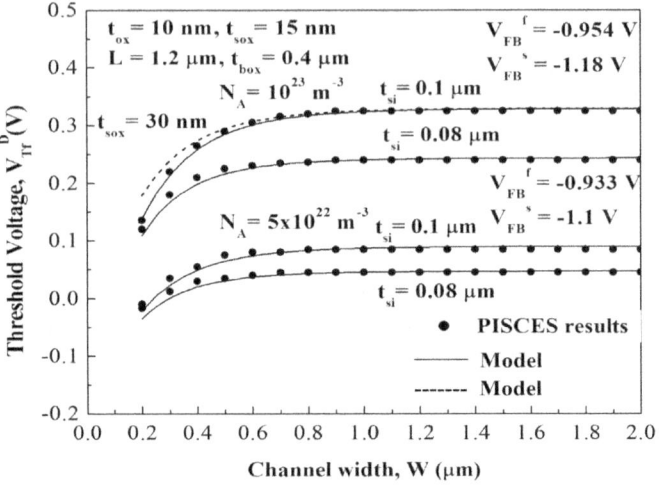

FIGURE 6.3 Comparison of analytical model of front-threshold voltage with PISCES [112] data for narrow width effect by varying silicon film doping and thicknesses.

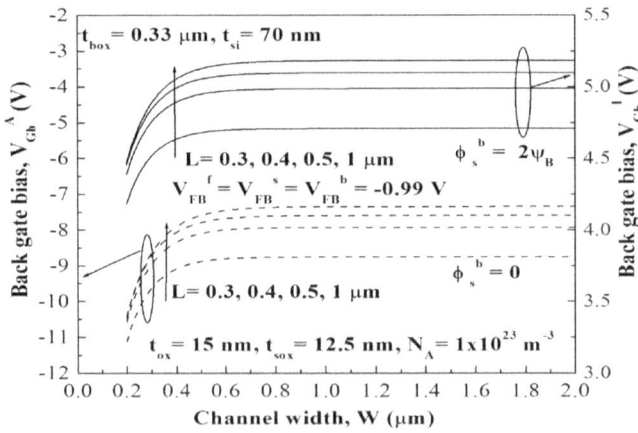

FIGURE 6.4 Back-gate bias variation at the onsets of back-interface accumulation ($\phi_s^b = 0$)V_{Gb}^A and inversion ($\phi_s^b = 2\psi_B$)V_{Gb}^I by applying inversion criteria ($\phi_s^f = 2\psi_B$) at front interface.

The DIBL effects on both the threshold voltages are calculated with the help of Eqs. (6.40) and (6.41) as depicted in Figure 6.5. Results of threshold voltages are matching well with the available simulation data [14]. As we

A 3D Analytic Modeling of Threshold Voltages

increase the drain voltage V_D, threshold voltage roll off increases. The charge sharing phenomena at drain end effectively reduces the doping concentration of the film, thereby increasing threshold roll off with increase of V_D.

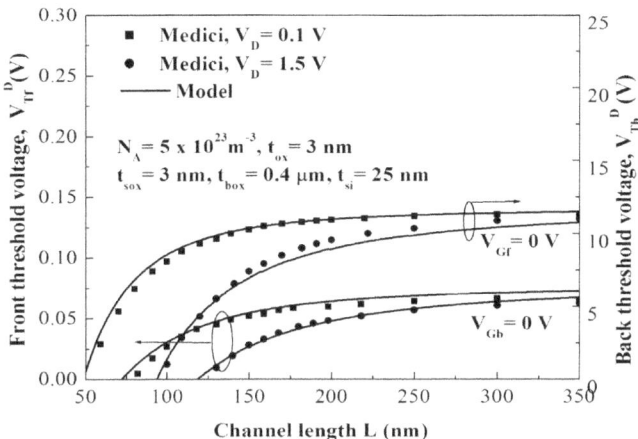

FIGURE 6.5 Effects of drain bias on threshold voltages with channel length and comparison with Medici [14] data $W = 1.2$ μm.

The small geometry effects on front-threshold voltage shift can be seen very clearly in Figure 6.6 when the device is operating at back interface in accumulation mode. The calculations are done by considering Eq. (6.38b), which has been derived from the simplified expression (6.33) (solid circles) by substituting $\phi_s^f = 2\psi_B$ and $\phi_s^b = 0$, whereas, solid line represents the threshold voltage shift, plotted by using generalized expression (6.26) under similar condition. As the device size shrinks laterally, the threshold voltage shift increases in the negative direction due to the significant enhancement of heavily inverted volume of SOI film which reduces the doping concentration which degrades the threshold voltage; resulting an increase in shift in negative side. At the source and drain ends the inversion is relatively high that results more pronounced short channel effect than narrow width effects (Figure 6.6).

The front-threshold voltage roll off when the device is operated in back interface depletion mode is shown in Figure 6.7. The results have been calculated using Eq. (6.41b) derived from Eq. (6.26) (solid line) and also evaluated from Eq. (6.33) (solid circle) for validating the simplification imposed. From this figure also, it is very clear that short channel effects are more pronounced than narrow width effects.

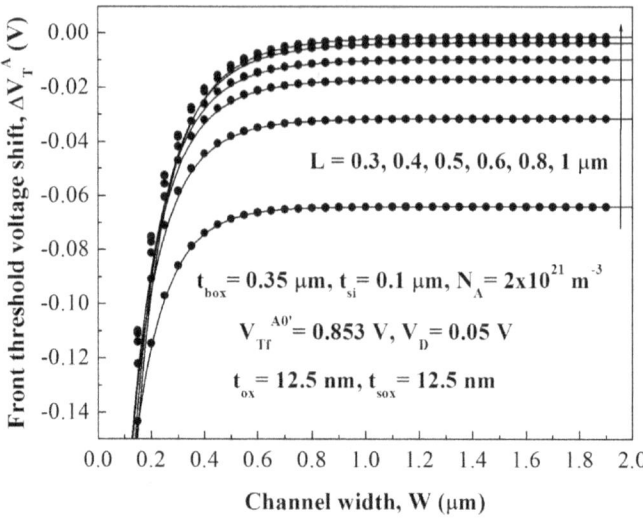

FIGURE 6.6 Narrow-width effects on front-threshold voltage shift at back-interface accumulation.

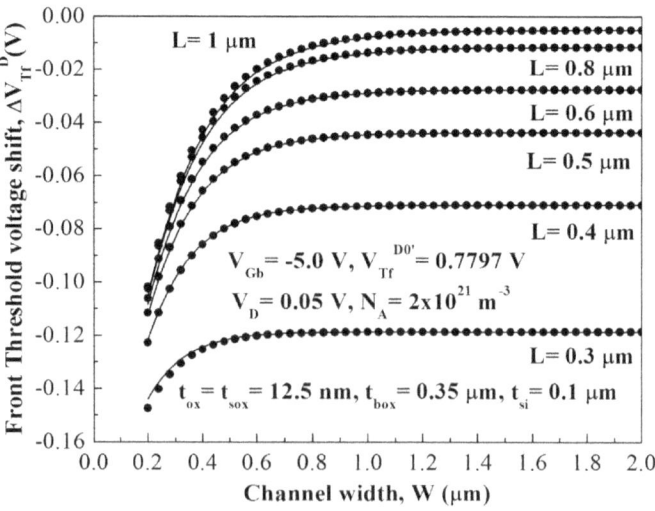

FIGURE 6.7 Narrow-width effects on front-threshold voltage shift at back-interface depletion.

By comparing Figures 6.6 and 6.7, it has been proved that the device operating under back-interface-accumulation mode is not so affected by small geometry as compared to back-interface-depletion mode. The lateral dimension scaling effects on back-gate threshold voltage shift is depicted in

Figure 6.8. The results have been calculated using Eq. (6.41b), (solid circle) and also compared with general expression (6.26) (solid line). Both the results are in good matching which again justifying our assumption.

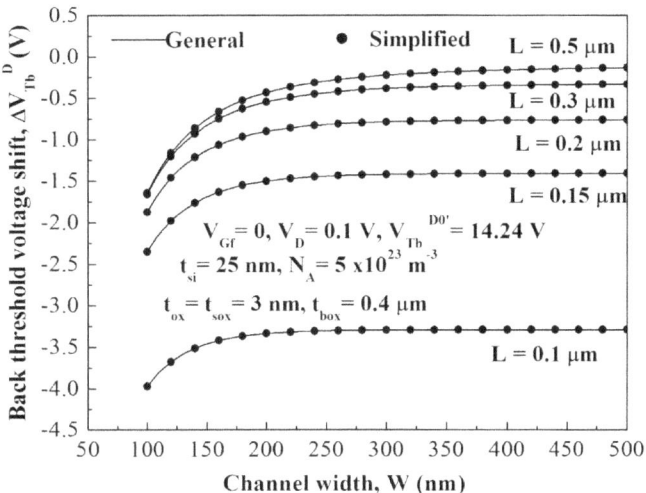

FIGURE 6.8 Narrow-width effects on back-threshold voltage shift at front-interface depletion.

6.4 CONCLUSION

A new approach for analytic modeling of threshold voltages for small geometry and fully depleted SOI MOSFETs has been presented in a simplified way. The new Green's functions have been derived for all the three zones by applying the real boundary conditions at the interfaces. By imposing some simplifications, the compact and closed form formulae of front- and back-gate threshold voltages along with their counterparts (back- and front-gate biases) for conditions have been derived in this chapter. The charge sharing phenomena within SOI as well as within front- and back-oxide regions under different gate and drain voltages coupled with device dimensions causes the degradation of threshold voltage. From the results of threshold voltages, it becomes evident that the lateral dimension of SOI MOSFETs can be scaled down up to submicron levels without exhibiting small geometry effects. Further, the immunity of device toward narrow width effect is more pronounced than short channel effect which can be reduced by increasing the thickness of the side oxide wall. Also a fact comes out that if the device is operated under the back interface at accumulation, its size can be further reducedup to deep submicrons without degrading the threshold voltage much. Now the subthreshold characteristics [15] can be studied by making use of surface potential expression obtained in this model.

KEYWORDS

- **FD**
- **SOI**
- **SOI MOSFET**
- **analytical model**
- **front-threshold voltage**
- **back-threshold voltage**
- **small geometry effect**

REFERENCES

1. Kamgar, A., Hillenius, S. J., Cong, H. I. L., Field, R. L., Lindenberger, W. S., Celler, G. K., Trimble, L. E., & Sheng, T. T.; Ultra-fast (0.5-µm) CMOS circuits in fully depleted SOI films. *IEEE Trans Electron Dev* **1992**; Vol. ED-39: 640–647.
2. Yan, R. H., Ourmazd, A., & Lee, K. F.; Scaling the Si MOSFET: from bulk to SOI to Bulk. *IEEE Trans Electron Dev* **1992**; Vol. 39, pp. 1704–1710.
3. Chai, K. T., Asada, K., & Sugano, T.; Modelling of 0.1µm MOSFET on SOI structure using Monte Carlo simulation technique. *IEEE Trans. Electron Dev* **1986**; Vol. ED-33, pp. 1005–1011.
4. Davis, J. R., Armstrong, G. A., Thomas, N. J., & Doyle, A.; Thin film SOI CMOS transistors with p+-polysilicon gates. *IEEE Trans Electron Dev* **1991**; Vol. ED-38, pp. 32–38.
5. Yoshimi, M., Hazama, H., Takahashi, M., Kambayashi, S., & Tango, H.; Observation of mobility enhancement in ultra-thin SOI MOSFETs. *Electron Lett,* **1988**; Vol. 24(17), pp. 1078–1079.
6. Tsao, S. S., Fleetwood, D. M., Weaver, H. T., Pfeiffer, L., & Celler, C. K.; Radiation tolerant sidewall-hardened SOI/MOS transistors. *IEEE Trans Nucl Sci,* **1987**; Vol. NS-34, pp. 1686–1691.
7. Sturm, J. C., Takunago, K., & Collinge, J. P.; Increased drain saturation current in the ultra-thin silicon-on-insulator (SOI) MOS transistors. *IEEE Electron Dev Lett* **1988**; Vol. EDl-9, pp. 460–463.
8. Matloubin, M., Sundaresan, R., & Lu, H.; Measurement and modeling of side wall threshold voltage of mesa isolated SOI MOSFETs. *IEEE Trans Electron Dev* **1989**; Vol. ED-36, pp. 938–942.

9. Meel, K., Gopal, R., & Bhatnagar, D.; Three-dimensional analytic modeling of front and back gate threshold voltages for small geometry fully depleted SOI MOSFET'. *Solid-State Electron* **2011**; Vol. 62, pp. 174–184.
10. Meel, K., Gopal, R., & Bhatnagar, D.; Three-dimensional analytical subthreshold current model of fully depleted SOI MOSFETs. *Int J Electron Commun Eng Technol (IJECET)* **2013**; Vol. 4, No. 7, pp. 74–79.
11. Sze, S. M.; Physics of semiconductor devices: 2nd ed. New Delhi: Wiley Eastern Limited. **1983**, p. 71.
12. Lim, H. K., & Fossum, J. G.; Threshold voltage of thin-film silicon-on-insulator (SOI) MOSFETs. *IEEE Trans. Electron Dev* **1983**; Vol. ED-30, pp. 1244–1251.
13. Su, K. W., & Kuo, J. B.; Analytical threshold voltage formula including narrow-channel effects for VLSI mesa-isolated fully depleted ultrathin silicon-on-insulator n-channel metal-oxide-silicon devices. *Jpn J Appl Phys* **1995**; Vol. 34 part1 (8A), pp. 4010–4019.
14. Meer, H. V., & Meyer, K. D.; A 2-D analytical threshold voltage model for fully-depleted SOI MOSFETs with halos or pockets. *IEEE Trans Electron Dev* **2001**; Vol. ED-48, pp. 2292–2302.
15. Saramekala, G. K., Santra, A., Kumar, M., Dubey, S., Jit, S., & Tiwari, P. K.; Analytical subthreshold current and subthreshold swing models of short-channel dual-metal-gate (DMG) fully-depleted recessed-source/drain (Re-S/D) SOI MOSFETs. *J Comput Electron.* **2014**; 13:467–476.

APPENDIX 6A

Here we describe the procedure to derive Green's functions, which have the combined effect of all the three zones (front oxide, SOI film, and back oxide). In this approach, we first deal with the set of differential equations (6.17) to arrive at the explicit expressions of Greens functions pertaining to silicon layer, other sets, (6.18) and (6.19), of differential equations can be tackled accordingly to achieve the solutions of Green's functions related to respective front and back oxide layers. Let us assume that the solutions of (6.17) are

$$G_{ox} = A_{ox}(x,y)\sin(\alpha z) + B_{ox}(x,y)\cos(\alpha z), \qquad (6A.1)$$

$$G_{si} = A_{si}(x,y)\sin(\alpha z) + B_{si}(x,y)\cos(\alpha z), \qquad (6A.2)$$

$$G_{bo} = A_{bo}(x,y)\sin(\alpha z) + B_{bo}(x,y)\cos(\alpha z), \qquad (6A.3)$$

For brevity, we have dropped the arguments of Green's functions. The application of homogeneous conditions of boundary values (6.7), (6.11) and interface boundary conditions (6.12)–(6.16) in (6A.1)–(6A.3), yields

$$G_{ox} = \eta \sum_{n=1}^{\infty} A_{si}^{(n)}(x,y) f_{ox}^{(n)}(z), \qquad (6A.4)$$

$$G_{si} = \sum_{n=1}^{\infty} A_{si}^{(n)}(x,y) f_{si}^{(n)}(z), \qquad (6A.5)$$

$$G_{bo} = \eta \sum_{n=1}^{\infty} A_{si}^{(n)}(x,y) f_{bo}^{(n)}(z), \qquad (6A.6)$$

The eigenfunctions representing respective layers are written as

$$f_{si}^{(n)}(z) = \sin(\alpha_n z) + \eta \tan(\alpha_n t_{ox}) \cos(\alpha_n z), \qquad (6A.7)$$

$$f_{ox}^{(n)}(z) = \frac{\sin \alpha_n (z + t_{ox})}{\cos(\alpha_n t_{ox})}, \qquad (6A.8)$$

$$f_{bo}^{(n)}(z) = Q_n \frac{\sin \alpha_n (t_{si} + t_{box} - z)}{\cos(\alpha_n t_{box})}, \qquad (6A.9)$$

where

$$Q_n = \eta \tan(\alpha_n t_{ox}) \sin(\alpha_n t_{si}) - \cos(\alpha_n t_{si}), \qquad (6A.10)$$

and eigen values α_n are the nonzero roots of the equation

$$\tan(\alpha_n t_{si}) = \frac{\eta \{\tan(\alpha_n t_{box}) + \tan(\alpha_n t_{ox})\}}{\eta^2 \tan(\alpha_n t_{box}) \tan(\alpha_n t_{ox}) - 1}. \qquad (6A.11)$$

Here n is the integer varying as, 1, 2, 3, ...,∞.
It may be noted that the series coefficients, $A_{si}^{(n)}(x,y)$, are common in all the series (6A.4)–(6A.6). Through this coefficient, Green's function includes the combined effect of all the regions. Besides, the series (6A.4)–(6A.6) are orthogonal in nature in the range, $-t_{ox} \leq z \leq t_{si} + t_{box}$. Now, we substitute (6A.4)–(6A.6) in respective differential equations of (6.17) and then take their Fourier series transform, which results in the single differential equation in 2D form as

$$\frac{\partial^2 A_{si}^{(n)}(x,y)}{\partial x^2} + \frac{\partial^2 A_{si}^{(n)}(x,y)}{\partial y^2} - \alpha_n^2 A_{si}^{(n)}(x,y)$$

$$= \frac{2 f_{si}^{(n)}(z')}{T_{sc} \Delta_n} \delta(x-x') \delta(y-y'). \qquad (6A.12)$$

The eigenfunction appeared in (6A.12) corresponds to silicon layer because the source point of Green's function is located in that layer. It is worth mentioning here that the series, (6A.4)–(6A.6), can also be used for

A 3D Analytic Modeling of Threshold Voltages

transformation purpose of sets (6.18) and (6.19). The series parameter Δ_n is defined as

$$\Delta_n = \frac{t_b}{T_{sc}} Q_n^2 \sec^2(\alpha_n t_{box}) + \frac{t_g}{T_{sc}} \sec^2(\alpha_n t_{ox})$$
$$+ \frac{t_{si}}{T_{sc}}\{1 + \eta^2 \tan^2(\alpha_n t_{ox})\},$$

where

$$t_g = \eta t_{ox}; \; t_b = \eta t_{box},$$

and the total scaled thickness of three-layer structure is

$$T_{sc} = t_g + t_{si} + t_b$$

Now (6A.12) can be further reduced to 1D form by assuming

$$A_{si}^{(n)}(x,y) = \sum_{n=1}^{\infty} A_{mn}^{(n)}(x) \sin \beta_m (y + L/2) \tag{6A.13}$$

By substituting (6A.13 in 6A.12) equation becomes

$$\frac{\partial^2 A_{mn}^{(n)}(x)}{\partial x^2} - \lambda_{mn}^2 A_{mn}^{(n)}(x) = \frac{4 f_{si}^{(n)}(z')}{LT_{sc}\Delta_n} \delta(x-x') \sin\left(\frac{n\pi}{L}\left(y' + \frac{L}{2}\right)\right) \tag{6A.14}$$

where

$$\lambda_{mn}^2 = \beta_m^2 + \alpha_n^2; \; \beta_m = \frac{m\pi}{L}$$

Here we will also apply the discontinuity of Green's function by integrating (6A.14) once about the source point ($x = x', y = y'$) along with their equality at the source point for obtaining the boundary conditions which are given as

$$\left.\frac{\partial^2 A_{mn}^+(x)}{\partial x^2}\right|_{x'^+} - \left.\frac{\partial^2 A_{mn}^-(x)}{\partial x^2}\right|_{x'^-} = \frac{4 f_{si}^{(n)}(z')}{LT_{sc}\Delta_n} \sin\left(\frac{n\pi}{L}\left(y' + \frac{L}{2}\right)\right) \tag{6A.15}$$

$$A_{mn}^{(-)}(x=x') = A_{mn}^{(+)}(x=x') \tag{6A.16}$$

$$A_{mn}^{(n)}(x) = A_{mn}^{(-)}(x) :(x<x'); \qquad A_{mn}^{(n)}(x) = A_{mn}^{(+)}(x) :(x>x').$$

The constants are evaluated by using above-mentioned boundary conditions along with boundary conditions at the side-wall interface (6.16)

$$A_{mn}^{(-)}(x) = -\frac{2f_{si}^{(n)}(z')}{\lambda_{mn}L\Delta_n T_{sc}}\sin\beta_m\left(y'+\frac{L}{2}\right)g_{mn}^{-}(x,x') \quad (x<x') \qquad (6A.17)$$

$$A_{mn}^{(+)}(x) = -\frac{2f_{si}^{(n)}(z')}{\lambda_{mn}L\Delta_n T_{sc}}\sin\beta_m\left(y'+\frac{L}{2}\right)g_{mn}^{+}(x,x') \quad x>x' \qquad (6A.18)$$

Thus the complete solution of Green's function can be expressed by (6.23).

CHAPTER 7

Fuzzy-Based Stratagem for Teleoperation of Robots in Incoherent Environments

SRIPARNA SAHA[1*], RIMITA LAHIRI[2], and AMIT KONAR[2]

[1]*Department of Computer Science and Engineering, Maulana Abul Kalam Azad University of Technology, West Bengal, India,*

[2]*Department of Electronics and Telecommunication Engineering, Jadavpur University, India*

Corresponding author. E-mail: sahasriparna@gmail.com

ABSTRACT

This chapter provides an interesting system for robot controlling in incoherent environments (like, a battlefield, space, or underwater) using human gestures. In this type of places where safety is a major concern, it is not feasible for any person to present there and perform some specified tasks. So to accomplish the given duties, robots can be employed as an alternative. But if the robots are asked to carry out the works by their own, then there is a high chance that the precise goals can be missed owing to the ever changing nature of the incoherent environments. As a solution to this problem, human intelligence can be imparted into the robots by sending gestural commands. Gestures depicting same command may differ not only from subjects to subjects, but also same command while displaying by the same person on different days can vary among them. So, gesture recognition technique employing Interval Type-2 fuzzy system is used. This chapter deals with a novel purpose of robot navigation in incoherent environments which are inaccessible to the human beings. The proposed system has propitious potentials for upcoming applications of robot maneuver based on well-accepted performance metrics when comparing with other existing literatures.

7.1 INTRODUCTION

In the late 1970s, after the concept of personal computing became popularized, every individual turned into a potential computer user with personal software (text editors, spreadsheets, etc.) and personal platforms (like operating system, programming language etc.). Day-by-day importance of computers on a daily basis felt badly. Human society becomes slave of computers [1]. Artificial intelligent agents are imparted with human intelligence more and more. Then comes a day [2] when the makers of robotic agents (i.e., the humans themselves) felt that whatever rigorous efforts may be put forward, but then also the agents lack in intelligence as compared to humans while pursuing jobs in dynamic and stochastic environments [3]. The nature of the environments is such that previous trainings cannot be supplied to the robots for accomplishing of tasks. As the shortcomings of computer as a sole sufficient tool became more prominent, the demand for an effective interactive system between a human and a robotic agent became more necessary.

Many robots are instructed for execution of crucial tasks based on some control commands from a computer. Conceptually, the instructions by a computer should have similar precision as compared to human instructions in order to complete that task efficiently. But computers lack in human intelligence [4], so to solve this problem, human commands are communicated to the computer through different modalities (e.g. voice, gesture, etc.) [5] and finally the computer instructs a robot after decoding the commands.

The work in this chapter deals with remote robot navigation in an incoherent environment, such as space [6], underwater [7], battle field [8], etc., for carrying out tasks where it is not feasible for humans to reach there either for safety issue or for inaccessible nature of the environments. Hence, the choice of communication modality for sending human instructions to the robot is of major concern [8]. Gestural commands outperform all the other modalities in terms of achieving better accuracy while transferring human intelligence to robotic agents [9], as compared to speech or emotions. "Gesture" is the different bodily movements of a human being while expressing a message [10, 11]. Du and Zhang develop a method to instruct a double-arm robot by double-hand movements from a distance and also without taking help from any marker-based approach [12]. Here the controlled robot is stationary, so how the robot will follow the controlling human being while moving from one place to another is unknown. But the proposed work described in this chapter is well acquaintance with dealing with robot maneuver. In a similar type of work, Makris et al. suggest an approach to manage dual-arm robot movement based on gestural commands using depth sensors [13]. Gestural command can also be mapped with robotic movements when the robot is static by Tsarouchi et al. [14]. Not only mapping with gestures, but also people following robots using depth images for real-time applications are also possible [15]. In all of the above cases, one major drawback is that none of the papers consider the robot maneuver in incoherent environment. As due to the unstructured nature of the environments, it is not possible that the robots could reach those places, so people following architectures do not hold ground there also.

As some from the works are there regarding robot movement using gestures, still detailed analysis and satisfactory reasoning are yet to be obtained. For example, gestural features corresponding to a specific movement of a specific subject at different time instances exhibit wide variety. Further, the gestural features of different subjects enacting the same pose also differ a lot. To deal with these uncertainties, in this article the proposed system uses Interval Type-2 fuzzy set (IT2FS) [16, 17] containing upper and lower membership functions corresponding to the different features, and after obtaining the directions from the membership values, the robot movement is controlled accordingly.

For this chapter, we have developed a novel technique of gestural-command-based robot maneuver procedure. For recognition of human gestures, Kinect sensor developed by Microsoft [18, 19] is used. It basically registers three-dimensional images of different users moving in front of it. Using software development kit (SDK) associated with the Kinect sensor, the images are analyzed and skeletons consisting of 20 different human body joints are generated. Further, it has included fuzzy membership functions to enhance the accuracy and also to keep all the available information intact. Suitable IT2FS membership curves are created from the gestural features. Since the robot is supposed to work in incoherent environment, the constrained framework for the robot movement is taken into account for enhanced performance.

In this chapter, without defuzzing the membership curves, empirical ways are used for better accuracy. For example, the experiment performed, does not allow the robot to turn more than 180° in either direction. So we did not derive an equation based on the feature set values which may generate angular values beyond the above mentioned range, instead a curve is generated depending on a range of membership values corresponding to different distance features. Another important improvement with respect to existing works is that in our proposed system, there are provisions for application of acceleration and brake. The acceleration and brakes are applied based on the movement of the user's right and left foot beyond a certain threshold value, which is calculated during the training session considering the information and readings generated by all the subjects and without loss of generality. After building a concrete theory, the experiment has been carried out on Khepera II [20] and it provided a convincing performance level, which justifies its usage in real-time applications.

The subsequent parts of the chapter are described as follows. Section 7.2 gives focus on preliminary technical background. In Section 7.3, the approach of the proposed work is outlined, while Section 7.4 highlights the findings of the experimental work. Finally, Section 7.5 concludes the chapter.

7.2 TECHNICAL BACKGROUND

7.2.1 MICROSOFT'S KINECT SENSOR

The Xbox 360 somatosensory peripheral developed by Microsoft in June, 2010 had been officially named as "Kinect." As shown in Figure 7.1, the Kinect sensor [18, 19] is a long bar like device to sense human body. The device has a unique set of IR and RGB cameras fixed within it. These cameras let the Kinect sensor to sense and track any subject present within a finite distance of 1.2–3.5 m and also generate 3D images of the corresponding subject irrespective of his/her attire. Apart from dynamic image capture and recognition, the Kinect sensor has provisions to carry out functions related to microphone input, speech recognition, etc. With the usage of the associated SDK, the captured images are analyzed and processed and a skeleton containing 20 different body joints in three dimensions (x, y, and z axes), is obtained. The skeleton information thus generated is based on depth (captured by IR sensor) and RGB (gathered by RGB camera) information.

Usually, the skeleton is obtained at a predefined 30 frames per second (fps) rate, which can be controlled according to the requirement of the application. So, at a rate of 30 fps for 20 joints, it will yield $30 \times 20 \times 3 = 1800$ real-time stick model coordinates per second. In the proposed work, to meet up to the speed of Khepera II, rather to accommodate the faster movements of the above-mentioned robot, the skeleton is generated at a rate of 5 fps. While dealing with data generated from humans (here, gestures), it is a crucial point to maintain the privacy of the subject. So, recognition based upon the skeleton generated by the Kinect sensor, provides a provision of maintaining subject privacy, it ensures generality also. Most importantly, it enables an analyst to deal with the joint coordinates only, thus fewer amounts of data are processed, and hence system complexity is reduced as well.

7.2.2 KHEPERA II

Khepera [20] enables a user to build a communication link with the real-world scenarios that are developed to serve various purposes. Basically, this particular mobile robot acts as an interface for various real-time applications. These days, the Khepera robot is used in many online simulations based upon real-world robotic applications due to its portability, robustness, and relatively low cost.

Khepera II can also communicate with the computer through a serial line; hence, the features obtained from the Kinect sensor can be analyzed and the motor speed of the robot wheels corresponding to different turns can be controlled [21]. Eight infrared (IR) sensors that are already present in the robot are used to avoid collision of the robot to any obstacle in every 20 ms [22]. For this particular feature, even in situations where may be due to human error (e.g., inattentiveness), the robot may collide with any obstacle. Then automatically brake is applied irrespective of the gesture of the subject, such that the robot can be halted at a safe distance of 50 mm. The unit for speed is 8 mm/s and the same for acceleration is 3.125 mm/s^2. At reset, these values are set as 20 and 64, respectively. Brake is negative of acceleration for Khepera II [23].

The navigational instructions are provided to the Khepera II robot wirelessly via robot operating system (ROS) topics. Khepera II has an inbuilt Linux operating system which is capable of networking through WiFi. Here, two different set of communicative programs are compiled and executed on the robot and the host device. The executable program on the host side connects to the ROS server running on the robot and exposes the sensors and motors of the robot as ROS topics [24].

7.2.3 TYPE-1 FUZZY SET

As mentioned earlier, the term "gesture" signifies to different human postures corresponding to various actions and emotions as well. Hence, it is quite obvious that gestures will vary according to ambiance of the surroundings, personal habit of the concerned subject and time also. Since, human beings are not always static at one position and even if they are static at a particular position that does not necessarily indicate that they will hold the same posture for the entire time duration taken under consideration, which leads to changes in the gestures at different time frames. These variations as discussed above give rise to uncertainty and hence pose ambiguities while correctly recognizing unknown gesture. Sometimes there are such huge variations in the datasets that a standard classifier may fail to perform accurately while there exists certain cases where the subtle changes that occur between two gestures may not be detected by a regular classifier, in these cases fuzzy-logic-based classifiers are used to handle such situations. Type-1 fuzzy sets (T1FS) [25] provides a researcher with an opportunity to deal with such classification problems by representing the ambiguities in data in different time instances with the help of a single membership function which is best suited for the problem.

In traditional set theory, binary memberships are given to different entities, in other words the membership values of either 0 or 1 is assigned depending on whether the concerned entity belongs to a set or not. But the problem with the binary membership values is that they do not provide any information about the extent of belonging to that particular set. Also if a certain value resides on the boundary between two unique sets, then it becomes a problem to decide to which set the concerned entity actually belongs. Fuzzy sets obey a different concept, where the membership value (μ) can take any value within the interval 0 and 1, including both the extreme limits. Each element (b) of the universal set is a member of a specified set Z, as $0 \leq \mu_b(Z) \leq 1$. While classifying using T1FS system, firstly the membership value of the unknown test sample is calculated using the required parameters for a particular class, likewise the same procedure is repeated for all the classes considered in the said experiment, and finally the test sample is assigned to the class having the highest membership value.

In this research, we require two types of membership functions described below.

7.2.3.1 γ FUNCTION

The γ function with two parameters, α and β can be presented as [26]

$$\gamma(l;\alpha,\beta) = \begin{array}{ll} 0 & \text{if } l \leq \alpha \\ \dfrac{l-\alpha}{\beta-\alpha} & \text{if } \alpha < l \leq \beta \\ 1 & \text{if } l > \beta \end{array} \qquad (7.1)$$

7.2.3.2 L FUNCTION

The L function with two parameters, α and β can be presented as [27]

Fuzzy-Based Stratagem for Teleoperation of Robots 155

$$L(l;\alpha,\beta) = \begin{cases} 0 & \text{if} \quad l \leq \alpha \\ \dfrac{\beta-l}{\beta-\alpha} & \text{if} \quad \alpha < l \leq \beta \\ 1 & \text{if} \quad l > \beta \end{cases} \quad (7.2)$$

7.2.4 INTERVAL TYPE-2 FUZZY SET

To avoid improper data recording due to excess stress on the subject or due to unavailability of subjects, data is often recorded during multiple sessions of a particular day or sometimes it is carried out on different days also. Despite having high performance, T1FS systems sometimes are not able to recognize variations in the membership values between several trials of a particular experiment over a number of days or over datasets corresponding to dissimilar subjects. As an obvious consequence, the performance is degraded. For example, given a situation, for a particular membership curve, the α and β are variable over a large range of observations, in other words, an environment where the parameter values are changed dynamically, T1FS system fails to provide satisfactory performance index. To avoid such problematic scenario, Interval Type-2 fuzzy sets (IT2FS) [16, 17] are used as a possible solution.

For IT2FS, the region formed by taking account of all the primary membership functions for alike set of observations, is called the Footprint of Uncertainty and the minimum and maximum values of the primary memberships over that many observations, are denoted as the lower membership function (LMF) and the upper membership function (UMF), respectively [28]. In IT2FS, the secondary membership function maintains uniformity and gets a continual value of 1 for all values between the LMF and UMF and it becomes zero otherwise.

Suppose in a dataset, we have N ($1 \leq n \leq N$) number of subjects and each subject is depicting a particular gesture for M ($1 \leq m \leq M$) number of times. From each gesture, we are calculating I ($1 \leq i \leq I$) number of features. Now for a particular feature i, for a particular subject n and for a particular instance m, we have a data point $l_i^{n,m}$. So, for all M instances for that particular subject n, we have $l_i^{n,1},\ldots,l_i^{n,m},\ldots,l_i^{n,M}$ data points. For these M data points, a membership curve (γ or L function) is determined based on the parameters α and β.

$$\alpha_i^n = \text{proc1}\left(l_i^{n,1},\ldots,l_i^{n,m},\ldots,l_i^{n,M}\right) \quad (7.3)$$

$$\beta_i^n = \text{proc2}\left(l_i^{n,1},\ldots,l_i^{n,m},\ldots,l_i^{n,M}\right) \quad (7.4)$$

where the definition of proc1 and proc2 functions are given in Tables 7.1 and 7.2. As here we are discussing about generalized IT2FS formation, so the specific meaning of those two functions are not described here. Based on these two parameters, a membership curve is generated, say γ_i^n.

For all N subjects, N number of membership curves $(\gamma_i^1, \ldots, \gamma_i^n, \ldots, \gamma_i^N)$ are produced. The LMF and UMF are determined using the following equations:

$$LMF_i = \min\left(\gamma_i^1, \ldots, \gamma_i^n, \ldots, \gamma_i^N\right) \tag{7.5}$$

$$UMF_i = \max\left(\gamma_i^1, \ldots, \gamma_i^n, \ldots, \gamma_i^N\right) \tag{7.6}$$

The footprint of uncertainty is obtained as

$$FOU_i = \bigcup\left(\gamma_i^1, \ldots, \gamma_i^n, \ldots, \gamma_i^N\right) \tag{7.7}$$

Suppose for an unknown gesture u for any frame number e, we get two memberships $\underline{\mu}_{i,e}^u$ and $\overline{\mu}_{i,e}^u$ from lower and upper membership curves where the x-axis value $l_{i,e}^u$ cuts the $LMF_{i,e}$ and $UMF_{i,e}$ at $\underline{\mu}_{i,e}^u$ and $\overline{\mu}_{i,e}^u$ respectively. Thus the support of that gesture u for that particular feature i is [29, 30]

$$S_{i,e}^u = \frac{\underline{\mu}_{i,e}^u + \overline{\mu}_{i,e}^u}{2} \tag{7.8}$$

This procedure is elaborated in Figure 7.1 for γ function. Similar process is carried out for L function.

Pseudocode for γ function

Procedure *it2fs* for feature i

Input: $l_i^{n,m}$ features for all N subjects and M instances
Output: Strength S_i
Procedure:
Begin
    For n = 1 to N %subject number
    For m = 1 to M %instance number
    Get $l_i^{n,m}$
    End.

$$\alpha_i^n = \text{proc1}\left(l_i^{n,1}, \ldots, l_i^{n,m}, \ldots, l_i^{n,M}\right)$$

$$\beta_i^n = \text{proc}\,2\left(l_i^{n,1},...,l_i^{n,m},...,l_i^{n,M}\right)$$

% proc1 and proc2 functions are defined in Tables 7.1 and 7.2.

Generate γ_i^n using Figure 7.2

End.

$$LMF_i = \min\left(\gamma_i^1,...,\gamma_i^n,...,\gamma_i^N\right)$$

$$UMF_i = \max\left(\gamma_i^1,...,\gamma_i^n,...,\gamma_i^N\right)$$

For unknown gesture u for eth frame,

$$\underline{\mu}_{i,e}^u \in LMF_i$$

$$\overline{\mu}_{i,e}^u \in UMF_i$$

$$S_{i,e}^u = \frac{\underline{\mu}_{i,e}^u + \overline{\mu}_{i,e}^u}{2}$$

7.3 PROBLEM FORMULATION AND APPROACH

The section gives a demonstrative explanation of the proposed gesture driven architecture for mobile robot movement. The proposed architecture has two dichotomies: background and foreground setups. The human subjects, who are going to give instructions in the form of gestures to the robots, are situated at the background [31, 32]. The remotely operated robots are performing the desired tasks in the foreground of the incoherent environment. Since the nature of the environment is stochastic in nature (e.g., industry where steel is molded in very high flame, battle ground where mines may have been placed, deep sea where underwater danger can happen, etc.), it is not feasible for the subject (i.e., human being) to go and perform the necessary actions, we have developed this system, where the robot takes the command based upon the human gestures and perform accordingly. For gathering the required knowledge about the status of the robot's current state, the robotic agent is attached with a surveillance camera, which is fixed upon the robot itself. The visual information captured by the robot is send to the human instructor, such that he/she can gaze the environment and decides which action need to be taken at that particular time. Based on his/her decision, justified gestural commands send to the robot wirelessly. Figures 7.2 and 7.3 show the schematic view and block diagram of the proposed technique, respectively. As the obstacles can change their positions and also external actions can be there to manipulate the environment where the robot works, this gives us the motivation to develop a gesture-driven robot control system for the said environment. Here as the subject can see the incoherent place by himself/herself and thus can direct the robot much more efficiently than the decisions taken by some algorithms already installed in the robot. In this case, Khepera II has been used because of its characteristics which seemed to be the most suitable option for this constrained setup, while any other mobile robots can be used. So the proposed framework is well suited to work in dynamically changing atmosphere. Different parts of the work are explained in the following sections.

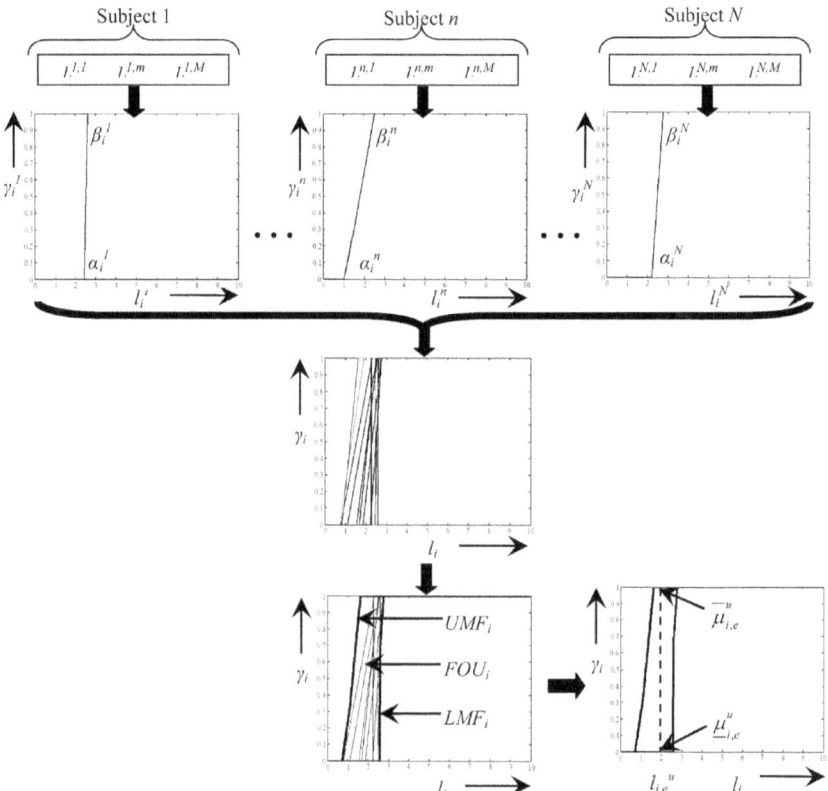

FIGURE 7.1 Flowchart for calculation of strength for ith feature for γ function.

Fuzzy-Based Stratagem for Teleoperation of Robots

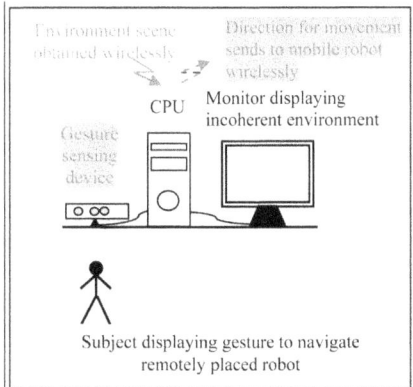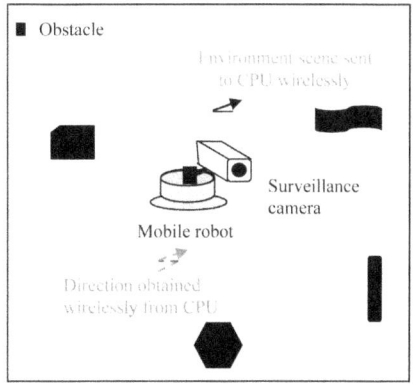

FIGURE 7.2 Overview of the proposed architecture, (a) Background setup from where gestural commands are given and (b) Foreground setup where the mobile robot operates.

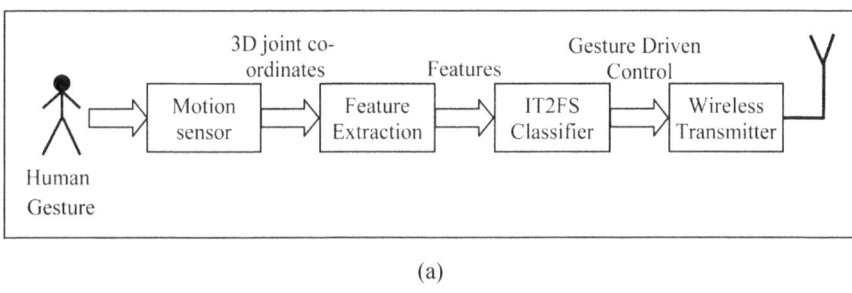

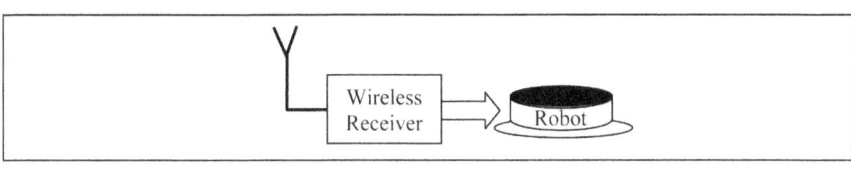

FIGURE 7.3 Block diagram of the robot manoeuvre system, (a) transmitter and (b) Receiver side.

7.3.1 FEATURE EXTRACTION

The various movements possible for the robot can be of nine types:

1. Direction : Straight (DS); Speed : Constant (DC)
2. Direction : Right (DR); Speed : Constant (DC)
3. Direction : Left (DL); Speed : Constant (DC)
4. Direction : Straight (DS); Speed : Acceleration (DA)

5. Direction : Right (*DR*); Speed : Acceleration (*DA*)
6. Direction : Left (*DL*); Speed : Acceleration (*DA*)
7. Direction : Straight (*DS*); Speed : Brake (*DB*)
8. Direction : Right (*DR*); Speed : Brake (*DB*)
9. Direction : Left (*DL*); Speed : Brake (*DB*)

Here, basically we are dealing with two important aspects of driving, one is direction of the robot (using *DS*, *DR*, and *DL*) and another one is the velocity of the robot (using *DC*, *DA*, and *DB*). Eight features (i.e., $I=8$) are extracted for this purpose. The features are the Euclidean distances with hip center (J_1): hand left (J_8), hand right (J_{12}), wrist left (J_7), wrist right (J_{11}), elbow left (J_6), elbow right (J_{10}), ankle left (J_{15}), and ankle right (J_{19}). The joint numberings (from the collected Kinetic skeletal data) for the above-mentioned joints are J_1, J_8, J_{12}, J_7, J_{11}, J_6, J_{10}, J_{15}, and J_{19}.

To normalize the effects of different person's body shapes, all the eight distances are divided by distance between J_1 and shoulder center (J_3). The features are as follows:

$$l_1 = \frac{\|J_1 - J_8\|}{\|J_1 - J_3\|} \tag{7.9}$$

$$l_2 = \frac{\|J_1 - J_{12}\|}{\|J_1 - J_3\|} \tag{7.10}$$

$$l_3 = \frac{\|J_1 - J_7\|}{\|J_1 - J_3\|} \tag{7.11}$$

$$l_4 = \frac{\|J_1 - J_{11}\|}{\|J_1 - J_3\|} \tag{7.12}$$

$$l_5 = \frac{\|J_1 - J_6\|}{\|J_1 - J_3\|} \tag{7.13}$$

$$l_6 = \frac{\|J_1 - J_{10}\|}{\|J_1 - J_3\|} \tag{7.14}$$

$$l_7 = \frac{\|J_1 - J_{15}\|}{\|J_1 - J_3\|} \tag{7.15}$$

$$l_8 = \frac{\|J_1 - J_{19}\|}{\|J_1 - J_3\|} \tag{7.16}$$

The skeletal joints and feature vector are depicted in Figure 7.4.

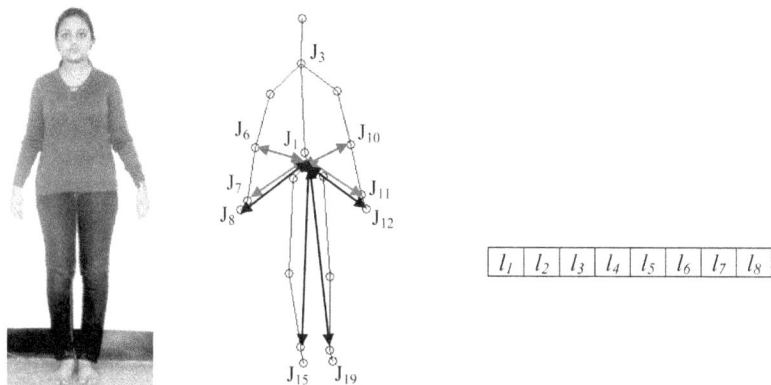

FIGURE 7.4 The required joints along with features: (a) RGB image and (b) skeleton image, (c) feature vector.

7.3.2 RECOGNITION OF DIRECTION OF ROBOT—DS GESTURE

For the training of the proposed system, the instructor is asked to provide *DS* gesture for the initial 2s. To treat a frame as a command for *DS*, two threshold values (τ_1 and τ_2) for l_3 and l_4 are measured, respectively. These calculations of thresholds are carried out after considering all *N* number of subjects and *M* number of instances. The calculation of τ_1 and τ_2 are done governing the following equations:

$$\tau_1^{n,m} = \max\left(l_{3,1}^{n,m},...,l_{3,f}^{n,m},...,l_{3,F}^{n,m}\right), \tag{7.17}$$

$$\tau_1^{n} = \max\left(\tau_1^{n,1},...,\tau_1^{n,m},...,\tau_1^{n,M}\right), \tag{7.18}$$

$$\tau_1 = \mathrm{mean}\left(\tau_1^{1},...,\tau_1^{n},...,\tau_1^{N}\right), \tag{7.19}$$

$$\tau_2^{n,m} = \max\left(l_{4,1}^{n,m},...,l_{4,f}^{n,m},...,l_{4,F}^{n,m}\right), \tag{7.20}$$

$$\tau_2^{n} = \max\left(\tau_2^{n,1},...,\tau_2^{n,m},...,\tau_2^{n,M}\right), \tag{7.21}$$

$$\tau_2 = \mathrm{mean}\left(\tau_2^{1},...,\tau_2^{n},...,\tau_2^{N}\right), \tag{7.22}$$

The flowchart for calculation of τ_1 is given in Figure 7.5. Similar procedure is carried out for calculation of τ_2 also.

Let, for *e*th ($1 \leq e \leq E$) frame number from unknown subject, the calculated length features are $l_{3,e}^{u}$ and $l_{4,e}^{u}$. If both of these distance measures are less than the thresholds τ_1 and τ_2, then that specific unknown gesture is considered as a command for "drive straight," otherwise the algorithm will look for "drive right" or "drive left" commands. After calculating the direction of the robot, we have to check for the velocity of the Khepera II.

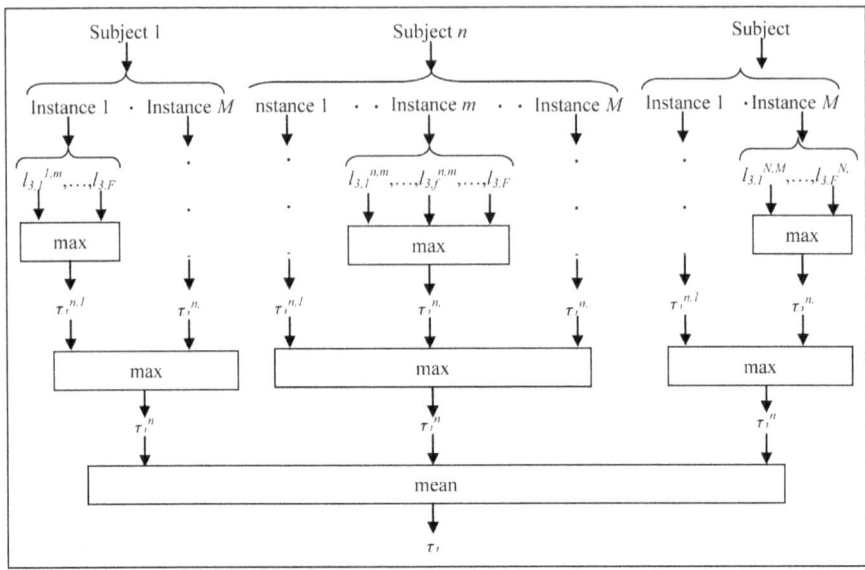

FIGURE 7.5 Flowchart for calculation of τ_1.

Pseudocode for *DS* gesture

Procedure *DS* for unknown subject *u* for frame number *e*

Input: $l_{3,e}^{u}$ and $l_{4,e}^{u}$ features for E frames of the unknown subject while giving direction to the robot and τ_1 and τ_2 already calculated from training dataset

Output: Check whether the gesture for *e*th frame is depicting *DS* or not

Procedure:

Begin

    For $e = 1$ to E

    If $l_{3,e}^{u} < \tau_1$ && $l_{4,e}^{u} < \tau_2$

        Drive straight

        Check for acceleration or brake

    End.

End.

7.3.3 RECOGNITION OF DIRECTION OF ROBOT—DR AND DL GESTURE

The choice of IT2FS membership functions plays a key role in the entire system framework, so the strategy behind the choice of each membership function needs to be explained well. It can be noticed from Figure 7.6 showing "drive right" command, the distance between the right elbow and the hip center joint is lesser than that of "drive straight" command, on the other hand for the left side of the body, the distance increases. So when the robot is needed to be rotated more towards right turn, the more turning of the virtual steering should be, that is, lesser is the distance between the right arm and the hip center. Hence, to represent this logic, a membership function for the right hand parameters should be such that for lesser values, the membership values should be larger. After much research, L membership function is chosen in this case and the parameters for the stated function are calculated while keeping all the constraints to incorporate all the information. Exact opposite scenario can be noticed for the left hand parameters and γ function becomes our choice here. These calculations of membership functions change completely for the "drive left" command.

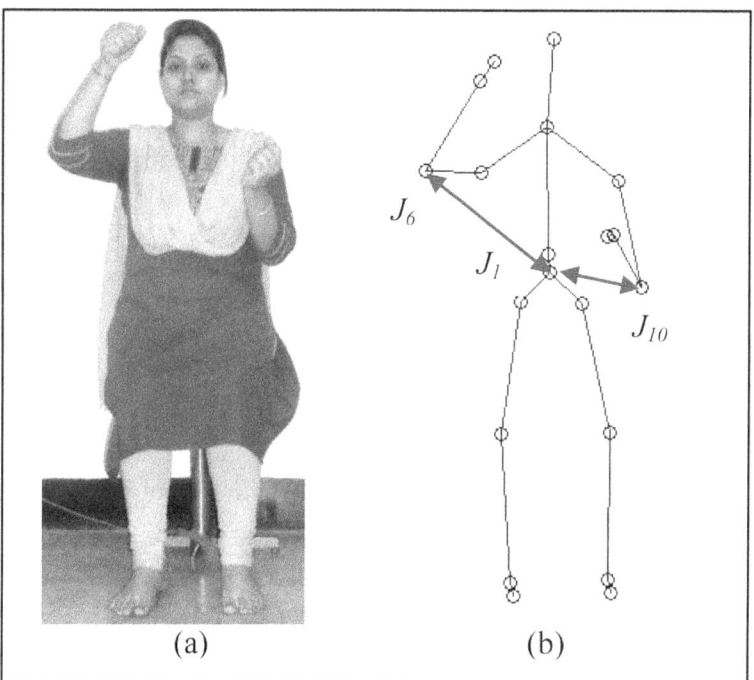

FIGURE 7.6 "Drive right" gesture: (a) RGB and (b) skeleton image depicting $l_{5,e}^u$ and $l_{6,e}^u$.

For dictating the robot about its direction, the other two experimentally chosen threshold values (τ_3 and τ_4) are calculated similar to that of τ_1 and τ_2.

$$\tau_3^{n,m} = \max\left(l_{5,1}^{n,m},\ldots,l_{5,f}^{n,m},\ldots,l_{5,F}^{n,m}\right) \quad (7.23)$$

$$\tau_3^n = \max\left(\tau_3^{n,1},\ldots,\tau_3^{n,m},\ldots,\tau_3^{n,M}\right) \quad (7.24)$$

$$\tau_3 = \text{mean}\left(\tau_3^1,\ldots,\tau_3^n,\ldots,\tau_3^N\right) \quad (7.25)$$

$$\tau_4^{n,m} = \max\left(l_{6,1}^{n,m},\ldots,l_{6,f}^{n,m},\ldots,l_{6,F}^{n,m}\right) \quad (7.26)$$

$$\tau_4^n = \max\left(\tau_4^{n,1},\ldots,\tau_4^{n,m},\ldots,\tau_4^{n,M}\right) \quad (7.27)$$

$$\tau_4 = \text{mean}\left(\tau_4^1,\ldots,\tau_4^n,\ldots,\tau_4^N\right) \quad (7.28)$$

Let, we are calculating for an unknown command obtained from *e*th frame number as captured by the Kinect sensor. The features obtained are $l_{5,e}^{\,u}$ and $l_{6,e}^{\,u}$. Whenever $l_{5,e}^{\,u}$ is greater than τ_3 and $l_{6,e}^{\,u}$ is less than τ_4, then the unknown driving instruction is taken as "drive right" command by the robot. In opposite case that command is considered as "drive left," Next we take to decide the proper degree of rotation (*dor*) for the robot using IT2FS for lengths l_1 to l_6. Tables 7.1 and 7.2 depict how the parameters α_i^n and β_i^n are decided for γ or L functions. In those tables, "min," "mean," and "max" are the functions to calculate minimum, average, and maximum values of the inputs within that functions.

TABLE 7.1 Calculation of IT2FS for *DR* Gesture

Feature	Membership Function	Parameters
l_1	γ	$\alpha_1^n = \min\left(l_1^{n,1},\ldots,l_1^{n,m},\ldots,l_1^{n,M}\right)$ $\beta_1^n = \text{mean}\left(l_1^{n,1},\ldots,l_1^{n,m},\ldots,l_1^{n,M}\right)$
l_2	L	$\alpha_2^n = \min\left(l_2^{n,1},\ldots,l_2^{n,m},\ldots,l_2^{n,M}\right)$ $\beta_2^n = \text{mean}\left(l_2^{n,1},\ldots,l_2^{n,m},\ldots,l_2^{n,M}\right)$
l_3	γ	$\alpha_3^n = \min\left(l_3^{n,1},\ldots,l_3^{n,m},\ldots,l_3^{n,M}\right)$ $\beta_3^n = \text{mean}\left(l_3^{n,1},\ldots,l_3^{n,m},\ldots,l_3^{n,M}\right)$
l_4	L	$\alpha_4^n = \min\left(l_4^{n,1},\ldots,l_4^{n,m},\ldots,l_4^{n,M}\right)$ $\beta_4^n = \text{mean}\left(l_4^{n,1},\ldots,l_4^{n,m},\ldots,l_4^{n,M}\right)$
l_5	γ	$\alpha_5^n = \min\left(l_5^{n,1},\ldots,l_5^{n,m},\ldots,l_5^{n,M}\right)$ $\beta_5^n = \text{mean}\left(l_5^{n,1},\ldots,l_5^{n,m},\ldots,l_5^{n,M}\right)$
l_6	L	$\alpha_6^n = \min\left(l_6^{n,1},\ldots,l_6^{n,m},\ldots,l_6^{n,M}\right)$ $\beta_6^n = \text{mean}\left(l_6^{n,1},\ldots,l_6^{n,m},\ldots,l_6^{n,M}\right)$

Fuzzy-Based Stratagem for Teleoperation of Robots 165

TABLE 7.2 Calculation of IT2FS for *DL* Gesture

Feature	Membership Function	Parameters	
l_1	L	$\alpha_1^n = \text{mean}\left(l_1^{n,1},...,l_1^{n,m},...,l_1^{n,M}\right)$	$\beta_1^n = \max\left(l_1^{n,1},...,l_1^{n,m},...,l_1^{n,M}\right)$
l_2	γ	$\alpha_2^n = \text{mean}\left(l_2^{n,1},...,l_2^{n,m},...,l_2^{n,M}\right)$	$\beta_2^n = \max\left(l_2^{n,1},...,l_2^{n,m},...,l_2^{n,M}\right)$
l_3	L	$\alpha_3^n = \text{mean}\left(l_3^{n,1},...,l_3^{n,m},...,l_3^{n,M}\right)$	$\beta_3^n = \max\left(l_3^{n,1},...,l_3^{n,m},...,l_3^{n,M}\right)$
l_4	γ	$\alpha_4^n = \text{mean}\left(l_4^{n,1},...,l_4^{n,m},...,l_4^{n,M}\right)$	$\beta_4^n = \max\left(l_4^{n,1},...,l_4^{n,m},...,l_4^{n,M}\right)$
l_5	L	$\alpha_5^n = \text{mean}\left(l_5^{n,1},...,l_5^{n,m},...,l_5^{n,M}\right)$	$\beta_5^n = \max\left(l_5^{n,1},...,l_5^{n,m},...,l_5^{n,M}\right)$
l_6	γ	$\alpha_6^n = \text{mean}\left(l_6^{n,1},...,l_6^{n,m},...,l_6^{n,M}\right)$	$\beta_6^n = \max\left(l_6^{n,1},...,l_6^{n,m},...,l_6^{n,M}\right)$

Thus proc1 and proc2 functions for (3–4) are min and max for γ function and same for *L* function are mean and max. Based on one T1FS curve from all *N* subjects, one IT2FS cure is obtained.

For *e*th frame number, let the feature space is $[l_{1,e}^u, l_{2,e}^u, l_{3,e}^u, l_{4,e}^u, l_{5,e}^u, l_{6,e}^u]$ and strength is S_e^u.

$$S_{e,\text{odd}}^u = \min\left(S_{1,e}^u, \min\left(S_{3,e}^u, S_{5,e}^u\right)\right) \quad (7.29)$$

$$S_{e,\text{even}}^u = \min\left(S_{2,e}^u, \min\left(S_{4,e}^u, S_{6,e}^u\right)\right) \quad (7.30)$$

$$S_e^u = \max\left(S_{e,\text{odd}}^u, S_{e,\text{even}}^u\right) \quad (7.31)$$

S_e^u is mapped with the *dor* as follows:

$$dor = \text{round}\left(dor_{\text{start}} + \frac{dor_{\text{end}} - dor_{\text{start}}}{S_{e,\text{end}}^u - S_{e,\text{start}}^u} \times \left(S_e^u - S_{e,\text{start}}^u\right)\right). \quad (7.32)$$

where x_{start} and x_{end} are the starting and ending ranges for *x*, respectively. As the range for S_e^u is from 0 to 1, so $S_{e,\text{start}}^u$ and $S_{e,\text{end}}^u$ are 0 and 1, respectively. Thus (7.32) becomes

$$dor = \text{round}\left(dor_{\text{start}} + \frac{dor_{\text{end}} - dor_{\text{start}}}{1 - 0} \times \left(S_e^u - 0\right)\right) \quad (7.33)$$

$$dor = \text{round}\left(dor_{start} + \left(\left(dor_{end} - dor_{start}\right) \times S_e^u\right)\right) \tag{7.34}$$

The values of dor_{start} and dor_{end} are calculated experimentally.

Pseudocode for *DR* and *DL* gesture:

Procedure *DR* and *DL* for unknown subject *u* for frame number *e*

Input: $l_{1,e}^u$ to $l_{6,e}^u$ features for all E frames of the unknown subject while giving direction to the robot and τ_3 and τ_4 already calculated from training dataset

Output: Rotate the robot to exact direction

Procedure:

Begin
    For $e = 1$ to E
        If $l_{5,e}^u > \tau_3$ && $l_{6,e}^u < \tau_4$
        Drive right
            For $i = 1$ to 8
            Choose proper IT2FS$_i$ curve generated using α_i^n and β_i^n from Table 7.1
            Determine S_e^u from (7.30)
            Determine *dor* from (7.33)
        End.
            Check for acceleration or brake
        Else if $l_{5,e}^u < \tau_3$ && $l_{6,e}^u > \tau_4$
        Drive left
        For $i = 1$ to 8
        Choose proper IT2FS$_i$ curve generated using α_i^n and β_i^n from Table 2
        Determine S_e^u from (7.30)
        Determine *dor* from (7.33)
        End.
            Check for acceleration or brake
        End.
    End.

7.3.4 RECOGNITION OF SPEED OF ROBOT—DC, DA, AND DB

The RGB image with the corresponding skeleton for "drive with acceleration" (*DA*) is shown in Figure 7.7 correspondingly.

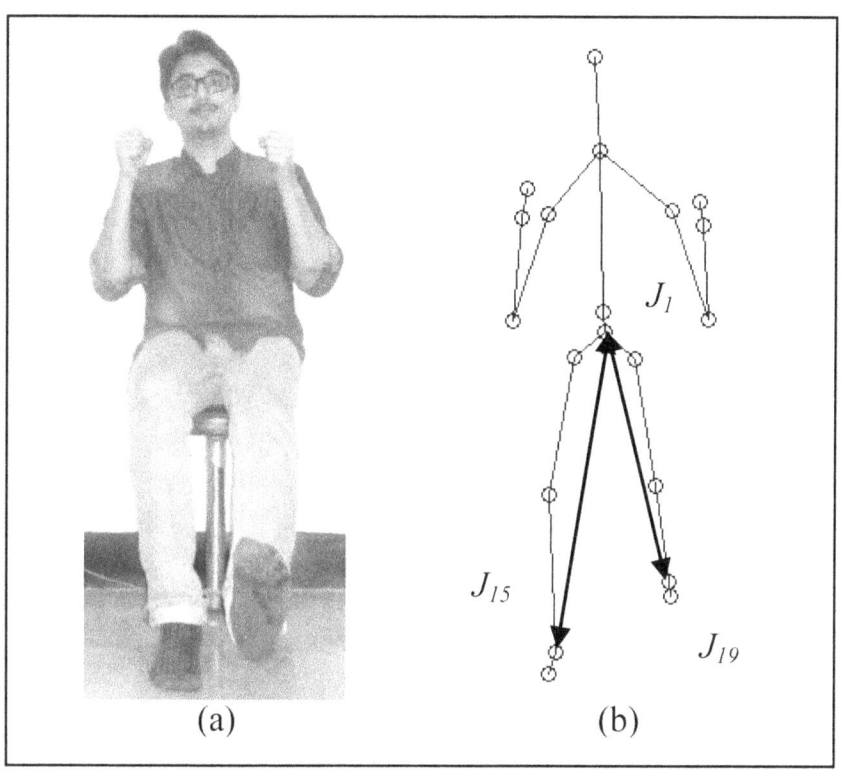

FIGURE 7.7 "Drive with acceleration" gesture: (a) RGB and (b) skeleton image depicting $l_{7,e}^u$ and $l_{8,e}^u$.

Two threshold values (τ_5 and τ_6) are experimentally calculated for "acceleration" or "brake," respectively, to navigate Khepera II robot

$$\tau_5^{n,m} = \max\left(l_{7,1}^{n,m}, \ldots, l_{7,f}^{n,m}, \ldots, l_{7,F}^{n,m}\right) \quad (7.35)$$

$$\tau_5^n = \max\left(\tau_5^{n,1}, \ldots, \tau_5^{n,m}, \ldots, \tau_5^{n,M}\right) \quad (7.36)$$

$$\tau_5 = \max\left(\tau_5^1, \ldots, \tau_5^n, \ldots, \tau_5^N\right) \quad (7.37)$$

$$\tau_6^{n,m} = \max\left(l_{8,1}^{n,m}, \ldots, l_{8,f}^{n,m}, \ldots, l_{8,F}^{n,m}\right) \quad (7.38)$$

$$\tau_6^n = \max\left(\tau_6^{n,1}, \ldots, \tau_6^{n,m}, \ldots, \tau_6^{n,M}\right) \tag{7.39}$$

$$\tau_6 = \max\left(\tau_6^1, \ldots, \tau_6^n, \ldots, \tau_6^N\right) \tag{7.40}$$

If the unknown distance $l_{7,e}^u$ is larger than τ_5, then brake is applied to the mobile robot and when $l_{8,e}^u$ is larger than τ_6, then the robot is accelerated. The overall flowchart of the proposed work is given in Figure 7.8.

Pseudocode for *DA* and *DB* gesture:

Procedure *DA* and *DB* for unknown subject *u* for frame number *e*

Input: $l_{7,e}^u$ and $l_{8,e}^u$ features for all E frames of the unknown subject while giving direction to the robot and τ_7 and τ_8 already calculated from training dataset

Output: Apply acceleration or brake to the robot

Procedure:

Begin

    For $e = 1$ to E

        If $l_{7,e}^u > \tau_5$

            Apply brake

        Else if $l_{8,e}^u > \tau_6$

            Apply acceleration

        Else if $l_{8,e}^u > \tau_6$

            Drive with same speed

    End.

End.

7.4 EXPERIMENTAL RESULTS

In this section, we are going to look into different parts of experimental paradigm.

Fuzzy-Based Stratagem for Teleoperation of Robots

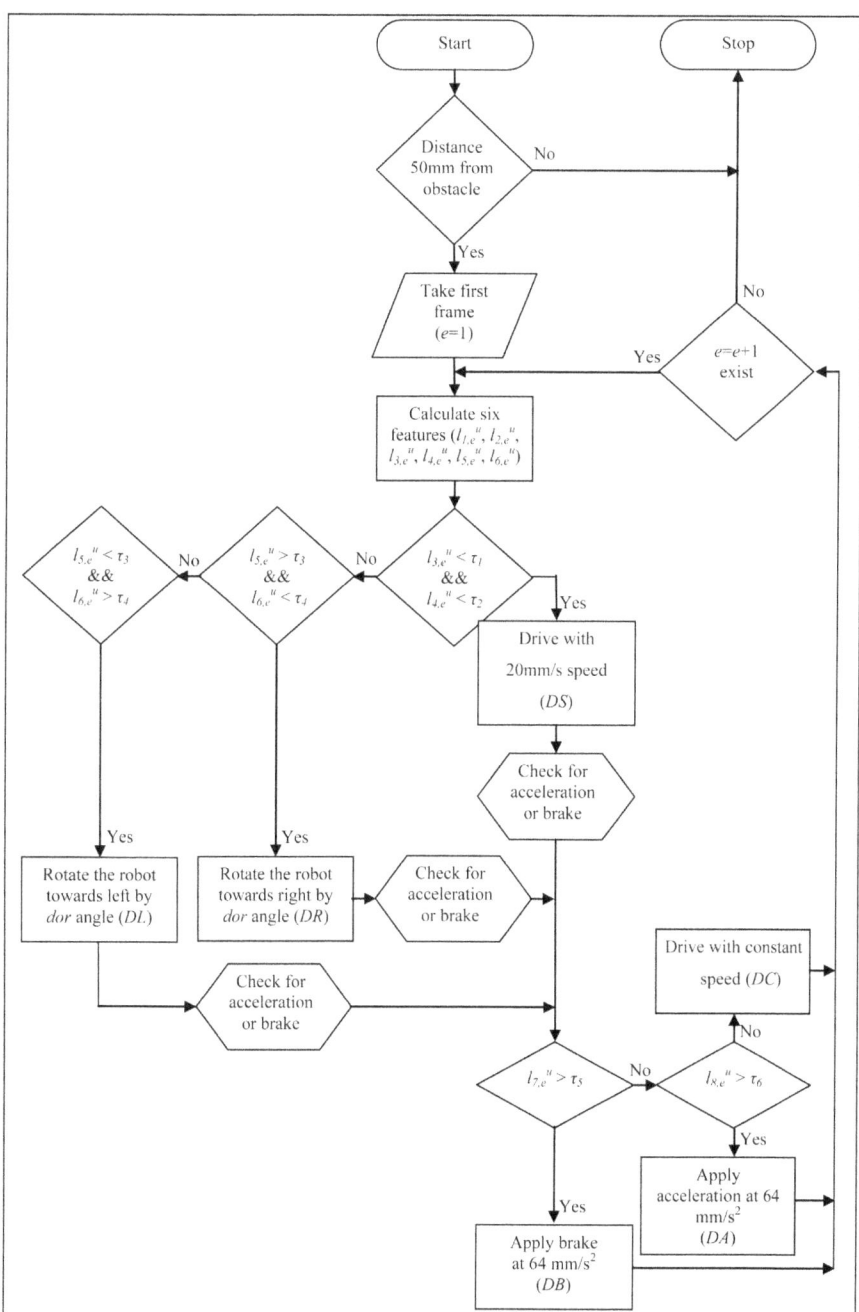

FIGURE 7.8 Complete flowchart of the proposed work.

3.4.1 PREPARATION OF TRAINING AND TESTING DATASETS

For the training purpose, we have acquired three datasets from research scholars as provided in Table 7.3. For the testing of the proposed work, we have collected data from 95 subjects.

TABLE 7.3 Training Dataset

Dataset Number	Age (years)	Number of Scholars (N)	Number of Times Data Collected from Each Scholar (M)
1	23 ± 3	60	40
2	24 ± 4	60	40
3	26 ± 5	60	40

The graphical relationship between S_e^u and dor is given in Figure 7.9.

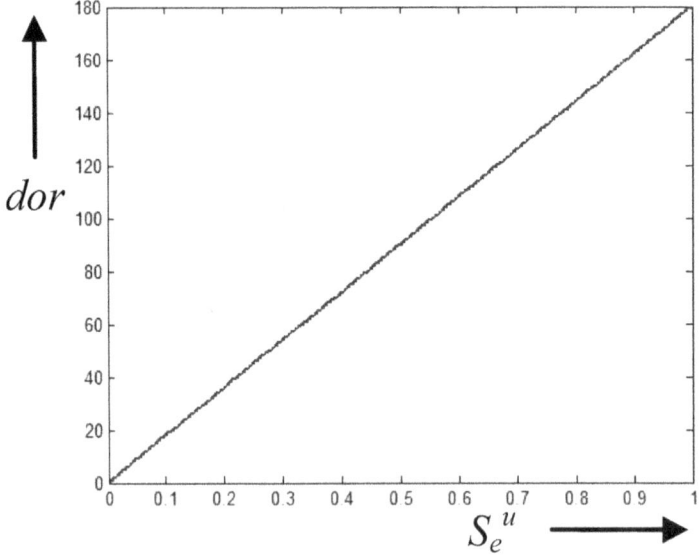

FIGURE 7.9 Relation between S_e^u and *dor*.

7.4.2 RESULTS GATHERED FROM THE TRAINING DATASET

The experimentally chosen threshold values for all the eight features are given in Table 7.4. As we are intending to rotate the remotely placed robot to a maximum of 180° in any direction, so the range for *dor* is $0 \leq dor \leq 180$. From the above (7.34), we can get

$$dor = \text{round}\left(180 \times S_e^u\right) \tag{7.41}$$

7.4.3 RECOGNITION OF GESTURAL COMMAND TO INSTRUCT THE ROBOT

For the space constraint, we are not able to demonstrate the whole procedure from initial state to the goal state. However, we are going to give idea how the proposed work runs for one particular unknown gesture. For 325th unknown gestural command, the robot navigation is presented in this subsection (Figure 7.10). The details about direction and speed calculation for Khepera II are given in Table 7.4 and calculation of *dor* is provided in Table 7.5. Based on these observations, we can easily say that our proposed work is capable of instructing the mobile robot correctly.

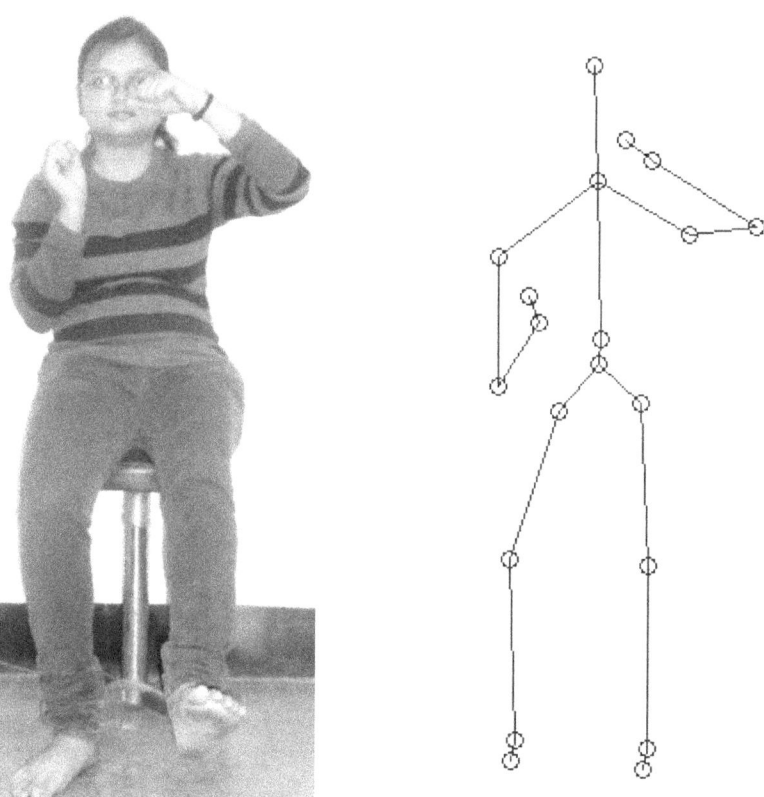

FIGURE 7.10 Unknown gesture: (a) RGB and (b) skeleton image.

TABLE 7.4 Calculation of Direction and Speed of Khepera II for Unknown Gestural Command from Figure 7.10

Unknown Features $(l_{i,325}{}^u)$				
1.79	Thresholds (τ) $l_{i,325}{}^u$		Direction	
2.58	$<\tau$			
1.49	2.71	No	Drive Left	
2.64	2.61	Yes	(DL)	
1.79	1.98	No		
3.46	2.04	Yes	Speed	
5.02	5.45	No	Drive with acceleration	
6.00	5.48	Yes	(DA)	

TABLE 7.5 Calculation of *dor*

LMF $\left(\underline{\mu}^u_{i,325}\right)$	UMF $\left(\overline{\mu}^u_{i,325}\right)$	Strength $\left(S^u_{i,e}\right)$	$S_{e,odd}{}^u$	$S_{e,even}{}^u$	$S_e{}^u$	dor
0.48	1.00	0.74	0.51	0.69	0.69	124
0.38	1.00	0.69				
0.78	1.00	0.89				
1.00	1.00	1.00				
0.01	1.00	0.51				
1.00	1.00	1.00				

7.4.4 PERFORMANCE ANALYSIS

The performance of the IT2FS-based gesture-driven robot movement mechanism is analyzed on the basis of three datasets that are recorded for the considered experiment. IT2FS has been performed here based on the "centroid" approach for evaluating class lengths [39]. There can be other two variants of IT2FS, "conservative" as well as "liberal" approaches by considering the lower bound and upper bound of the interval respectively [38]. To justify the performance of the proposed system, the said algorithm has been compared with seven other widely accepted standard algorithms in terms of accuracy, error rate, F1 score, etc. The above-mentioned comparative framework includes Type 1 fuzzy-system-based classifier T1FS [33, 34], support vector machine (SVM) classifier [35–37], k-nearest neighbor (kNN) classification [38, 39], ensemble decision tree (EDT) [40, 41] and

Levenberg–Marquardt algorithm induced neural network (LMA-NN) [42, 43]. The T1FS classifier assumes γ and L membership functions depending on the concerned variables and turning directions (*dor*). Since for two different directions, the pattern of the membership curves corresponding to left- and right-hand features vary, so to incorporate all the information it is preferable to choose membership curve with different abscissa and ordinate relationship. The required parameters of all other above-mentioned classifiers are set after observing their best performance among all the trials taken under consideration. For SVM, the radial basis function kernel is chosen with kernel parameter value of 1 and cost value of 100. The performance of *k*NN has been analyzed while considering *k*=5 using Euclidean distance as the similarity measure with taking help of Majority Voting technique for the determination of classification results. For LMA-NN, the number of neurons in hidden layer is 10, the value of the blending factor is 0.01, the increase and decrease factors of the blending factors are 10 and 0.1, respectively, and the stopping condition is considered when the attainment of minimum error gradient value reaches 1e−6. Ensemble decision tree classifier considers adaptive boosting principle taking maximum iterations as 100.

All the classifications have been performed in a multiclass basis, with SVM considered as an exception to the above-stated strategy since it can only perform binary classification. A binary confusion matrix is calculated and all the performance metrics are obtained. Further, to obtain the final performance index, the average of the performance metrics over all the classes is calculated. The performance metrics consist of positive predicted value, negative predicted value, sensitivity, specificity, accuracy, error rate and F1 score. For a binary confusion matrix, True Positive, True Negative, False Positive and False Negative samples are denoted by *TP*, *TN*, *FP* and *FN*, respectively.

$$\text{PPV} = \frac{TP}{TP + FP} \tag{7.42}$$

$$\text{NPV} = \frac{TN}{TN + FN} \tag{7.43}$$

$$\text{Sensitivity} = \frac{TP}{TP + FN} \tag{7.44}$$

$$\text{Specificity} = \frac{TN}{TN + FP} \tag{7.45}$$

$$\text{Accuracy} = \frac{TP + TN}{TP + TN + FP + FN} \tag{7.46}$$

$$\text{Error Rate} = \frac{FP + FN}{TP + TN + FP + FN} \qquad (7.47)$$

$$\text{F1 Score} = 2\frac{\text{Precision} \times \text{Recall}}{\text{Precision} + \text{Recall}} \qquad (7.48)$$

To further illustrate, the average and the standard deviation of the performance metrics are shown in Figure 7.11. It is clearly observed that IT2FS is producing better performance in terms of above-mentioned parameters when compared to other standard algorithms, which motivates us to establish our stand to choose IT2FS over other classifiers for the constrained framework and also provides confidence to use the proposed system in other real-time research applications in future also.

Figure 7.12 is dedicated to show the time requirement for all the competitive algorithms, where unit in y-axis is millisecond. It is evident that T1FS has lowest time for recognition of unknown gesture. But combining the results from Figures 7.11 and 7.12, IT2FS is the best choice for the proposed work.

Figure 7.13 shows the receiver operating curves (ROC) for all the concerned using proposed technique. The areas under curves for the three datasets are 0.7599, 0.8272, and 0.7410, respectively. It is evident that for all the three datasets equally good results are obtained.

The work captures Kinetic data at 5 fps, so the difference between two successive frames is 200 ms. The initial values for Khepera II robot are set at 20 mm/s for speed and 64 mm/s^2 for acceleration. Figure 7.14 pictorially gives the timing diagram, where x and y axes values with units are also given. Here, theoretical and experimental speed values are shown in blue and red color, respectively. The delay between those two speed values is obtained as 0.03 s. To have a clearer view the time axis is taken in millisecond unit.

These parametric advantages of the system are described here:

1. *Robustness analysis:* The proposed framework has been checked with three datasets taken from a large population of subjects, having varying body types. Despite of all the mentioned factors, the proposed framework provided equally promising results over all those datasets to justify the robustness of the algorithm.
2. *Convenience:* The proposed system is well adaptable also as it has minimal hardware requirements; hence, it is cost effective too. It requires a Kinect sensor, a CPU for capturing and analyzing human postures. Kinect sensor is preferred over other variations because of its easy availability and its capability of working in any surroundings and lighting conditions. Further the image and skeleton information

generated by the Kinect sensor in independent of the subject's attire. A single Kinect sensor is adequate for a room area; hence it is quite convenient to use this device in any industrial area. Because of the large coverage area, it reduces the total number of devices required for a large space in comparison with other sensor; hence the cost gets reduced too.

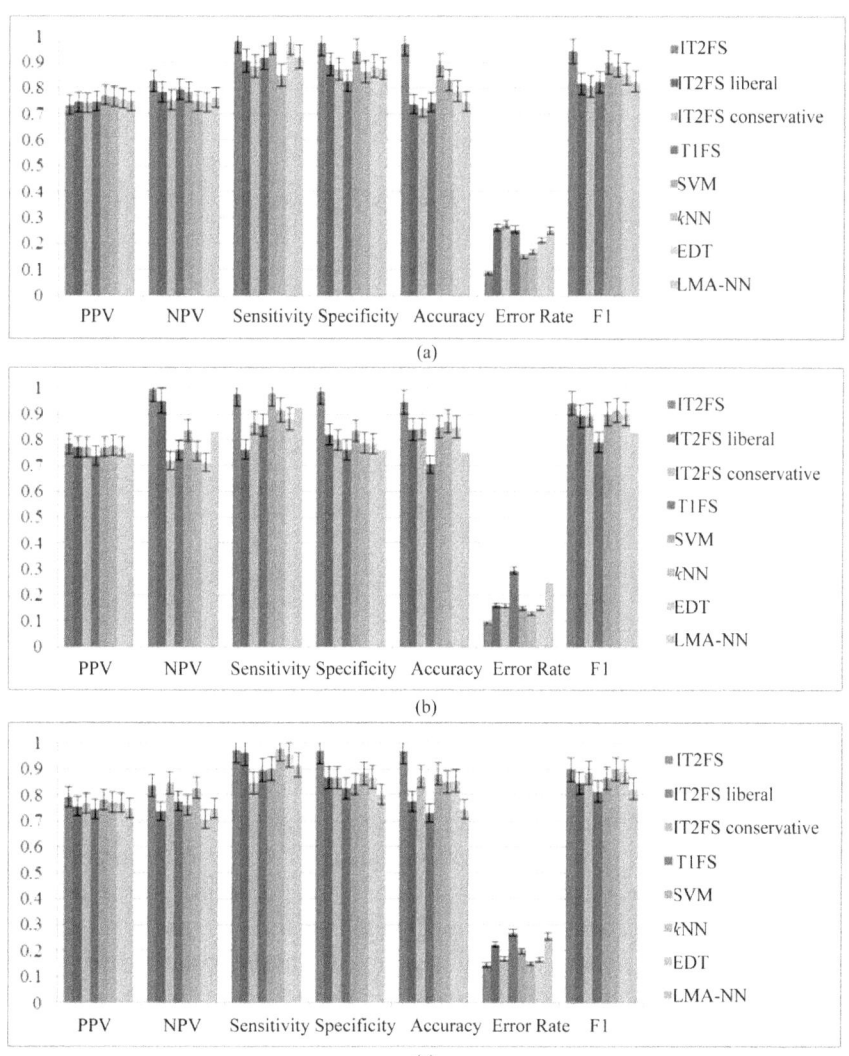

FIGURE 7.11 Performance analysis for competitive algorithms for three training datasets as given in Table 7.3: (a) dataset number 1, (b) dataset number 2 and (c) dataset number 3.

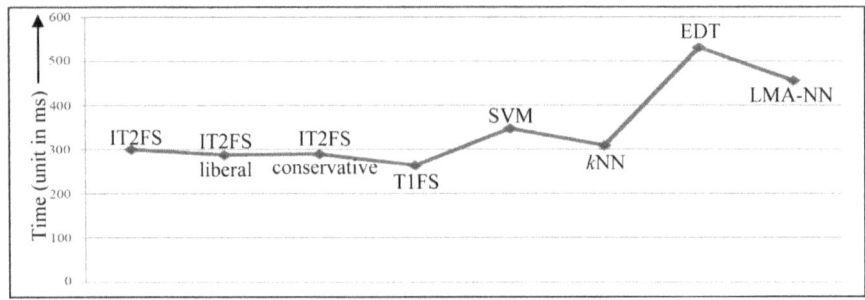

FIGURE 7.12 Time requirement of the algorithms.

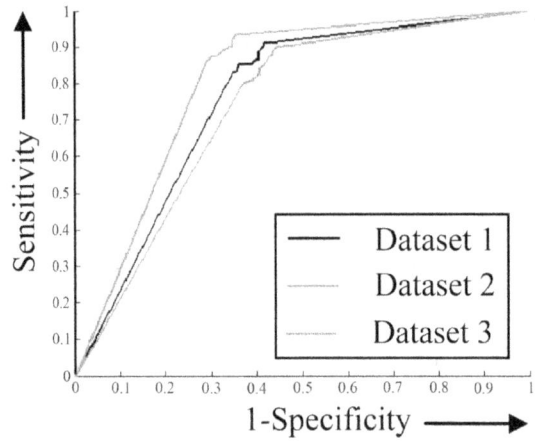

FIGURE 7.13 ROC curves.

3. *Benefits:* The presented work is to direct any mobile robot (here Khepera II robot is used) using body gestures in incoherent environments. Here both the speed and direction of the robot have been controlled using the gestures recognized by Kinect sensor.
4. *Productivity:* The said system detects and recognizes accurate Kinect generated gestures to instruct the robot according to the environmental requirements by analyzing the gestures for skeletal features.
5. *Convergence:* The time complexity of the proposed system is also quite satisfactory, which means it requires lesser or nearly equal time to produce better performance when compared to other standard systems in this domain.
6. *Flexibility:* The above-formulated strategy has been tested on three datasets, obtained from different subjects having largely varying

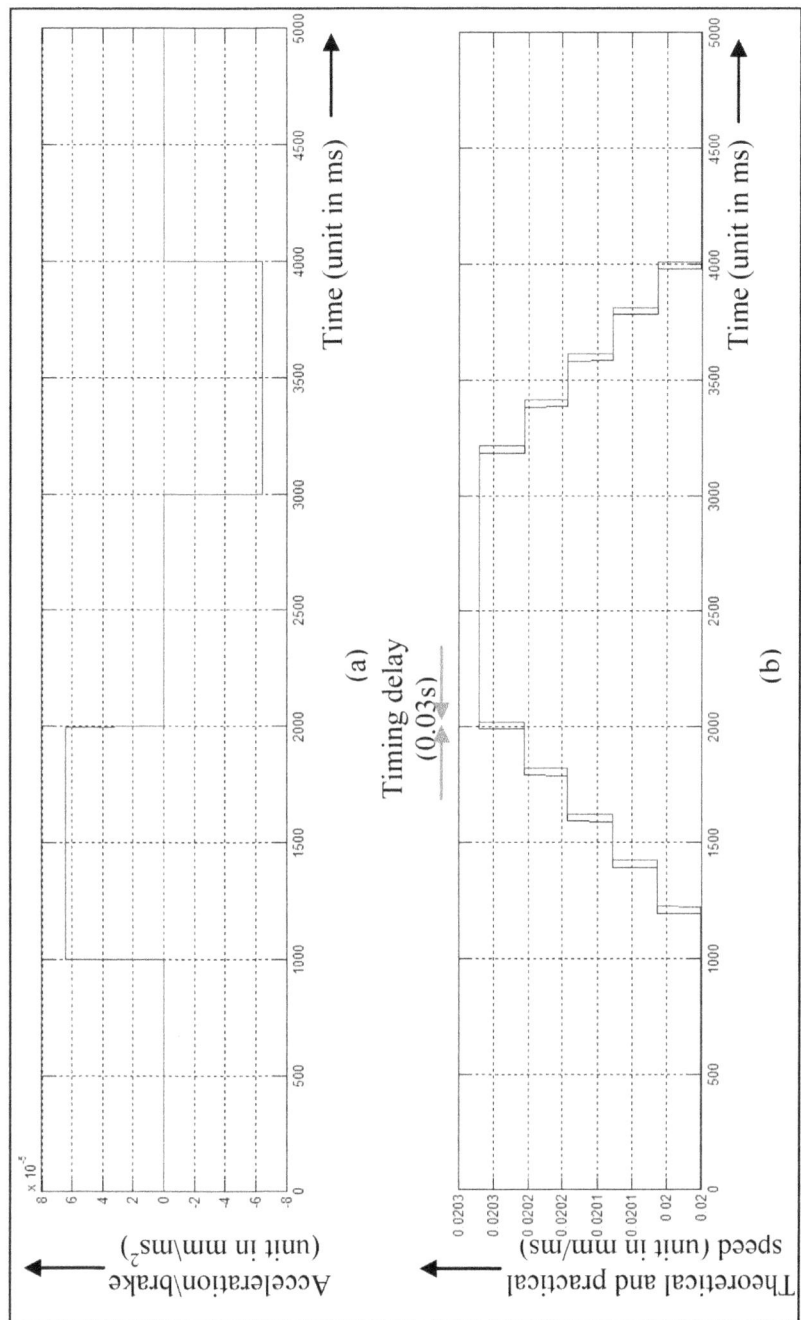

FIGURE 7.14 Time required to navigate robot using the proposed work: (a) for acceleration/brake values obtained from gestural command and (b) theoretical and practical speed values.

physical features and the system can be modified quite easily just by changing a mere code in the simulating software used for this purpose, which proves that the system is flexible enough to be used in real world scenarios.
7. *Feasibility:* The system that has been discussed so far has been implemented on research scholars and the online sessions are conducted in university laboratory. As the framework is designed for remote mobile robot control, so there is no need for the subjects to go to the incoherent environment, hence it can be concluded that feasibility is not an issue; the proposed system can be realisable in reality.
8. *Efficiency:* The proposed system shows an average accuracy of 96.8% for correctly classification of the gestures.
9. *Computational time:* The time required for recognizing an unknown gesture is 0.03 s for an Intel Core 2 Duo processor @ 1.60 GHz and 1 GB RAM with MATLAB R2012b.
10. *Diversity:* The proposed system maintains diversity also, since the system has been tested on datasets acquired from subjects having different physical features.
11. *Reliability:* Reliability is also a major issue that should be kept in mind always. The concept utilizes the Kinect's property of detecting 3D skeletons of different gestures belonging to the different subjects, who were present within a finite distance, in front of the sensor, irrespective of the colour of the skin or the subject's dress or the background. So even in terms of reliability the proposed framework can be used in any dynamically varying real-time situation.
12. Two statistical tests are evaluated to prove that the proposed work shows better performance over the existing ones.

7.4.4.1 FRIEDMAN TEST

If there are total C algorithms contending for a specific problem solution. Then the best performing algorithm among all others is given a rank of 1 and the worst in that scenario is assigned the rank of C. Let D be the total number of datasets. If R_c is the average ranking acquired by the cth ($1 \leq c \leq C$) algorithm over all d ($1 \leq d \leq D$), then the Friedman's statistic is [44]

$$\chi^2 = \frac{12D}{C(C+1)} \left[\sum_{c=1}^{C} R_c^2 - \frac{C(C+1)^2}{4} \right] \qquad (7.49)$$

Fuzzy-Based Stratagem for Teleoperation of Robots

In this chapter, $D = 3$ and $C = 8$. Table 7.6 reports that the null hypothesis is cancelled, as $\chi^2_F = 17.00$ is greater than the critical value of 14.067 of the χ^2 distribution for 7 ($=C - 1$) degrees of freedom at probability of 0.05 [45].

TABLE 7.6 Results Obtained From Friedman Test

Algorithm	Age Group 20–25	Age Group 25–30	Age Group 30–35	R_c	Friedman Test χ^2	Comment
IT2FS	1	1	1	1.00	17.00	Reject
IT2FS liberal	7	6	6	6.33		
IT2FS conservative	8	3	5	5.33		
T1FS	6	8	8	7.33		
SVM	2	2	3	2.33		
kNN	3	5	2	3.33		
EDT	4	4	4	4.00		
LMA-NN	5	7	7	6.33		

7.4.4.2 BONFERRONI–DUNN TEST

For Bonferroni–Dunn test, depicted in Figure 7.15, a critical difference (CD) [46] is 2.606 for $\alpha = 0.05$ for the proposed work. The performance of two algorithms is considerably distinct, only if the average ranks between those two algorithms differ by at least a CD.

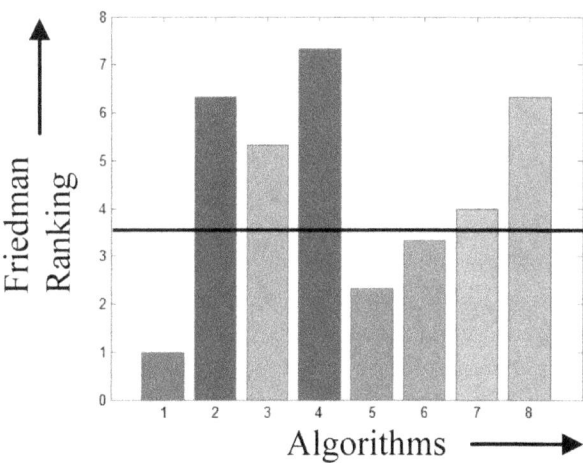

FIGURE 7.15 Bar chart view on of Bonferroni–Dunn's procedure.

7.5 CONCLUSIONS AND FUTURE DIRECTIONS

The explained system can be implemented for a teleoperation for robots using a gesture sensing device (a Kinect sensor), a computer, a wirelessly accessed robot (Khepera II) and a surveillance camera. It is useful for any incoherent environment where feasibility of human reaching that place is not possible, so his/her gestural commands are communicated to the robot for the necessary actions. If the said environment is static, then at times autonomous robot can be used for the same purpose, as the robot can be trained in an artificially built similar environment to perform the required task and then asked to perform the same in the originally constrained environment. But for a dynamically changing environment, the robot has to be provided with some sort of intelligence by transferring the necessary instructions, which are derived from an operator, who can monitor the entire scenario while sitting in a remote place.

Also in a multiagent scenario, if the goal has already been achieved, then aiming for that specific goal is no longer required. In such cases, the robots must be able to sense whether the target is already achieved or not, if so it should stop at that position, realign to the reference orientation and move back to the reference position and wait for the next target. In this way, not only extra effort will be saved but the time complexity can also be improved. The robots are generally designed to sense obstacles, but in a platform having multiple robots, it is necessary to sense other robots residing in close proximity to avoid collisions and faster achievement of targets. In such cases, the proposed work can provide better accuracy than the traditionally developed systems of automated robot path planning.

Gesture-based teleoperation is the best choice to counter those problems, not only because it maintains a high accuracy and provides a large number of options for robotic movements are concerned, but it also enables the mobile robot to act smoothly with higher degrees of freedom. Interval Type-2 fuzzy logic is used for the classification of gestural commands. We achieved an accuracy close to 100% which validated our reasoning to use the said system in different online experiments. The said algorithm has been compared with other standard classification algorithms and it provided better accuracy in terms of most precision parameters.

For the earlier works based on Kinect sensor, the feature set always included angular features between two planes, which can dense calculations for moderately configured personal computers. Moreover, confusion can also arise as the simulation software (MATLAB R2012B) always considers the acute angle between two planes which poses an ambiguity regarding whether to deal with the original angle or the alternate one (e.g., acute value can be obtained instead of obtuse value). In this chapter, we developed a completely distance-based normalized feature set, which are easy to deal with and those features also made it easier to formulate the strategies for solving the problem.

Not only robot control, this system is equally useful for designing a gesture commanding gaming where usual techniques use mouse or joystick, but the pleasure of playing virtual games using owns commands is way better. In this chapter, there are only mere provisions of application of acceleration and brakes, but a constant value is assumed for those parameters, later further research can be carried out to incorporate variable acceleration and brakes. The said mechanism can be extended and tested for multiple robot platforms in future as well.

KEYWORDS

- **gesture recognition**
- **incoherent environment**
- **interval Type-2 fuzzy set**
- **Khepera II**
- **Kinect sensor**
- **robot movement**

REFERENCES

1. Card, S. K., *The Psychology of Human-Computer Interaction*. CRC Press, FL, USA, 2018.
2. McClelland, J. L., "Is a machine realization of truly human-like intelligence achievable?," *Cognit. Comput.*, vol. 1, no. 1, pp. 17–21, 2009.
3. Du Toit, N. E., & Burdick, J. W., "Robotic motion planning in dynamic, cluttered, uncertain environments," *2010 IEEE Int. Conf. Robot. Autom.*, 3–7 May 2010, pp. 966–973, IEEE.
4. Murphy, R. R., "Human-robot interaction in rescue robotics," *IEEE Trans. Syst. Man, Cybern. Part C (Applications Rev.)*, vol. 34, no. 2, pp. 138–153, 2004.
5. Jaimes, A., & Sebe, N., "Multimodal human–computer interaction: A survey," *Comput. Vis. Image Underst.*, vol. 108, no. 1, pp. 116–134, 2007.

6. Diftler, M. A., et al., "Robonaut 2—the first humanoid robot in space," *2011 IEEE Conf. Robot. Autom.*, May 9, 2011, pp. 2178–2183, IEEE.
7. Zhao, S., & Yuh, J., "Experimental study on advanced underwater robot control," *IEEE Trans. Robot.*, vol. 21, no. 4, pp. 695–703, 2005.
8. Fields, M., Haas, E., Hill, S., Stachowiak, C., & Barnes, L., "Effective robot team control methodologies for battlefield applications," *2009 IEEE/RSJ Int. Conf. Intell. Robot. Syst.*, 2009, pp. 5862–5867.
9. Ono, T., Imai, M., & Ishiguro, H., "A model of embodied communications with gestures between human and robots," *Proceedings of the Annual Meeting of the Cognitive Science Society*, 2001, vol. 23, no. 23.
10. Konar, A. & Saha, S., *Gesture Recognition—Principles, Techniques and Applications*, vol. 724. Springer, 2018.
11. Kendon, A., *Gesture: Visible Action as Utterance*. Cambridge University Press, 2004.
12. Du, G., & Zhang, P., "Markerless human–robot interface for dual robot manipulators using Kinect sensor," *Robot. Comput. Integr. Manuf.*, vol. 30, no. 2, pp. 150–159, 2014.
13. Makris, S., Tsarouchi, P., Surdilovic, D., & Krüger, J. "Intuitive dual arm robot programming for assembly operations," *CIRP Ann. Technol.*, vol. 63, no. 1, pp. 13–16, 2014.
14. Tsarouchi, P., Athanasatos, A., Makris, S., Chatzigeorgiou, X., & Chryssolouris, G., "High level robot programming using body and hand gestures," *Proc. CIRP*, vol. 55, pp. 1–5, 2016.
15. Xing, G., Tian, S., Sun, H., Liu, W., & Liu, H., "People-following system design for mobile robots using kinect sensor," in *Control and Decision Conference (CCDC), 2013 25th Chinese*, 2013, pp. 3190–3194, Guiyang, China.
16. Mendel, J. M., & Rajati, M. R., "On computing normalized interval type-2 fuzzy sets," *Fuzzy Syst. IEEE Trans.*, vol. 22, no. 5, pp. 1335–1340, 2014.
17. Bustince Sola, H., Fernandez, J., Hagras, H., Herrera, F., Pagola, M., & Barrenechea, E., "Interval type-2 fuzzy sets are generalization of interval-valued fuzzy sets: towards a wider view on their relationship," 23(5), 1876–1882, 2015.
18. Correa, D. S. O., Sciotti, D. F., Prado, M. G., Sales, D. O., Wolf, D. F., & Osorio, F. S., "Mobile robots navigation in indoor environments using kinect sensor," in *2012 Second Brazilian Conference on Critical Embedded Systems*, 2012, pp. 36–41, Campinas, Brazil.
19. El-laithy, R. A., Huang, J., & Yeh, M., "Study on the use of Microsoft Kinect for robotics applications," in *Proceedings of the 2012 IEEE/ION Position, Location and Navigation Symposium*, 2012, pp. 1280–1288, Myrtle Beach, SC, USA.
20. Mondada, F., Franzi, E., & Guignard, A., "The development of khepera," in *Experiments with the Mini-Robot Khepera, Proceedings of the First International Khepera Workshop*, 1999, no. CONF, Paderborn, Germany.
21. Das, P. K., Behera, H. S., & Panigrahi, B. K., "Intelligent-based multi-robot path planning inspired by improved classical Q-learning and improved particle swarm optimization with perturbed velocity," *Eng. Sci. Technol. Int. J.*, vol. 19, no. 1, pp. 651–669, 2016.
22. Michel, O., "Khepera simulator version 2.0 user manual," *Univ. Nice–Sophia Antipolis. Lab. I3S-CNRS, Fr. Swiss*, 1996.
23. Prasad, B., *Soft Computing Applications in Business*, vol. 230. Springer Science & Business Media, 2008.
24. Ooi, C. C., & Schindelhauer, C., "Minimal energy path planning for wireless robots," *Mob. Netw. Appl.*, vol. 14, no. 3, pp. 309–321, 2009.

25. Mendel, J. M., "Uncertain rule-based fuzzy logic system: introduction and new directions," Springer International Publishing, p. 684, 2001.
26. Konar, A., *Computational Intelligence: Principles, Techniques and Applications*. Springer, 2005.
27. Konar, A., *Artificial Intelligence and Soft Computing: Behavioral and Cognitive Modeling of the Human Brain*, vol. 1. CRC press, FL, USA, 1999.
28. Halder, A., et al., "General and interval type-2 fuzzy face-space approach to emotion recognition." *IEEE Trans. Syst. Man. Cybern. Syst.*, vol. 43, no. 3, pp. 587–605, 2013.
29. Mendel, J. M., "On the importance of interval sets in type-2 fuzzy logic systems," in *IFSA World Congress and 20th NAFIPS International Conference, 2001. Joint 9th*, 2001, vol. 3, pp. 1647–1652.
30. Lee, C.-H., Hong, J.-L., Lin, Y.-C., & Lai, W.-Y. "Type-2 fuzzy neural network systems and learning," *Int. J. Comput. Cogn.*, vol. 1, no. 4, pp. 79–90, 2003.
31. Cupertino, F., Giordano, V., Naso, D., & Delfine, L., "Fuzzy control of a mobile robot," *Robot. Autom. Mag. IEEE*, vol. 13, no. 4, pp. 74–81, 2006.
32. Hamel, W. R., Murray, P., & Kress, R. L., "Internet-based robotics and remote systems in hazardous environments: review and projections," *Adv. Robot.*, vol. 16, no. 5, pp. 399–413, 2002.
33. Zhu, Y., & Ji, X., "Expected values of functions of fuzzy variables," *J. Intell. Fuzzy Syst.*, vol. 17, no. 5, pp. 471–478, 2006.
34. Pal, N. R., & (nee Dutta), K. P., "Handling of inconsistent rules with an extended model of fuzzy reasoning," *J. Intell. Fuzzy Syst.*, vol. 7, no. 1, pp. 55–73, 1999.
35. Parajuli, M., Tran, D., Ma, W., & Sharma, D., "Senior health monitoring using Kinect," in *2012 Fourth International Conference on Communications and Electronics (ICCE)*, 2012, pp. 309–312, **Hue**, Vietnam.
36. Le, T.-L., Nguyen, M.-Q., & Nguyen, T.-T.-M. "Human posture recognition using human skeleton provided by Kinect," in *2013 International Conference on Computing, Management and Telecommunications (ComManTel)*, 2013, pp. 340–345.
37. Theodoridis, S., Pikrakis, A., Koutroumbas, K., & Cavouras, D., *Introduction to Pattern Recognition: A Matlab Approach: A Matlab Approach*. Academic Press, 2010.
38. Oszust, M., & Wysocki, M., "Recognition of signed expressions observed by Kinect sensor," in *2013 10th IEEE International Conference on Advanced Video and Signal Based Surveillance (AVSS)*, 2013, pp. 220–225.
39. Mitchell, T. M., "Machine learning and data mining," *Commun. ACM*, vol. 42, no. 11, pp. 30–36, 1999.
40. Stone, E., & Skubic, M., "Fall detection in homes of older adults using the Microsoft Kinect," *IEEE J. Biomed. Health Inform.*, vol. 19, no. 1, pp. 290–301, 2014.
41. Dietterich, T. G., "An experimental comparison of three methods for constructing ensembles of decision trees: Bagging, boosting, and randomization," *Mach. Learn.*, vol. 40, no. 2, pp. 139–157, 2000.
42. Saha, S., Pal, M., Konar, A., & Janarthanan, R., "Neural network based gesture recognition for elderly health care using kinect sensor," in *Swarm, Evolutionary, and Memetic Computing*, Springer, 2013, pp. 376–386.
43. Vasant, P., Ganesan, T., Elamvazuthi, I., Barsoum, N., Faiman, D., & Vasant, P., "Solving deterministic non-linear programming problem using Hopfield artificial neural network and genetic programming techniques," in *AIP Conf. Proc.*, 2012, vol. 1499, no. 1, p. 311.

44. S. García, Molina, D., Lozano, M., & Herrera, F., "A study on the use of non-parametric tests for analyzing the evolutionary algorithms' behaviour: a case study on the CEC'2005 special session on real parameter optimization," *J. Heuristics*, vol. 15, no. 6, pp. 617–644, 2009.
45. Zar, J. H., *Biostatistical Analysis*. Pearson Education India, 1999.
46. Picek, S., Golub, M., & Jakobovic, D., "Evaluation of crossover operator performance in genetic algorithms with binary representation," in *Bio-Inspired Computing and Applications*, Springer, 2012, pp. 223–230.

CHAPTER 8

Sensor Architecture, Coverage, and Connectivity: A Comprehensive Study

SUSHREE B. B. PRIYADARSHINI[1*], D. SINGH[1], and R. SHARMA[2]

[1]*Department of Computer Science and Information Technology, Institute of Technical Education and Research, Siksha 'O' Anusandhan (Deemed to be University), Bhubaneswar, Odisha, India*

[2]*Department of Electronics and Communication Engineering, SRM University, NCR Campus, Ghaziabad, Uttar Pradesh, India*

*Corresponding author. E-mail: bimalabibhuprada@gmail.com.

ABSTRACT

In this modern era, the adoration of sensors is increasing rapidly with the peregrination of effective technologies. In this context, the issues of sensing coverage and network connectivity stand as the two major aspects in the context of environmental sensing and robust data reporting. Our current chapter elaborates on the fundamental studies on sensor architecture, coverage types, and connectivity while infusing the various types of coverage encountered in sensor networks. The aim of the chapter is to discuss the various concepts such as area coverage, barrier coverage, point coverage, target coverage, and *k*-coverage. Finally, we conclude our chapter while giving hints on future work.

8.1 INTRODUCTION

A sensor network is defined as a network consisting of a set of sensor nodes that are capable of sensing, computing, and communicating to different components in a specific environment—either a physical or environmental. A wireless sensor network (WSN) [1, 2] contains a number of sensor nodes equipped with storage devices that are monitored by either electricity, humidity, vibration, pressure, heat, or temperature. These sensor nodes can sense information and are capable of communicating and processing information to other neighbor nodes wirelessly. WSNs are self-organized information-retrieval networks where all the sensor nodes aggregate the data, information, and subsequently transfer to the sink that is controlled by a base station (BS).

Sensor nodes are arbitrarily sprinkled in a network. For any event occurring in the network, these sensor nodes send the required signals to the BS through the sink. BSs serve as a gateway through which communication with other networks become possible [3]. The most important fact is that the "supplied energy" is limited to a particular node. Thus, in order to transmit the data to other nodes in the network, how much coverage area and how much energy are available at those nodes are always considered as the important aspects.

8.1.1 WIRELESS SENSOR NETWORKS

In a WSN, sensor nodes are densely deployed. The nodes at the neighborhood may be deployed close to each other. Hence, the multihop communication has been regarded as one of the most efficient ways to consume less of power supply. Mostly all the sensor networks are data-centric in nature. The data-centric routing protocols are mainly dependent on the data aggregation and data association, which helps to solve the overlap problems with implosion. The protocols associated with WSN are also data-centric in nature, as well as it requires attribute-based naming. The data-centric approaches are performed in the following ways:

1. Sensor node broadcast the advertisement for the concerned data and wait for a request.
2. Sink broadcast the information to all nodes associated with it.

Sink node collects the information from all the sensor nodes associated with it and acts as a gateway as well as a backbone of all other networks [4]. The routing protocols are very often considered as a reverse multicast tree. So, the sink collects all concerned aggregated information from multiple sensor nodes as they are using the same routing way back to sink [5].

Sensor nodes get deployed arbitrarily in a large geographical area called the deployed area [6], which provides a robust and scalable performances. Due to the above reason, it is broadly used in various applications, that is, area monitoring, health monitoring, environmental sensing, and industrial monitoring. Environmental/earth sensing includes air pollution tracking, forest fire tracking, landslide tracking, agriculture automation [7], water quality ensnaring, and natural disaster avoidance [8]. Industrial tracking includes structural security [9], emergency response [10], machine health monitoring, data center, waste waters, structural health monitoring, and wine production.

The properties of a sensor network are characterized as combinations of localized or distributed sensors in an interconnection network and a group of computing resources connected to the central point (CP) of a cluster (group of similar types of sensor nodes). The major advantages of a WSN over conventional sensing systems are as follows:

1. Power expenditure constraints for nodes employing either batteries or harvesting system
2. Capability to handle with node failure
3. Mobility nature of sensor nodes
4. Ability to withstand harsh environmental conditions
5. Homogeneity and heterogeneity of nodes
6. Easy to use
7. Effective cross layer design.

The major challenge in this network (WSN) represents a longer period of network survival and high consumption of energy. The sensor nodes are driven by the supplied battery, and due to high consumption, the structure and low power design techniques cannot give an adequate solution [11]. These nodes normally depend upon the finite operating life-time batteries. To power a WSN node, the energy at that node can be harvested through the availability of potential ambient energy sources. Ambient energy harvesting is the process of accumulating and utilizing the energy [12] from the environment such as solar, mechanical, and thermal energy, and radiofrequency energy [13].

8.2 SENSOR ARCHITECTURE

The components of an energy-harvesting system architecture of a wireless sensor node are given below (Figure 8.1):

1. Sensor nodes and their equipments
2. An analog-to-digital converter that digitizes the analog signal produced through the sensors. The converter is connected with a microcontroller for further processing
3. A microcontroller
4. A low/high-power radio transceiver for receiving and transmitting the data and information

5. One memory to store the data (application), information (sensed), and source code
6. Ambient sources (external energy sources)
7. The energy harvesters and the systems
8. A power management system that helps in storage or transmit the energy from the harvesters for use
9. A harvesting energy storage device for future use.

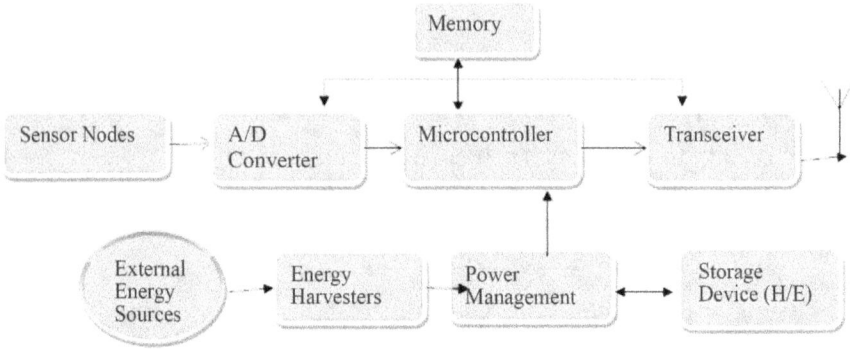

FIGURE 8.1 WSN architecture.

The architecture of WSN is important in the design of networking protocols. We can generally classify WSN architectures into single-hop, multi-hop, and two-tier hierarchical clusters.

8.2.1 SINGLE-HOP EH-WSN

In the single-hop architecture, all the sensor nodes are within the direct transfer range of the sink as illustrated in Figure 8.2. Although this architecture is simple, it is commonly used to achieve the tractable analysis of networking protocols.

8.2.2 MULTIHOP EH-WSN

In the multihop architecture (illustrated in Figure 8.3), except for a few nodes, data from the source nodes have to be relayed through intermediate sensor nodes. This is the most commonly assumed architecture in the WSN literature.

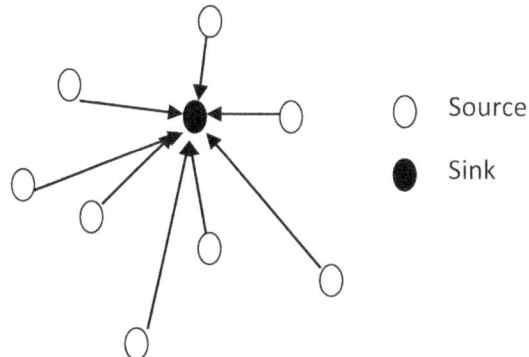

FIGURE 8.2 Single-hop architecture.

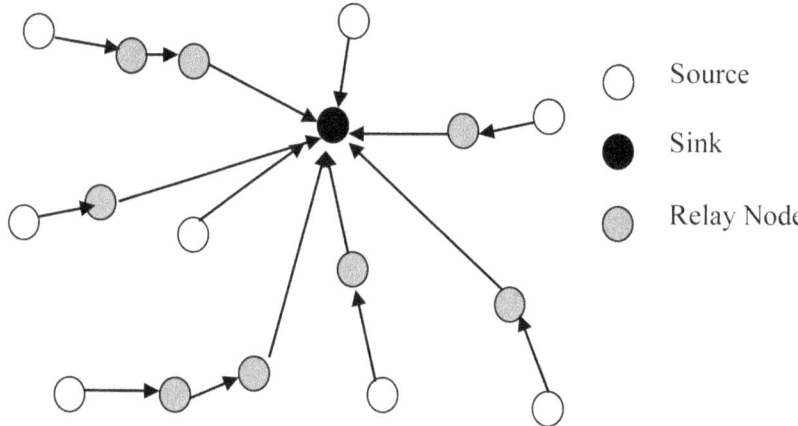

FIGURE 8.3 Multihop architecture.

8.2.3 TWO-TIER HIERARCHICAL CLUSTER

In WSN, the multiple nodes are deployed within a specified region and make a number of clusters and one cluster head (CH) from the clusters. There are different ways in which hierarchical architecture may be implemented in a heterogeneous network. The hierarchical cluster structure naturally decomposes a large network into smaller networks, containing the smaller number of cluster members, and creates different zones where data aggregation as well as processing can be accomplished locally. Single-hop or multihop information exchange may be present within the cluster members. Once the data reach at CH, it is routed through the two-tier network produced by another CH. The two-tier network may be a wired network and utilize a higher bandwidth. The two-tier nodes get connected by the wired framework. Having a wired network for the two-tier network is comparatively easier in building-like ambiance, however not for arbitrary deployments in distant positions.

8.3 CLASSIFICATION AND APPLICATIONS OF SENSORS

An appliance that converts a physical or chemical signal into an electronic signal is generally called a sensor node. It is an adaptor that is formed in large quantities by means of general microtechnologies. It is also called a compact measuring unit that converts chemical/biological, binary, physical parameters through transducers into an electrical outcome. Due to the maximum availability, most sensors have limited accuracy and low price.

As illustrated in Table 8.1, sensors can be classified on the basis of the input signals, applications, materials used in sensors, production technologies, conversion mechanism, cost, accuracy, coverage range, and characteristics.

TABLE 8.1 Types of Sensors

Types	Detection Properties
Thermal sensors	Temperature, specific heat, heat flow, etc.
Electrical sensors	Charge, current, voltage, resistance, inductance, etc.
Magnetic sensors	Magnetic flux density, magnetic moment, etc.
Optical sensors	Light intensity, wavelength, polarization, etc.
Mechanical sensors	Length acceleration flow, force, pressure, etc.
Chemical sensors	Composition, concentration, pH, etc.

Various applications of sensors are as follows:
1. Food and beverage processing
2. Health care
3. Combustion control
4. Waste water treatment
5. Automobiles
6. Customer product
7. Defense
8. Biosensors (chemical sensors in medicines)

9. Toxic and combustibles gas monitoring—residential use, that is, clothes dryer, dishwasher, etc.

8.4 COVERAGE ISSUE IN WSN

8.4.1 COVERAGE CLASSIFICATION

To monitoring the targets within the WSN, coverage is divided into three types:
1. Target coverage
2. Area coverage
3. Barrier coverage.

8.4.1.1 TARGET COVERAGE

It is otherwise called as point coverage. It is a target coverage scenario in which eight targets can be monitored by three sensor nodes in the deployment area. Targets t1, t2, and t3 are covered by the s1 sensor node; targets t3, t4, and t5 are covered by the s2 sensor node; and targets t5, t6, t7, and t8 are camouflaged by the s3 sensor node (Figure 8.4). The target coverage diminishes the energy expenditure due to deployed overlapping areas in the deployment area.

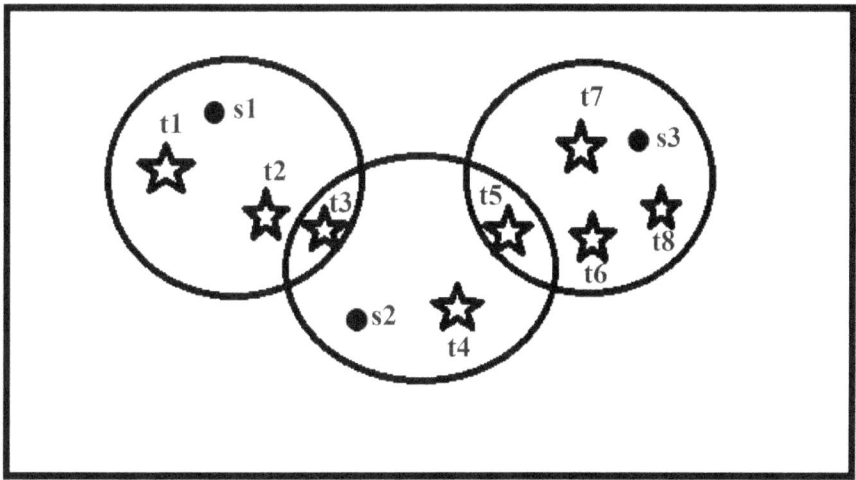

FIGURE 8.4 Target coverage.

8.4.1.2 AREA COVERAGE

It is otherwise called blanket coverage. In the deployment area, n numbers of sensor nodes get randomly sprinkled to track a given field of study. S1, S2, ..., S5 are the deployed sensor nodes in the network, and the circles represent the sensing range of each sensor nodes. A scenario of area coverage is portrayed in Figure 8.5.

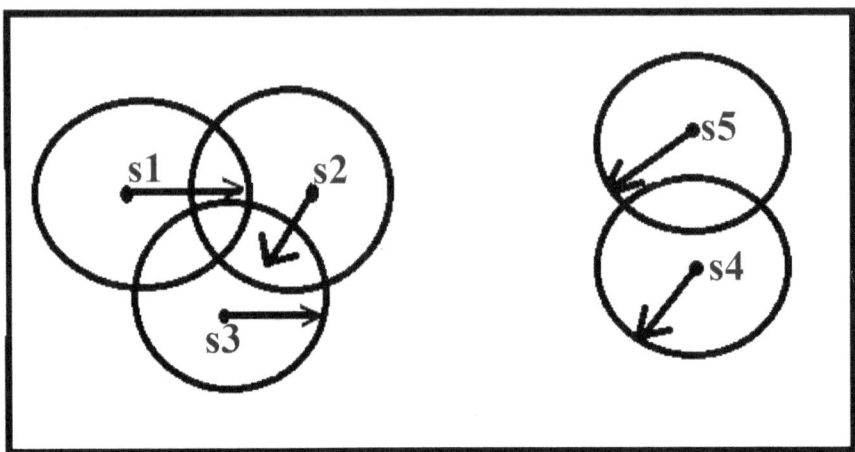

FIGURE 8.5 A scenario of area coverage.

8.4.1.3 BARRIER COVERAGE

Constructing a barrier for intrusion detection within a coverage area called barrier coverage. The sensor nodes can easily detect the intrusion if any intrusion prevails along the barrier. It can be divided into two categories, that is, strong and weak barrier coverage. In strong barrier coverage, the intruders must be ensnared through the sensor nodes, whereas in weak barrier coverage, either some uncovered zones or holes are present that helps in tracking the target. Figure 8.6 shows a situation of barrier coverage.

8.4.2 COVERAGE MODELS

In WSN, the tracking capability of the prevailing events can be measured by a coverage model. The coverage model forms the relationship between the sensitivity of the sensor nodes and the Euclidian distance of the concerned

Sensor Architecture, Coverage, and Connectivity

sensor from the physical point of interest. The coverage model can be classified into two categories according to the detection probability of the events occurred in the network.

1. Binary coverage model
2. Probabilistic coverage model.

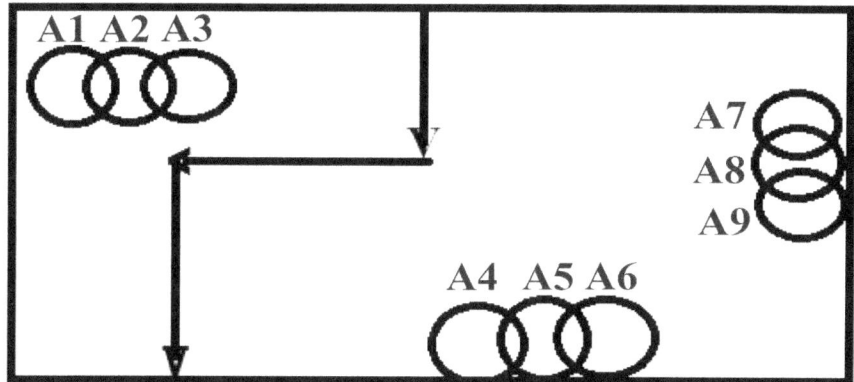

FIGURE 8.6 A scenario of barrier coverage.

8.4.2.1 BINARY COVERAGE MODEL

In WSN, monitoring of an event in the sensing zone of a sensor nodes is constant. It is otherwise called binary disk sensing (BDS), or the Boolean coverage model, or the deterministic disk coverage model. Further, the possibility of coverage of a sensor node S_n on a point P in the BDS model can be represented by Equation (8.1) as follows:

$$\text{Cov}(P, S_n) = \begin{cases} 1 & \text{if } d(p, \in_n) \leq S_n \\ 0 & \text{Otherwise} \end{cases}, \tag{8.1}$$

where S_n is the sensing range of a sensor node, $\in_n$ represents the position of a sensor node among S_n, and $d(p, \in_n)$ is the Euclidean distance between the positions of X and Y.

8.4.2.2 PROBABILISTIC COVERAGE MODEL

The binary coverage model may be further modified by the probability of tracking the corresponding events, known as the probability sensing coverage

(PSC) model. It reflects the real behavior of a sensor node. The probability of coverage of a sensor node $Cov(P,S_n)$ on a point P in the PSC model can be represented by Equation (8.2) as follows:

$$Cov(P,S_n) = \begin{cases} e^{-wd(p,\epsilon_n)^a} & \text{if } d(p,\epsilon_n) \leq S_n \\ 0 & \text{Otherwise} \end{cases}, \quad (8.2)$$

where the sensor node S_n can ensnare an object at point P with the probability $e^{-wd(p,\epsilon_n)^a}$ at a distance lesser than equal to the concerned sensing range, w is the physical features of S_n, and a represents the path loss of the system.

8.5 RELEVANT TERMINOLOGIES USED IN SENSOR NETWORKS

The following are the relevant terminologies and definitions that are used in the ensuing discussion:

8.5.1 EVENT

Event represents any sort of activity prevailing in the ensnared zone under consideration.

8.5.2 EVENT REGION

Event region indicates the specific area within which the event prevails. Initially, *camera sensors* and *scalar sensors* are sprinkled arbitrarily throughout the tracked event region.

8.5.3 INNER AND OUTER CAMERA SENSORS

Based on the event region location, the *camera sensors* are categorized as *inner cameras* and *outer cameras*. *Inner cameras* represent the *camera sensors* those reside completely within the purview of the prevailing event and *outer cameras* are the *camera sensors* those reside fully outside the prevailing event zone.

8.5.4 SENSING RANGE

Sensing range refers to the distance within which a *sensor* senses the occurring event(s). Basically, in conventional WSNs, the deployed *scalar sensors* gather information from the environment within a predetermined *sensing range* (generally a circular region characterized by the kind of *sensor* used) [15-18]. However, interactive *camera sensors* normally have greater detecting ranges. Specifically, *camera sensors* can ensnare the images of objects or parts of them which are not essentially closer to them. Moreover, every *camera sensor* perceives the corresponding environment from a different and unique viewpoint known as the *field of view* (FoV).

8.5.5   FIELD OF VIEW

FoV indicates the angle at which a *camera sensor* can ensnare the accurate image of any kind of object [15]. Depending on such angle, a *camera sensor* can be of the following two main types:

1. **Omni-directional camera sensor**: *Omni-directional camera sensor* is the *sensor* that ensnares the image of objects uniformly along all the directions and thus provides a panoramic view of the prevailing events.
2. **Directional camera sensor:** *Directional camera sensor* is the *sensor* that traps image of objects along a specified direction.

8.5.6   DEPTH OF FIELD

DoF indicates the distance within which a *camera sensor* can ensnare the perfect image of any object [15].

8.5.7   SENSING NEIGHBORS

Any two *sensors* SE_p and SE_q are called the *sensing neighbors* of each other, if the *Euclidian distance* between them is lower than the double (i.e., two times) of their *sensing ranges* [17].

8.5.8   SENSING REGION

Normally, the *sensing field* (i.e., the region where an event is sensed by the *sensors*) is camouflaged through the *camera sensors*. The term *sensing zone* represents a subregion within the *sensing field*, which is a collection of points. If and only if any two points are pertaining to the same *sensing zone*, they are camouflaged by the same set of *sensors*.

8.5.9 TARGET REGION

Such region indicates the *sensing region* where the *scalar sensors* track the prevailing event(s) [18]. At a particular point of time, we can represent the set of *target regions* in the entire *sensing field* [19].

8.5.10 SENSING MODEL RELATIONSHIP

There exist three types of *sensing model relationships* [15, 18] based on which *scalar sensors* are categorized into three types:

1. **Fringe scalar sensor:** If the disk sensing zone of a *scalar sensor* gets partially camouflaged by the DoF of a *camera sensor*, it is regarded as a *fringe scalar sensor*.
2. **Inner scalar sensor:** If the disk sensing zone of a *scalar sensor* gets completely within the DoF of a *camera sensor*, it is regarded as an *inner scalar sensor*.
3. **Outer scalar sensor:** If the disk sensing zone of a *scalar sensor* gets completely outside the DoF of a *camera sensor*, it is regarded as an *outer scalar sensor* [19].

8.5.11 SCALAR COUNT

Scalar count (SC) of a *camera sensor* refers to the number of event ensnaring *scalars* lying within DoF of the corresponding *camera sensor* [18-19]. The number of event ensnaring *scalar sensors* those reside within the purview of the *camera sensors* represents the SC value of the corresponding *camera sensor*.

8.5.12 SCALAR PREMIER

Scalar premier (SP) (scalar leader) refers to the representative of *scalar sensors* that acts as an informant for event information reporting to its corresponding *camera sensor(s)* within whose DoF(s) the SP is positioned.

8.5.13 CONNECTIVITY

Two *sensors*, SE_p and SE_q, located within a *two-dimensional* region are said to be connected if they can communicate with each other [16].

8.6 DATA REDUNDANCY ISSUE

This section rigorously analyzes the past reviews and discusses the threads of work carried out in the field of event zone coverage as well as redundant data diminishing. Currently, investigation on sensors advances toward becoming more prominent because of its popularity and presence of effectually powerful embedded platforms with high facility at diminishing expenses. With the development in technology, multimedia facility has been appended to *sensor nodes* [20, 23]. Therefore, currently, many research analysts have started working on WMSNs while investigating the various challenges and issues in the field. In this context, the comprehensive picture of both coverage and redundancy issues individually, and in some cases conjointly, involving the various techniques and strategies suggested by numerous researchers are outlined as follows.

8.6.1 SCALAR COUNT-BASED METHOD

One of the crucial contributions involving distributed camera actuation can be attributed to the work presented by Newell and Akkaya, where a major collaborative camera actuation scheme, namely, "Distributed Collaborative Camera Actuation based on Scalar Count (DCA-SC)" has been proffered. This scheme aims at lowering the number of *camera sensors* activated for averting possible redundancy in multimedia data transmission while enhancing the event region coverage. On occasion of a prevailing event, the *scalars* coming under the ambit of the *camera sensors* communicate them regarding the event occurrence.

Subsequently, the *camera sensors* being communicated by the *scalars* collaborate among each other by counting the number of event ensnaring *scalar sensors* residing within its DoF. Basically, in DCA-SC, the *camera sensors* are activated based on the decreasing sequence of their *scalar count* values (*scalar count* indicates the number of event ensnaring *scalar sensors* which reside within the DoFs of *camera sensors*) while matching the *ids* of *scalar sensors* residing within their respective DoFs.

8.6.2 EVENT BOUNDARY METHOD

A strategy namely the "Event Boundary (EB)" approach is proposed in [28] where the *scalar sensors* those reside at the boundary of the prevailing event can inform the *camera sensors* regarding the prevailing event instead of all the event detecting *scalar sensors* as used in the case of DCA-SC. As a result, the EB information becomes available to the corresponding *camera sensors* that will provide more accuracy in decision-making. At the beginning, every *sensor* exchanges its binary event measurement value (0 or 1) with its neighboring *sensors*. Afterward, each *sensor* independently decides whether it is a boundary *sensor* or not. Finally, each of the *sensors* verifies the number of 1s and 0s fetched. Being informed by the *scalar sensors*, the EB information becomes available to the *camera sensors* that help them to decide whether to be actuated or not.

8.6.3 SENSING REGION MANAGEMENT METHOD

A novel scheme called "Distributed Collaborative Camera Actuation Scheme based on Sensing Region Management (DCCA-SM)." In this approach, the entire network [19] is assumed to be consisting of two layers of *sensors*: *scalars* and *cameras*. The complete monitored zone is segregated into a number of *sensing zones* that are covered by various sets of *camera sensors* and *scalar sensors*. In each of the sensing regions, representatives of *scalars* called *scalar CHs* are selected by forming a cluster of *scalar sensors* those are periodically determined according to the remaining energy among the *scalar sensors*. These scalar CHs report their corresponding *camera*(s) regarding the event occurrence instead of all the *scalars*. Thereafter, being informed from the *scalar CHs*, the *camera sensors* can find out the superimposing zones exactly without any event coverage calculation algorithm during the whole coordination phase.

Three types of sensing model relationships exist in this approach based on the position of *scalars* with respect to FoV as well as DoF of the *camera sensors*. Accordingly, the *scalar sensors* can be categorized as the *inner scalar sensor*, *fringe scalar sensor*, and *outer scalar sensor*. Both *inner* and *fringe scalar sensors* take part in event information communication. The *fringe scalar sensors* always convey the event information to their nearest *camera sensors*. Further, the events prevailing in every *sensing zone* can be effectively monitored through the selected *scalar CHs*. Further, the *outer scalar sensor* that does not reside within the FoV of any of the *cameras* never take part in information exchange.

8.6.4 K-COVERAGE, LIFETIME EXTENSION, AND SCHEDULING-ORIENTED COVERAGE METHOD

A particular point is called as *k-covered* if it lies within the sensing ranges of *k-sensors*. A dynamic *k*-coverage scheduling scheme (DKCS) is proposed in which the aim is at prolonging the network lifetime while satisfying the required *k*-coverage. In this approach, a *virtual hexagon topology* is utilized to initialize the *sensor* members of each of the layers. The whole area is segregated into a set of virtual equal-sized hexagonal cells termed *redundancy cells* (RCs) by following the concept used by Xiaofei [19]. DKCS builds a maximal number of layers where every layer is *1*-covered and *1*-connected. Besides, it provides two types of *k*-coverage: *static k-coverage* and *dynamic k-coverage*. In *static k-coverage*, each point in the zone is *k*-covered, whereas in the case of *dynamic k-coverage*, *k*-coverage is provided merely for the intruder nodes.

Further, the research in [21] addresses the scheduling problem where a set of *sensors* and targets are presented in a Euclidean plane. A *sensor* can entrap merely one *target* at a given moment. In this proposal, the *sensors* are planned to track the *targets* so that the lifetime of the whole framework is amplified, where the lifetime is the entire duration within which all the intended *targets* are to be viewed. Moreover, a distributed mechanism for maintaining full coverage of an environment by using deployed *mobile sensors* is demonstrated in [22].

The coverage issue represents a crucial predicament for *sensor networks* and thus, various research contributions are dedicated to this problem. Further, since the energy of *sensors* is constrained and it is infeasible to supplant them, conserving the energy of the *sensors* while ensuring the coverage of targets/areas is a pivotal issue in practical applications. Extensive spectrum of investigations about the coverage issue exists in omni-directional *sensor* frameworks [24,25]. First, the coverage problem discussed in [24] considers that a large number of *sensors* are scattered randomly near to a set of *targets* and they report the detected data to a central processing *sensor*.

8.6.5 GRAPH-BASED APPROACHES

In [26], efficient algorithms are presented for finding a path with maximum observability under a general assumption of the sensing model. Further, it is justified to be the same as the best coverage problem, which can be solved by an efficient distributed algorithm using the relative neighborhood graph to be constructed locally. In this approach, the way of finding an optimum best coverage path that travels a low distance is discussed. Another work [27] advocates the coverage issue from various points of views and defines the best- and worst-case coverage in *sensor networks*. Moreover, the major highlights of the paper have been established by incorporating computational geometry and graph theoretic methods, specifically the *Voronoi diagram* and graph search algorithms. Furthermore, various potential applications have been analyzed in the same paper for enhancing coverage.

8.6.6   QUALITY-BASED COVERAGE APPROACH

The coverage problem in directional sensor networks is discussed in [28], where the *targets* need various coverage qualities. In this paper, a set of directions are regarded as a feasible cover set if it can gratify the coverage quality for each *target*. Moreover, the work is aimed at maximizing the network lifetime of a directional sensor network which is accomplished through organizing the directions of *sensors* into nondisjoint subsets, each of which represents a feasible cover set.

8.6.7   GRID-BASED APPROACH

A grid-based working node (WN) choice method has been demonstrated that considers the area coverage problems for WSNs. In this approach, a minimal subset of nodes serve as WNs, and rest of the nodes are deactivated for conserving power and to bring down their interference. Every vertex on the grid denotes a point in the checked territory. The primary motto of the proposed solution is to present the coverage of *sensors* by various sample points (i.e., the intersection points of the established grids).

8.6.8   PRIORITY-BASED COVERAGE APPROACH

A priority-based *target* coverage approach is presented in [29] where all the *targets* get attached with different priorities. This approach is aimed at determining the minimal subset of directional *sensors* that can track all the desired *targets* gratifying the concerned priorities. By proffering the direction partition strategy, the priority augmented graph and leveraging the genetic strategy, the minimal subset of sensors gets well defined.

8.6.9 COVER SET-BASED APPROACHES

To attain effective tracking of the targets by *sensors*, distinct coverage schemes have been developed. Such approaches segregate the *sensors* into cover sets, where every cover set is capable of ensnaring all the desired targets. A new coverage methodology is advocated [16] that can generate both disjoint cover sets (i.e., cover sets having no common sensor nodes) and nondisjoint cover sets (i.e., cover sets having common sensor nodes). Tracking a set of discrete targets simultaneously is a crucial issue in WSNs. One approach to solve such predicament is framing an effective scheduling strategy that is capable of organizing *sensors* into various cover sets so that every cover set can track all the intended targets. Further, several pruning rules get designed for averting the determination of redundant *sensors* while conjointly managing the concerned sensors.

8.6.10 ART-GALLERY-BASED COVERAGE METHOD

Art gallery problem [30] is basically used for determining the least number of *sensors* and their positions to afford 100% coverage of the zone under speculation, once the FoVs of *camera sensors* are known. However, such a problem cannot be applied to the situation of the real-life random placement of *sensors*, because for the art gallery solution, the prior manual placement of *camera sensors* is to be accomplished considering that the topology for *scalar sensors* is known in advance.

Similarly, various papers are developed in [31, 32] that aim at diminishing the redundant data transmitted while maximizing the coverage of the monitored zone under consideration. In [31], a centralized cum subcentralized scheme is addressed where a BS along with a substation is present. Further, the paper [32] elaborates a hexagonal scheme that determines SPs in a hexagonal fashion that operate as the nominee of scalars for conveying the prevailing event information.

8.7 CONCLUSIONS

This chapter presented a systematic study of existing investigation sensor architecture, coverage, connectivity, and redundancy in data transmission. To accomplish this goal, we have discussed the details of coverage types and coverage models. Subsequently, the relevant terminologies have been elaborated while elaborating the concepts of sensing and target zones. Finally, we have discussed the redundancy issue and various work done concerning it.

KEYWORDS

- sensors
- coverage
- connectivity
- k-coverage

REFERENCES

1. Karl, H.; Willig, A., *Protocols and Architectures for Wireless Sensor Networks*, John Wiley & Sons, **2005**.
2. Yick, J.; Mukherjee, B.; Ghosal, D., Wireless sensor network survey, *Computer Networks Journal*, **2008**, vol. 52, no. 12, pp. 2292–2330.
3. Dargie, W.; Poellabauer, C., *Fundamentals of Wireless Sensor Networks: Theory and Practice*, John Wiley & Sons, **2010**.
4. Bajaber, F. G., Design, analysis and performance evaluation of communication protocols under various topologies to enhance the lifetime of wireless sensor networks, *PhD Dissertation*, University of Bradford, **2011**.
5. Sudevalayam, S.; Kulkarni, P., Energy harvesting sensor nodes: Survey and implications, *IEEE Communications Surveys and Tutorials*, **2010**, vol. 13, no. 3, pp. 443–461.
6. Sonam, M.; Jain, K. V., Fuzzy based energy efficient sensor network protocol for precision agriculture, *Computers and Electronics in Agriculture*, **2016**, vol. 130, pp. 20–37.
7. Anastasi, G.; Conti, M.; Francesco, M. D.; Passarella, A., Energy conservation in wireless sensor networks: A survey, *Ad Hoc Networks Journal*, **2009**, vol. 7, no. 3, pp. 537–568.
8. Paradiso, J. A.; Starner, T., Energy scavenging for mobile and wireless electronics, *IEEE Pervasive Computing*, **2005**, vol. 4, no. 1, pp. 18–27.
9. Arms, S. W.; Townsend, C. P.; Churchill, D. L.; Galbreath, J. H.; Mundell, S. W., Power management for energy harvesting wireless sensors, in *SPIE International Symposium on Smart Structures and Smart Materials*, **2005**, vol. 5763, pp. 267–275.
10. Alippi, C.; Galperti, C., An adaptive system for optimal solar energy harvesting in wireless sensor network nodes, *IEEE Transactions on Circuits and Systems*, 2008, vol. 55, no. 6, pp. 1742–1750.
11. Anastasi, G.; Conti, M.; Francesco, Di; Passarella, A., Energy conservation in wireless sensor networks: A survey, *Ad Hoc Networks*, **2009**, vol. 7, no. 3, pp. 537–568.

12. Stefano, B.; Naderi, M. Y.; Petrioli, C.; Spenza, D., Wireless sensor networks with energy harvesting, *Mobile Ad Hoc Networking: The Cutting Edge Directions*, **2013**, pp. 701–736.
13. Hande, A.; Polk, T.; Walker, W.; Bhatia, D., Indoor solar energy harvesting for sensor network router nodes, *Microprocessors and Microsystems*, **2007**, vol. 31, no. 6, pp. 420–432.
14. Newell, A.; Akkaya, K., Distributed collaborative camera actuation for redundant data elimination in wireless multimedia sensor networks, *Ad Hoc Networks*, **2011**, vol. 9, no. 4, pp. 514–527.
15. Naumowicz, T.; Freeman, R.; Kirk, H.; Dean, B.; Calsyn, M.; Liers, A.; Braendle, A.; Guilford, T.; Schiller, J., Wireless sensor network for habitat monitoring on Skomer Island, In *Proceedings of 35th Annual IEEE Conference on Local Computer Networks* (*LCN*), Denver, CO, USA, **October 10–14, 2010**.
16. Ghosh, A.; Das, S. K., Coverage and connectivity issues in wireless sensor networks: A Survey, *Pervasive and Mobile Computing*, **2008**, vol. 4, no. 3, pp. 303–334.
17. Al-Shalabi, A.; Manaf, M., DkCS: An efficient dynamic k-coverage scheduling algorithm for wireless sensor networks, *2012 International Symposium on Telecommunication Technologies* (*ISTT*), Kuala Lumpur, Malaysia, November **2012**.
18. https://cs.wmich.edu/~gupta/teaching/cs603/wsnSp04/habitatMontor%20analysis%20bookchapter.pdf (Last date of access: April 30, 2017).
19. Priyadarshini, Sushree B. B., Adequate Coverage of Event Region based on Optimum Camera Actuation in Redundant Data Elimination for Wireless Multimedia Sensor Networks, **2018**, *PhD Thesis*, Veer Surendra Sai University of Technology.
20. https://www.defit.org/data-redundancy/
21. Liang, J.; Liu, M.; Kui, X., A survey of coverage problems in wireless sensor networks, *Sensors & Transducers*, **2014**, vol. 163, no. 1, 240–246.
22. Hung, L.-L.; Huang, Y.-W.; Lin, C.-C., Temporal coverage mechanism for distinct quality of monitoring in wireless mobile sensor networks, *Ad Hoc Networks*, **2014**, vol. 21, pp. 97–108.
23. Guvensan, M. A.; Yavuz, A. G., On coverage issues in directional sensor networks: A survey, *Ad Hoc Networks*, **2011**, vol. 9, no. 7, 1238–1255.
24. Cardei, M.; Thai, M. T.; Li, Y.; Wu, W., Energy-efficient target coverage in wireless sensor networks, *Proceedings IEEE INFOCOM*, **2005**, vol. 3, pp. 1976–1984.
25. Huang, C-F; Tseng, Y-C., A survey of solutions to the coverage problems in wireless sensor networks, *Journal of Internet Technology*, **2005**, vol. 6, no. 1, pp. 1–8.
26. Li, X-Y.; Wan, P-J; Frieder, O., Coverage in wireless ad hoc sensor networks, *IEEE Transactions on Computers*, **2003**, vol. 52, no. 6, pp. 753–763.
27. Megerian, S.; Koushanfar, F.; Potkonjak, M.; Srivastava, M., Worst and best-case coverage in sensor networks, *IEEE Transactions on Mobile Computing*, **2005**, vol. 4, no. 1, pp. 84–92.
28. Yang, H., Li, D.; Chen, H., Coverage quality based target-oriented scheduling in directional sensor networks, In: *Proceedings of 2010 IEEE International Conference on Communications* (*ICC*), Cape Town, South Africa, **2010**.
29. Wang, J.; Niu, C.; Shen, R., Priority-based target coverage in directional sensor networks using a genetic algorithm, *Computers and Mathematics with* Applications, **2009**, vol. 57, no. 11–12, pp. 1915–1922.

30. O'Rourke, J., Open problem from art gallery solved, *International Journal of Computational Geometry and Applications*, **1992**, vol. 2, pp. 215–217.
31. Priyadarshini, Sushree B. B.; Panigrahi, S., Centralised cum sub-centralised scheme for multi-event coverage and optimum camera activation in wireless multimedia sensor networks, *Special Issue on Creating a Smarter Environment through Advancement of Communication Systems, Networks and Applications, IET Networks, Published in IET and IEEE Xplore Digital Library*, **2015**, vol. 4, no. 6, pp. 314–328.
32. Priyadarshini, Sushree B. B.; Panigrahi, S., Redundant data minimization using hexagonal scalar premier neighbourhood for optimum camera actuation, *Journal of Engineering*, **2016**, vol. 2016, no. 3, pp. 1–11.

CHAPTER 9

Smart Antennas for Contemporary Wireless Communication Systems: Concepts, Challenges, and Performance

GARIMA SRIVASTAVA[1*], NEETA SINGH[1], and SACHIN KUMAR[2]

[1]Department of Electronics and Communication Engineering, Ambedkar Institute of Advanced Communication Technologies and Research, Delhi, India

[2]School of Electronics Engineering, Kyungpook National University, Daegu, Republic of Korea

*Corresponding author. E-mail: garima.shrivastav@gmail.com.

ABSTRACT

The emerging wireless communication systems need an antenna configuration with a large coverage area, substantial system capacity, and improved spectral efficiency. All these requirements are only possible if one makes use of smart antennas, the antennas with signal processing capability. The smart antenna can adjust its beam pattern according to the system requirements, to decrease the signal of interference and enhance the signal of interest. Smart antennas can overcome the problem of signal fading, interference due to frequency reuse, and limited battery life of handheld terminals. The main functions of smart antennas are beamforming and direction of arrival estimation, which has been described in detail in this chapter. The applications of smart antennas for satellites, radars, acoustic signal processing, cellular systems, and GPS/Wi-Fi/WLAN/Wi-MAX are also presented in the further sections.

9.1 INTRODUCTION

An antenna is a device through which electrical signals from the transmitter are radiated into free space in the form of radio frequency (RF) energy. The contemporary wireless applications need versatile and dynamic antennas that can adapt according to the system requirements. The smart antenna is composed of steerable transmitting/receiving systems that dynamically make changes in the antenna radiation pattern to encounter channel fading effects [1]. In this way, the smart antenna solves the issue of multipath fading in the band of interest, thereby achieving an output with a better signal-to-noise ratio. The smart antenna senses electromagnetic (EM) waves in an adaptive fashion by using signal processing algorithms [2]. The signal processing algorithms and steerable mechanism in smart antennas improve the performance/capacity of the wireless system, without increasing the channel bandwidth or transmit power.

Basically, smart antennas are metal arrays that are terminated to a sophisticated digital signal processor. Due to their digital signal processing (DSP) capability, these antennas are called "smart." The digital signal processors integrated with these antennas make them capable of adjusting or adapting their beam pattern, to enhance the signal of interest and suppress the interfering signals [3–6]. The combination of digital electronics based hardware and signal processing tools made smart antennas a reality for modern and forthcoming wireless communications systems.

The smart antennas are usually surrounded by a switched beam formed by several adaptive systems. The switched beam arrangement has a fixed beam pattern and depending upon the requirements, the beam can be accessed at a given point of time. In such systems, the beam can be directed in any desired path and interfering signals can be canceled easily. The smart antenna systems achieve improved performance either by combining diversity techniques/multiple-input multiple-output (MIMO) or by the help of adaptively weighted excitations to antenna elements, for optimizing antenna pattern performance [7, 8]. Earlier, the smart antennas were known as adaptive or digital beamforming arrays but these days they are famous as MIMO. The traditional system is neither intelligent nor adaptive. On the other hand, the smart antennas are designed to adapt changing signals environment, accordingly optimizing the digital processing algorithms [9, 10].

9.2. NEED FOR SMART ANTENNAS

The major problems faced by the radio communication system are as follows:

1. A small bandwidth is allocated for uplink and downlink.
2. The indoor and outdoor multipath signal fading and spreading of a signal.
3. Small battery life of portable devices.
4. Frequency reuse interference.

To overcome the above-mentioned challenges many techniques, such as multiple access, channel coding, equalization, and smart antennas, have been devised [11].

In conventional communication systems, only one antenna is used at the transmitter or receiver. This method is popularly known as a single-input single-output (SISO) system. When an EM wave comes across to obstacles such as mountains, buildings, or any other movable/immovable objects, the wavefront scatters and signals take numerous paths to reach the terminal. The multipath fading factors reduce the speed of transmission and a degraded signal is received at the destination. These effects can be reduced by means of smart antennas and diversity techniques [12, 13]. A base station with smart antennas eliminates cochannel effects of the nearby base stations, in contrast to base stations that use omnidirectional antennas [6], as depicted in Figure 9.1.

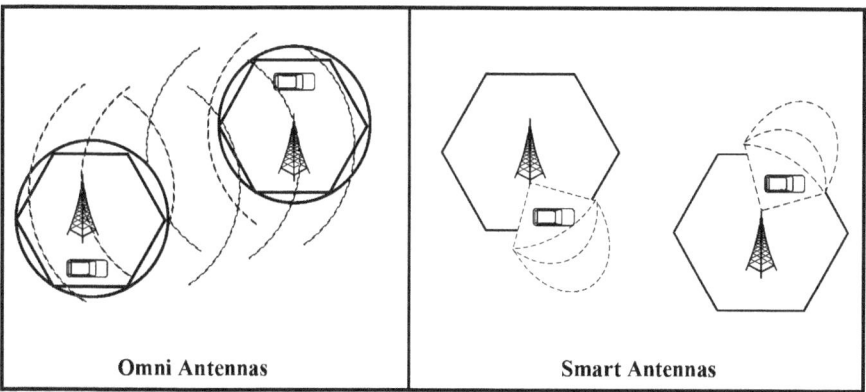

FIGURE 9.1 Interference reduction using smart antennas [6].

Source: Adapted from http://lib.unipune.ac.in:8080/xmlui/bitstream/handle/123456789/6991/12_chapter%203.pdf?sequence=12&isAllowed=y

9.3 CLASSIFICATION OF SMART ANTENNAS

The classification of smart antennas is shown in Figure 9.2.

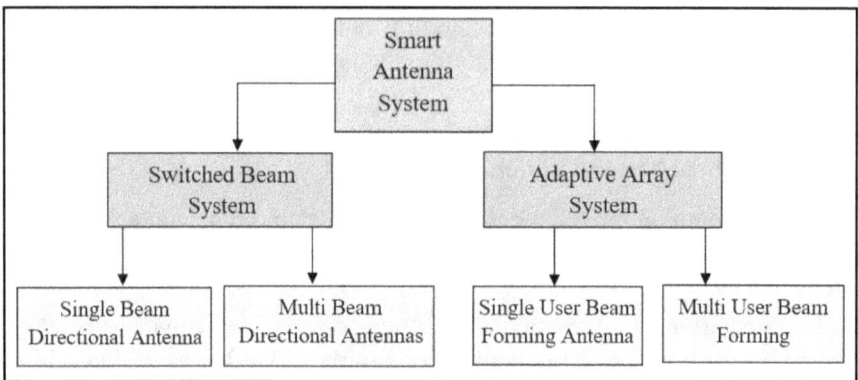

FIGURE 9.2 Classification of smart antennas.

Depending on the type of environment and requirement of the system the smart antennas are described below.

9.3.1 SWITCHED BEAM/PHASE ARRAY/BEAM SMART/MULTIBEAM ANTENNA

The switched beam smart antenna schematic is shown in Figure 9.3. In this type of antenna, there are several fixed beam patterns, out of which one beam is selected and steered in the direction of the desired output. This can be accomplished by correcting the phase of the signals. In other words, the beam will be steered with the movement of wanted targets [3].

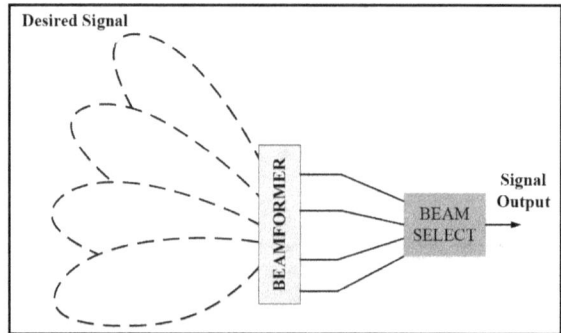

FIGURE 9.3 Schematic of switched beam smart antenna [3].

Source: Adapted from https://www.circuitstoday.com/smart-antennas

9.3.2 SINGLE BEAM DIRECTIONAL ANTENNA

In this antenna, only one beam is used at a specific time. The simultaneous transmission of beams is not permitted in this system [5].

9.3.3 MULTIBEAM DIRECTIONAL ANTENNA

In this antenna, simultaneous transmission of beams is permitted. It is a type of spatial division multiple access (SDMA) system [5].

9.3.4 ADAPTIVE ARRAY SMART ANTENNA

In this type, the beam shape will be changed following the movement of the wanted user and interference. The received signal will be weighted and combined to increase the wanted signal to interference ratio. This antenna can easily steer the beam in the preferred direction and simultaneously canceling the interfering signals. The direction of arrival (DOA) estimation method can be used to find the direction of the beam [14, 15]. The adaptive array smart antenna is shown in Figure 9.4.

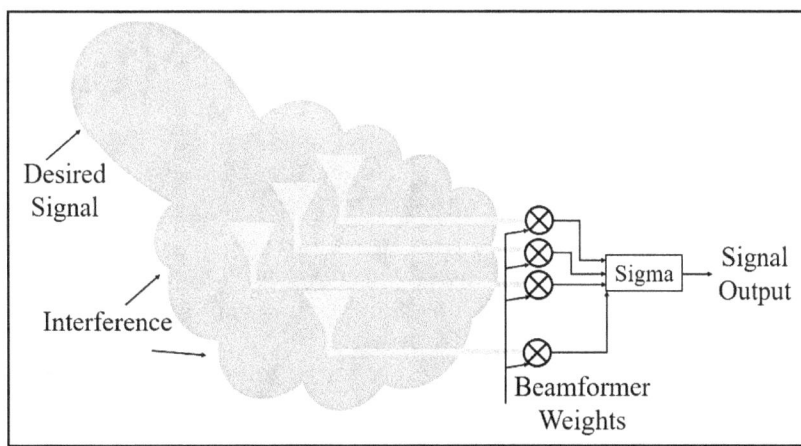

FIGURE 9.4 Adaptive array smart antenna.

9.3.5 SINGLE USER BEAMFORMING

In this antenna, as shown in Figure 9.11, the antenna beam is tuned to catch the desired signal and cancel the undesired signals [5].

9.3.6. MULTIUSER BEAMFORMING

In this antenna, as shown in Figure 9.12, there are various beam patterns, which are used for the tracking of many users. Thus, simultaneous transmissions are permitted and SDMA is realized. It can have multiple transceiver beam pairs [5].

9.4 TYPES OF SMART ANTENNAS DEPENDING ON THE NUMBER OF INPUT/OUTPUT

9.4.1 SINGLE-INPUT MULTIPLE-OUTPUT

This type of smart antenna, as shown in Figure 9.5, has only one transmitter at the source and multiple receivers at the terminus [4].

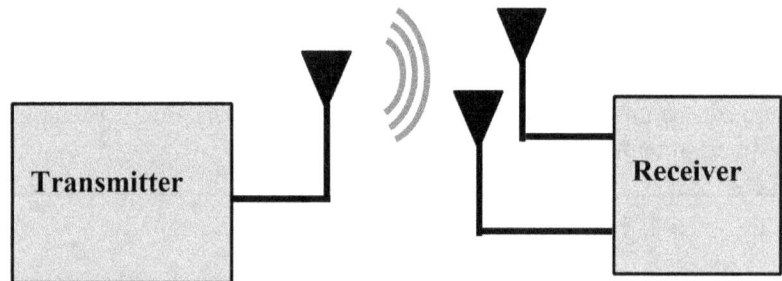

FIGURE 9.5 Single-input-multiple-output.

9.4.2 MULTIPLE-INPUT SINGLE-OUTPUT

In this type of smart antenna, as shown in Figure 9.6, there are multiple antennas at the source (transmitter), and there is only one antenna at the destination (receiver) [4].

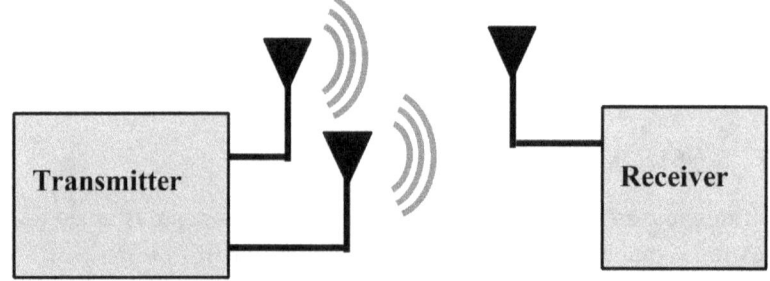

FIGURE 9.6 Multiple-input single-output.

Smart Antennas for Contemporary Wireless 211

9.4.3 MULTIPLE-INPUT MULTIPLE-OUTPUT

In this type of smart antenna, as shown in Figure 9.7, there are multiple antennas at source (transmitter) and destination (receiver) [4]. The space-time coding is used with, which does not require channel information at the source [14].

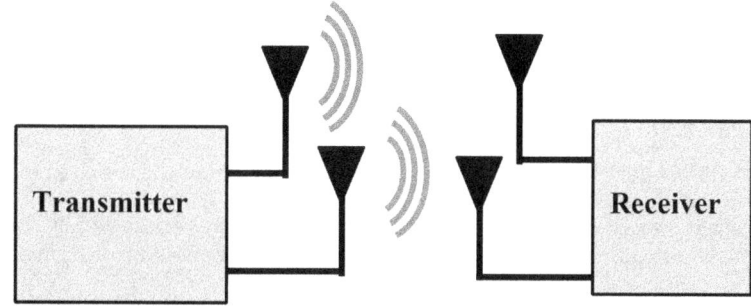

FIGURE 9.7 Multiple-input multiple-output.

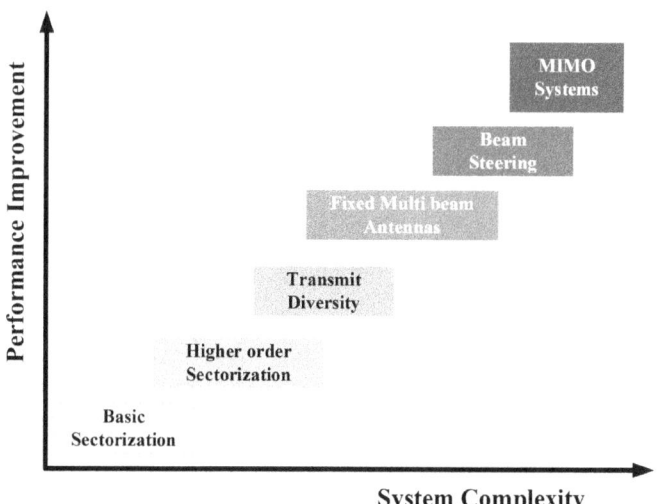

FIGURE 9.8 Comparison of major spatial techniques [4].

In Figure 9.8, the major spatial techniques are compared, where the system complexity is changed with performance improvements. From this, it is observed that the MIMO system has superior performance and higher system complexity than other systems. The comparison between the switched beam antenna and adaptive array antenna is given in Table 9.1.

TABLE 9.1 Difference Between Switched Beam Antenna and Adaptive Array Antenna

Switched Beam Antenna	Adaptive Array Antenna
• Numerous fixed directional beams with narrow beam widths	• Steers the beam in the direction of wanted signals
• The necessary phase shifts are given by phase shift networks such as the Butler matrix	• Requires implementation of DSP technology
	• Requires complex adaptive algorithms to direct the beam. It is difficult to implement in current systems
• Simple algorithms are used for beam selection	
• Integration into the existing cellular system is easy	• Requires complex adaptive algorithms to direct the beam
• The switched beam antenna does not ensure that the main beam receives maximum enhancement while the interfering signals receive maximum suppression	• It offers more coverage area and better capacity
	• The adaptive array model ideally ensures that the main signal receives a maximum enhancement

9.5 FUNCTIONS OF SMART ANTENNA

There are mainly two functions of a smart antenna: DOA estimation and beamforming method [16].

9.5.1 DOA ESTIMATION

There are three techniques available for the estimation of DOA, which are as follows.

1. Multiple signal classification. This technique estimates a set of constant parameters from measurements. The received signals are dependent on these constant parameters. This method requires a lot of computations and algorithms.
2. ESPRIT algorithm. In this technique, the signal parameters are estimated via the rotational invariance technique. It also requires a lot of computations and algorithms.
3. Matrix pencil method. This technique is generally used for real-time systems. It is much efficient than the other two techniques. In this method, the radiator behaves like a sensor that selects the spatial bandwidth of the array [17]. The DOA is calculated from the peaks of the spectrum.

9.5.2 BEAMFORMING METHOD

In this method, the mobile or targets are first searched, then the pattern of the antenna array is created by summing the phases of the signals in the desired direction of mobile or targets. The undesired radiation pattern of the mobile and targets are canceled. This method is accomplished by finite impulse response (FIR) tapped delay line filters. The weights of FIR filters are changed accordingly to the signal used.

This method provides optimal beamforming and also decreases the minimum mean square error between required and beam pattern designed. But this method is quite complicated as the steepest descent algorithm and least mean square algorithms were used for beamforming. The digital antenna arrays with multichannel use digital beamforming usually discrete Fourier transform or fast Fourier transform.

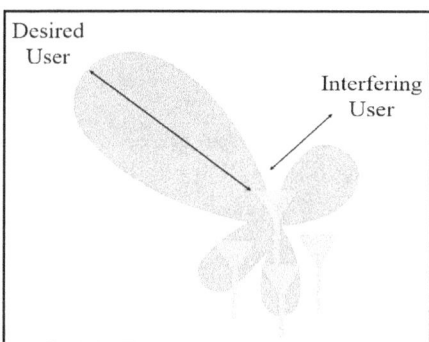

FIGURE 9.9 Beamforming method [4].

In Figure 9.9, the digital signal processor justifies the magnitude of the phase shifter and identifies the desired direction/user in which it radiates with maximum gain [4].

9.5.3 COVERAGE AREA COMPARISON

In Figure 9.10, it is seen that an adaptive smart antenna has a large coverage area as compared to the switched beam smart antenna and conventional sectorization. Therefore, the adaptive smart antenna works well in both low interference and high interference environments. The switched beam antenna works very well in a low interference environment but not in a high interference atmosphere. In comparison, conventional sectorization does not work well in both low interference and high interference environments [4].

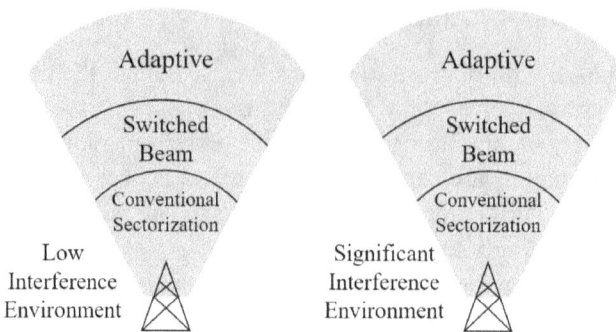

FIGURE 9.10 Coverage area comparison [4].
Source: Redrawn from Ref. [4].

9.6 ADVANTAGES

9.6.1 COVERAGE EXTENSION

Both N element switched beam and adaptive array smart antennas offer N fold rise in antenna gain with a small angular spread, which is given by the following equation:

$$G_a = 10\log_{10} N dB.$$

This extra gain can be utilized for the range extension of the base station. The smart antenna range (Rs) is more than the traditional antenna (Rc) and range extension factor (REF) is given by the following equation:

$$\text{REF} = \frac{R_s}{R_c} = N^{1/n}$$

where n is path loss exponent. The area extension factor (AEF) is the ratio of the area enclosed by smart antenna cell (As) to the area enclosed by traditional antenna element given by the following equation:

$$\text{AEF} = \left[\frac{R_s}{R_c}\right]^2 = N^{2/n}$$

Therefore, if Nc is the number of conventional base stations required for the area coverage, the same area can be covered using base stations with smart antennas. Thus, with smart antennas, the number of base stations needed to offer a similar cell area will be reduced and the base station reduction factor (BSRF) is given by the following equation:

$$\text{BSRF} = \frac{N_s}{N_c} = N^{-2/n}$$

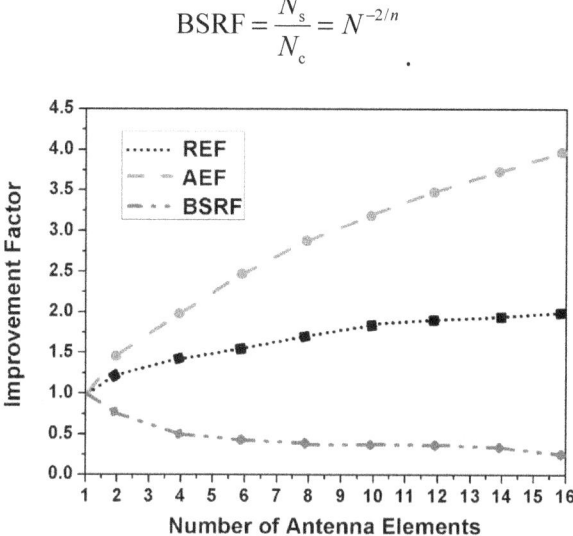

FIGURE 9.11 Variation of REF, AEF, and BSRF with antenna elements for a smart antenna array with path loss exponent n = 4 [6].

Source: Redrawn from http://lib.unipune.ac.in:8080/xmlui/bitstream/handle/123456789/6991/12_chapter%203.pdf?sequence=12&isAllowed=y

Figure 9.11 shows that a 10 antenna element array provides 78% range extension and the area coverage increases to 3.17 times that of a single antenna element. The number of base stations can be decreased to 32% of the original number.

9.6.2 SYSTEM CAPACITY IMPROVEMENT

The number of users maintained by each base station depends on the processing gain, interference from adjacent sectors, and other cells in a CDMA system. However, the N element smart antennas can cancel interferers, which affect the capacity. The empirical formula for the most number of subscribers that can be maintained by each cell for uniform path loss exponent $n = 4$ is [6]:

$$K_{max} = \frac{F \times N \times M}{G_i(N) \times v \times \text{SINR}}$$

where M is processing gain, N is the number of elements in an array, F is reuse factor, $G_E(N)$ is interference gain of an array, SINR is signal to interference and noise ratio, and v is voice activity factor.

A cell with an IS-95 system ($M = 128$), path loss exponent ($n = 4$), comprised of a single tier of adjacent CDMA cells, has reuse factor $F = 0.694$ and $v = 0.6$. The maximum number of subscribers maintained by each sector as a function of the array size N is plotted in Figure 9.12 for SINR = 9 dB.

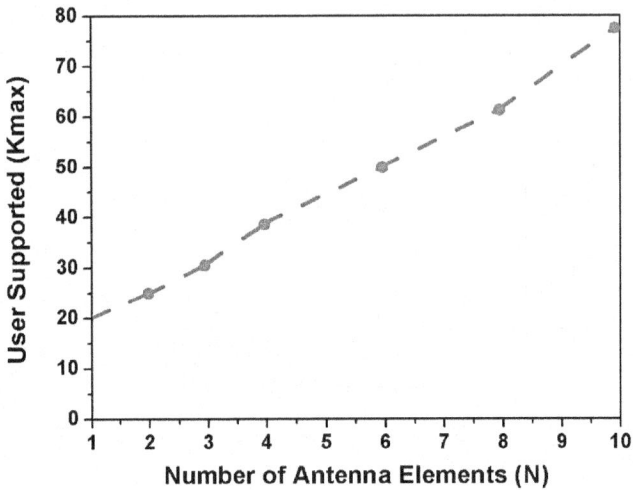

FIGURE 9.12 Variation of the number of antenna elements [6].

Source: Redrawn from http://lib.unipune.ac.in:8080/xmlui/bitstream/handle/123456789/6991/12_chapter%203.pdf?sequence=12&isAllowed=y

In Figure 9.12, the omnidirectional antenna supports 19 subscribers whereas the smart antenna with four elements supports 38 subscribers in a CDMA cell on the reverse link. Thus, the utilization of smart antennas provides more capacity improvement for CDMA system in a nominal amount of spectrum [18, 19].

9.6.3 SPECTRAL EFFICIENCY IMPROVEMENT

The normalized channel capacity with the adaptive array at the base station is given by the following equation:

$$C = \log_2 [1 + \text{SINR} \times N] \text{ bps/Hz}$$

where N is the number of antenna radiators in an adaptive array.

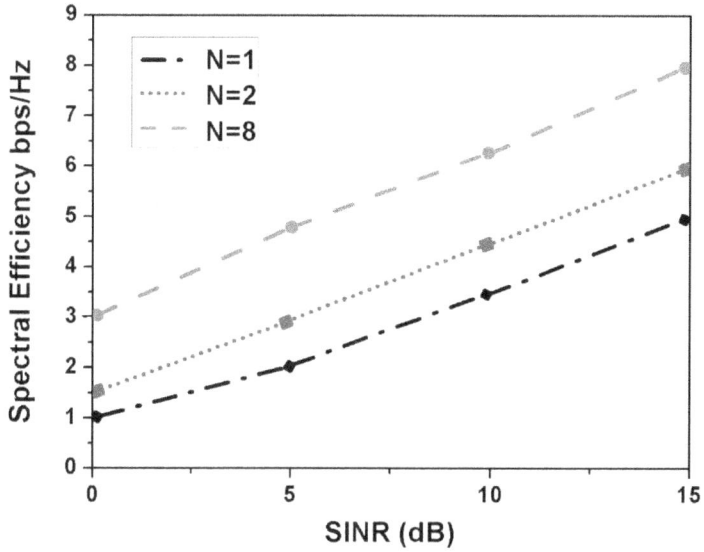

FIGURE 9.13 Variation of spectral efficiency and SINR of adaptive array smart antenna [6].

Source: Redrawn from http://lib.unipune.ac.in:8080/xmlui/bitstream/handle/123456789/6991/12_chapter%203.pdf?sequence=12&isAllowed=y

In Figure 9.13, the spectral efficiency and SINR as a function of N are plotted. The use of a smart antenna at the base station provides higher spectral efficiency compared to the omnidirectional antenna. The improved spectral efficiency provides a high data rate in wireless communication [20, 21].

9.7 DISADVANTAGES

1. The cost of smart antennas is very high and they consume more power, especially MIMO smart antennas decreases the battery life of mobile terminals. It is because of the use of distinct RF electronic devices and A/D converter circuitry for all antenna elements.
2. Smart antennas in wireless communication need large base stations and multiple antenna elements at each terminal. However, the dual-polarization is used to reduce the overall design size.
3. For suppressing multipath fading effects, the terminal and base stations must have multiple antennas with different positions and

orientations (for spatial, polarization, and angle diversity), which makes the system complex and impractical.

9.8 APPLICATIONS

The smart antennas could be useful for many applications like:

1. Multiband systems covering several Wi-Fi/WLAN standards.
2. Satellite communication.
3. Acoustic signal processing.
4. Surveillance and tracking through radars.
5. Radio astronomy.
6. Cellular system: smart antennas are in function for 2.5 (GSM-EDGE), third (IMT 2000) and fourth generation (LTE) communication.
7. GPS and Wi-MAX applications.

9.8.1 SMART ANTENNA APPLICATION STANDARDS

Smart antennas are appropriate for almost all the major wireless communication standards comprising the following schemes.

9.8.1.1 ACCESS METHOD

Analog-FDMA: The total bandwidth is divided among M users and each user is allocated a separate channel.

Digital-TDMA: Smart antennas can be used for PCs, cellular, and WLL networks to obtain a substantial rise in quality of service. To increase the range, the adaptive array may be preferable with TDMA, in large angular spread environments.

CDMA: In switched beam smart antennas, CDMA is preferred and applied to downlink to increase the performance. The adaptive array with TDMA increases the capacity considerably than that of switched beam smart antenna with CDMA. The adaptive array with TDMA is used for uplink as the base station has many interferers. While the switched beam smart antenna with CDMA is used for downlink because the signals from interfering base station are not much stronger seeing that the mobile selects the base station having the strongest signal.

9.8.1.2 DUPLEX METHOD

Duplex method is one of the major achievements in this wireless world. Duplex method can be of two types half duplex and full duplex but full-duplex configuration is most commonly used. It consists of a transceiver that can receive and transmit the signal simultaneously. To avoid interference uplink and downlink bands are used and the same subcarriers are allotted to user equipment for communication. Full-duplex architecture work in two modes: frequency division method and time division method.

9.8.1.2.1 Frequency Division Duplex

This communication system uses distinct frequency bands for transmitting and receiving information signals. In this scheme, uplink channel state information is required to accomplish spatially selective transmission.

9.8.1.2.2 Time Division Duplex

This communication system uses same frequency for the transmission and reception. The uplink and downlink channels are considered reciprocal.

KEYWORDS

- **cellular system**
- **RF energy**
- **signal-to-noise ratio**
- **digital signal processing**
- **spatial division multiple access**

REFERENCES

1. Frank, B. Gross. *Smart Antennas for Wireless Communications With MATLAB*, McGraw-Hill, New York, NY, 2005.
2. Ahmed El, Zooghby. *Smart Antenna Engineering*, Artech House, Norwood, MA, 2005.

3. WWW.circuitstoday.com/smart-antennas.
4. https://www.sabanciuniv.edu/mdbf/telecom/eng/comnet/cisco/
5. https://www.sabanciuniv.edu/mdbf/telecom/eng/comnet/cisco/overview.htm.
6. http://lib.unipune.ac.in:8080/xmlui/bitstream/handle/123456789/6991/12_chapter%203.p df?sequence=12&isAllowed=y.
7. Rabideau, D., & Parker, P. Ubiquitous MIMO Multifunction Digital Array Radar, *IEEE Signals, Systems, and Computers*, 37th Asilomar Conference, Vol. 1, pp. 1057–1064, 2003.
8. Fishler, E., Haimovich, A., Blum, R. et al. MIMO Radar: An Idea Whose Time Has Come, Proceedings of the IEEE Radar Conference, pp. 71–78, 2004.
9. Litva, J., & Kwok-Yeung Lo, T.. *Digital Beamforming in Wireless Communications*, Artech House, Boston, MA, 1996.
10. Weisman, C. *The Essential Guide to RF and Wireless*, 2d ed., Prentice Hall, New York, NY, 2002.
11. Shivapanchakshari, T. G., & Aravinda, H. S.. Review of Research Techniques to Improve System Performance of Smart Antenna, *Open Journal of Antennas and Propagation*, Vol. 5, pp. 83–98, 2017.
12. Abdallah, A., Kadry, S., & Joumaa C. Design and Performance Study of Smart Antenna Systems for WIMAX Applications. In: Yang D. (eds), Informatics in Control, Automation and Robotics. Lecture Notes in Electrical Engineering, Vol. 133. Springer, Berlin, Heidelberg, 2011.
13. http://shodhganga.inflibnet.ac.in/bitstream/10603/72806/12/11.%20chapter%202.pdf.
14. Jain, R. K., Katiyar, S., & Agrawal, N. K.. Smart antenna for cellular mobile communication, VSRD-IJEECE, Vol. 1, No. 9, pp. 530–541, 2011.
15. Balaji, G., Hogade, Shrikant K Bodhe. Effect of Wideband Signals on Smart Antenna, *International Journal of Advancements in Technology*, Vol. 3, pp. 55–63, 2012.
16. Ertan, S., H. Griffiths, & Wicks, M. et al. Bistatic Radar Denial by Spatial Waveform Diversity, *IEE RADAR*, Edinburgh, pp. 17–21, 2002.
17. Talwar, S., Viberg, M., & Paulraj, A.. Blind Estimation of Multiple Co Channel Digital Signals Using an Atnenna Array, *IEEE Signal Processing Letters*, Vol. 1, No. 2, 4673807, 1994.
18. Holma, H., & Toskala, A. *WCDMA for UMTS: Radio Access for Third Generation Mobile Communications*, 3rd ed., John Wiley & Sons, New York, NY, 2004.
19. Ross, A. H. M., & Gilhousen, K. S. CDMA technology and the IS-95 North American Standard. In: *The Mobile Communications Handbook*, CRC Press and IEEE Press, Boca Raton, FL, pp. 430–448, 1996.
20. Simon, M. K., et al. *Spread Spectrum Communication Handbook*, McGraw-Hill, New York, NY, 1994.
21. Compton, R. T., Jr. *Adaptive Antennas: Concepts and Performances*, Prentice-Hall, Englewood Cliffs, NJ, 1988.

CHAPTER 10

Introduction to Metamaterials

RAGINI SHARMA[1], VANDANA NIRANJAN[2], and VIBHAV K. SACHAN[1]

[1]*KIET Group of Institutions, Ghaziabad, Uttar Pradesh, India*

[2]*Indira Gandhi Delhi Technical University for Women, Delhi, India*

ABSTRACT

Metamaterial or left-handed metamaterial (LHM) is an artificial structure with unique properties of negative permittivity and permeability. Usually, permittivity and permeability of natural materials are positive. In 1967, V. G. Veselago, a Russian scientist, introduced a theoretical phenomenon of the negative refraction index. Later in 2000, J. B. Pendry work reopened this topic of the negative refraction index. Afterward metamaterial became the topic of interest for many researchers. Metamaterial can be applied in the electromagnetic field, acoustics, and optical physics. Metamaterial is widely embodied with microstrip antennas to get better results. The low gain of the microstrip antenna is one of its major drawbacks. The array of antenna can be used to overcome this problem, but it suffers from mutual coupling. Also, the array of patch antenna increases size. LHM can be the solution of above-said problems of the microstrip patch antenna and array of antenna. Metamaterial enhanced the gain of the microstrip patch antenna and reduced the dimension of antenna. LHM with a microstrip patch antenna also provides a wide band. Hence, LHM integrates with the microstrip patch antenna, thereby boosting the performance of the antenna. In this chapter, history, basic concept, and applications of metamaterial are illustrated. Further, characteristics and design equations of metamaterial are explained. This chapter also describes simulation, characterization, incorporation, and fabrication of metamaterial with the help of examples.

10.1 INTRODUCTION

Metamaterial is a composite structure that exhibits different electromagnetic properties not found in a natural material. Metamaterials are also known as artificial material. Characteristics of metamaterial are very unusual as compare to the material found in nature; therefore, metamaterial became the subject of new research topics around the world. Metamaterial is an artificial structure. Its permittivity and permeability are negative; therefore, it is also known as left-handed (LH) materials [1]. With these unique properties of metamaterial, characteristics of the microstrip filter and microstrip antenna can be improved. Incorporation of metamaterial with a microstrip antenna gives advantages such as increased bandwidth, reduces radiation losses, and reduces dimensions of the microstrip antenna.

The classification of materials based on the value of permittivity and permeability has four possibilities.

1. *Right-handed materials (RHMs) ($\mu > 0$ and $\varepsilon > 0$):* RHM also known as a double-positive (DPS) material consists of a positive value for permittivity (ε) as well as for permeability (μ). Mostly material found in nature is RHM.
2. *Epsilon negative material ($\mu > 0$ and $\varepsilon < 0$):* Epsilon negative (ENG) material consists of the negative value of permittivity; however, permeability is positive in it.
3. *Mu-negative (MNG) material ($\mu < 0$ and $\varepsilon > 0$):* Mu-negative (MNG) material has a positive value of permittivity and a negative value of permeability.
4. *Double-negative (DNG) material ($\mu < 0$ and $\varepsilon > 0$):* DNG also known as LHM. DNG possesses negative value for permittivity as well as for permeability.

LHM generates a focusing effect due to the negative value of permittivity and permeability. Since negative refraction occurs due to the structure of LHM, it will ensure that the radiation of the antenna leads to an increase in the gain of the antenna.

10.2 HISTORY OF METAMATERIAL

In 1967, V. G. Veselago, a Russian scientist, gave theoretical explanations about artificial material whose properties are very different from the material available in nature. This artificial material is a composite structure that gives a negative refractive index, that is, the values of permittivity and permeability are negative [1]. He explained that if a slab will focus a light beam, provided the condition $\varepsilon = -1$ and $\mu = -1$, a diverged beam of light can be collected at one point. Although at that time no LHM existed there to support his theory, the paper of Veselago inspired many researchers to design such a lens. Later in 2000, J. B. Pendry published a paper "Negative refraction makes a perfect lens" based on a perfect lens to obtain negative refraction [2]. This research paper triggered the development of the artificial metallic structure, which possesses negative value for permittivity as well as for permeability. First experimental design was given by Shelby, Smith, and Schultz at the University of California in 2001 [5]. The LHM structure composed of the group of a split ring resonator (SRR) and a thin wire (TW). Thereafter many researchers started working on designing different kinds of metamaterials for different frequency ranges. Metamaterials can work for megahertz to optimum frequency ranges. Due to their focusing effect, metamaterials are among very popular techniques to enhance the characteristics of microwave planar circuits such as antenna, filter, and circulator. Metamaterial also reduces the size of the antenna and filter, which is very useful for today's compact portable wireless devices [6-12].

In 2002-2004, interdisciplinary scientific conferences for radio and optical engineers gave the term "metamaterials." Now, metamaterials are considered as a branch of electromagnetics.

10.3 APPLICATION OF METAMATERIAL

1. Metamaterial is used to make super lenses. These lenses will work above the diffraction limit.
2. Metamaterial is used in antennas to enhance the gain and bandwidth of the microstrip antenna and to reduce the dimension of the antenna.
3. Concept of metamaterial is utilized in making of the Hidden Cloak, that is, make something disappear. If the electric field and magnetic field generated by an object get cancelled, then it is possible to make a cloak. It is based on coordinate transformation.
4. Metamaterials are also used in sensors as they enhance the resolution and sensitivity of the sensors.
5. Metamaterials are also used in acoustics. New structures of metamaterials are developing in the field of ultrasonic and supersonic waves.

10.4 STRUCTURE OF LEFT-HANDED METAMATERIAL

A very first structure of metamaterial comprises an SRR and a TW or capacitance-loaded strip (CLS) [5]. SRR generates the negative value of permeability. CLS and TW generate negative permittivity.

10.4.1 SPLIT RING RESONATOR

An SRR which is part of the LHM structure that causes negative permeability. A magnetic dipole moment will generate providing excitation of the magnetic field orthogonal to the plane of the LHM structure. The structure of SRR is immensely conductive in nature whose capacitance across the two rings balances inductance [13–15]. The SRR generates a high current density structure that generates a huge magnetic moment.

The structures of CLS and TW, respectively. The current is induced along the structure when the electric field propagates parallel through the TW or CLS, respond like dielectric. This will produce an electric dipole moment with in structure [16, 17].

10.5 CHARACTERISTICS OF LEFT-HANDED METAMATERIAL

10.5.1 NEGATIVE REFRACTION

The unusual features of metamaterial (negative value of ε and μ) cause changes of other characteristics of the material. The refractive index of the material will change due to change in the permittivity and permeability of the material. The relation of the refractive index with ε and μ is given below:

$$N^2 = \varepsilon\mu \tag{10.1a}$$
$$N = \pm \sqrt{\varepsilon\mu} \tag{10.1b}$$

From Equation (10.1b), it is derived that when ε and μ are positive, the value of the refractive index is positive, whereas ε and μ are negative; we take the negative sign of square root that makes the refractive index negative.

As shown in Figure 10.1(a), wave propagation takes place in the right-handed (RH) medium where both ε and μ are positive.

In Figure 10.1(b), the refractive index of the LH medium is N2¢ = –N2. Due to the above condition, the wave will be refracted in contrast to the propagation of the wave in the RH medium. Furthermore, if the negative

Introduction to Metamaterials

value of the refractive index is substituted into the equation of Snell's, Snell's law will still be justified despite the fact that the wave bends toward the opposite direction. The equation of Snell's law is

$$N1 \sin \theta_1 = N2 \sin \theta_2, \theta_2 < 0 \text{ is obtained} \tag{10.2}$$

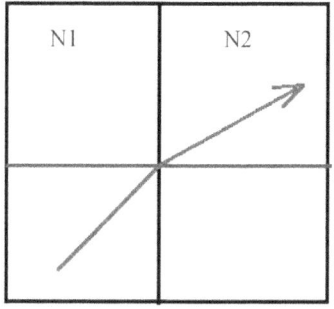 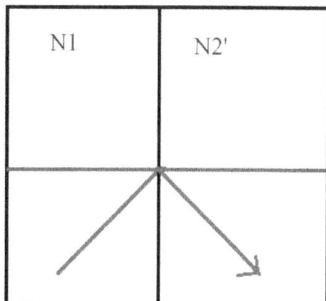

FIGURE 10.1 (a) Behavior of the refracted beam in the RH medium and (b) behavior of the refracted beam in the LH medium.

10.5.2 BACKWARD WAVE PROPAGATION

Backward wave propagation is the other atypical characteristic of metamaterial.

Behavior of the electromagnetic waves in the RH medium is shown in Figure 10.2(a), whereas the behavior of the electromagnetic waves in the RH medium is shown in Figure 10.2(b).

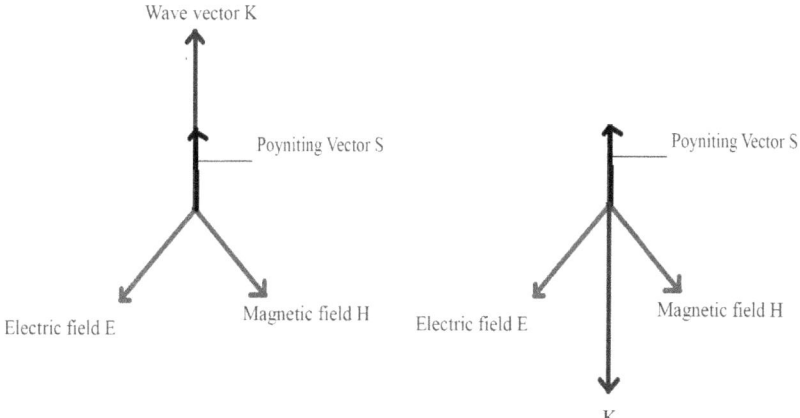

FIGURE 10.2 E, H, K, and the Poynting vector S for an electromagnetic wave. (a) Conventional RH medium and (b) LH medium.

Consider that the wave is propagating in a lossless medium. Then, according to Maxwell's equations,

$$\nabla \cdot \mathbf{D} = \rho \tag{10.3a}$$

$$\nabla \times \mathbf{E} = -j\omega\mu\mathbf{H} \tag{10.3b}$$

$$\nabla \cdot \mathbf{B} = 0 \tag{10.3c}$$

$$\nabla \times \mathbf{H} = \mathbf{J} + j\omega\varepsilon\mathbf{E} \tag{10.3d}$$

With the help of Maxwell's equations, we derive the following equations for plane waves:

$$\mathbf{k}\,\mathbf{E} = \omega\mu\mathbf{H}, \tag{10.3e}$$

$$\mathbf{k} \times \mathbf{H} = -\omega\varepsilon\mathbf{E} \tag{10.3f}$$

where **E** denotes the electric field, **H** denotes the magnetic field, and **k** denotes the wave vector.

Equations (10.3e) and (10.3f) make an RH orthogonal system where μ, **E**, **H**, and **k** are positive.

For the negative values of μ and $\varepsilon < 0$,

$$\mathbf{k} \times \mathbf{E} = -\omega\mu\mathbf{H}, \tag{10.4a}$$

$$\mathbf{k} \times \mathbf{H} = -\omega\varepsilon\mathbf{E} \tag{10.4b}$$

The Poynting vector **S** which can be described as

$$\mathbf{S} = \mathbf{E} \times \mathbf{H}^*. \tag{10.5}$$

The Poynting vector is associated with the power flow $P0$, and therefore is oriented toward the direction of the propagation of energy over time.

Equations (10.1a) and (10.1b) make an LH orthogonal system where μ and ε are negative. Subsequently, it is found that the observe direction of the wave vector **k** is opposite to the direction of **k** in the RH medium, so it can be said that **k** is negative. The phase velocity of the wave is defined by the following relation:

$$\upsilon p = \frac{\omega}{k}. \tag{10.6}$$

From Equation (10.6), it can also be justified that the value of **k** is negative as the frequency has always the positive value.

Subsequently, S is parallel to the group velocity (velocity of a modulated signal in a distortionless medium),

$$v_g = \nabla_k \cdot \omega \qquad (10.4a)$$

After the investigation of all of the above equations, we get the following conclusion:

RH medium: $\upsilon p > 0$ ($k > 0$) and $\upsilon g > 0$,
LH medium: $\upsilon p < 0$ ($k < 0$) and $\upsilon g > 0$.

10.6 FEATURES OF METAMATERIAL

1. Improvement in the performance of a small monopole antenna, realized via the use of an ENG envelope that compensates for its high capacitive reactance.
2. Lens effect produced by DNG slabs that are useful for enhancing the directivities of a small antenna, for example, dipole and microstrip patches, by collimating the cylindrical waves emanating from these antennas and focusing them at infinity.
3. Creation of super-lenses that can have a spatial resolution below that of the wavelength.

10.7 PROCEDURE TO OBTAIN THE VALUE OF PERMITTIVITY AND PERMEABILITY

The modified Nicolson-Ross-Wier method commonly known as the NRW approach is used to find the accurate approximation of permittivity and permeability [18-20].

The NRW method used the reflection and transmission parameters to derive the value of permittivity and permeability.

The transmission measurement T is obtained from the following equation:

$$T = \frac{v1 - \Gamma}{1 - v1\Gamma}. \qquad (10.8)$$

And the reflection coefficient Γ is given by

$$\Gamma = \frac{T - v2}{1 - v2T}, \qquad (10.9)$$

where

$$V_1 = S_{21} + S_{11} \qquad (10.10)$$

$$V_2 = S_{21} - S_{11}. \qquad (10.11)$$

From (10.9) and (10.10), we can obtain

$$1-T = \frac{(1-v1)(1+\Gamma)}{1-v1\Gamma} \tag{10.12}$$

$$\eta = \frac{1+\Gamma}{1-\Gamma} = \frac{(1+T)(1-V2)}{(1-T)(1+V2)} \tag{10.13}$$

where T is the transmission coefficient, Γ is the reflection coefficient, and η is the wave impedance.

Consider that the electrical thickness of the LH material slab is not large (i.e., $k_{real} d < 1$) and the wave number k is

$$k = \frac{\omega\sqrt{\mu\varepsilon}}{c} = k0\sqrt{\mu\varepsilon} \tag{10.14}$$

where,
ω (angular frequency) = $2\pi f$
c (speed of light) = 2.998×10^8 m/s.

The approximate value of the transmission coefficient is $T \approx 1 - jkd$.

From Equations (10.13) and (10.14), the approximate values of the permittivity and permeability can be derived as follows:

$$\mu_r = \frac{2(1-V2)}{j \cdot k_0 \cdot d(1+V2)} \tag{10.15}$$

$$\varepsilon_r = \left(\frac{k}{k_0}\right)^2 \frac{1}{\mu_r}, \tag{10.16}$$

where d is the thickness of the substrate. The refraction index can be given by

$$n = \sqrt{\mu\varepsilon} = \frac{k}{k_0} \tag{10.17}$$

and the wave impedance,

$$\eta^2 = \frac{\mu}{\varepsilon} = \frac{(1+V1)(1-V2)}{(1-V1)(1+V2)} = \frac{(S11+1)^2 - S21^2}{(S11-1)^2 - S21^2} \tag{10.18}$$

Since issue of square root will be obtained in Equations (10.16) and (10.18). Figure 10.12 shows the fabricated metamaterial.

The following equation can be used to get the accurate value of permittivity:

$$\varepsilon_r = \frac{2 \cdot (1-V1)}{j \cdot k0 \cdot d(1+V1)} \tag{10.19}$$

Introduction to Metamaterials 229

The value of permeability can be found out from Equation (10.15). Similarly, the value of permittivity for LHM can be found out from Equation (10.19).

An alternative approach is MathCAD software. This software can be used to obtain the value of the permittivity and permeability of the metamaterial structure [20]. This can be achieved by S-parameters of the antenna from (HFSS, CSTMW Studio, IE3D, etc.) to MathCAD software.

10.8 FUNDAMENTAL CONCEPT OF RECTANGULAR MICROSTRIP PATCH ANTENNA

Microstrip patch antennas are widely used antennas owing to their advantages such as compact size, easy to fabricate, and low cost. A microstrip patch antenna comprises a radiating patch on one side of a dielectric substrate and a ground plane on the other side. The patch is generally made up of a conducting material such as copper or gold. The patch can be of different shapes, for example, square, elliptical, inverted F, rectangular, circular, and triangular. Microstrip lines or coaxial lines are used for providing feed to the microstrip patch antenna. A rectangular microstrip patch antenna is shown in Figure 10.3. Microstrip patch antennas are used in wireless communication and mobile industries, and in medical and scientific research fields. The microstrip patch antenna suffered from disadvantages such as low gain and narrow bandwidth. To improve these characteristics, metamaterial can be embodied with the patch antenna. Metamaterial also reduces the dimension of the antenna [21, 22].

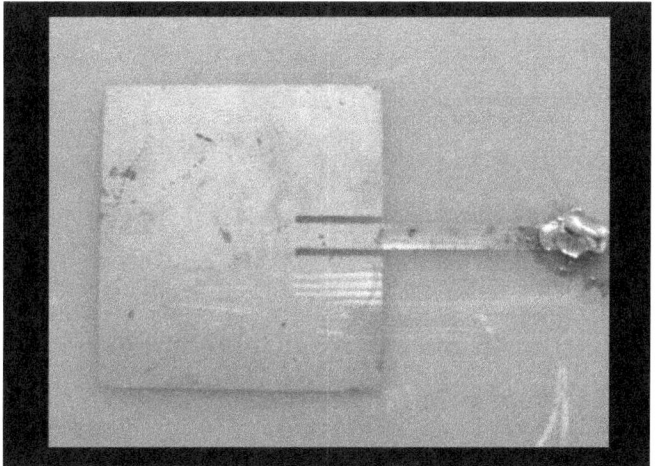

FIGURE 10.3 Structure of a rectangular microstrip patch antenna with inset feed.

Radiation through microstrip patch antennas occurs due to the generation of fringing fields between the ground plane and patch structure. To get the better performance of patch antenna, the dielectric constant of the substrate should be low, and the thickness of the dielectric should be high. This arrangement provides wide bandwidth and better radiation, although this will lead to an increase in the size of the antenna. Higher dielectric constants can be used while designing a microstrip patch antenna, although it gives a narrower bandwidth and a lower gain. To design a microstrip antenna, we need to deal with antenna dimensions and characteristics as per the requirements.

10.8.1 RESONANT FREQUENCY OF MICROSTRIP PATCH ANTENNA

The resonance frequency for the (1, 0) mode is given by

$$f_o \frac{c}{2L_e \sqrt{\varepsilon_r}}, \tag{10.20}$$

where c is the speed of light in the vacuum. Considering the fringing of the cavity fields occurred at the edges of the patch and the length, the effective length L_e is given by

$$L_e = L + 2\Delta L.$$

The Hammerstad formula for the fringing extension is

$$\frac{\Delta L}{h} = 0.412 \frac{(\varepsilon_{eff} + 0.3)\left(\frac{w}{h} + 0.264\right)}{(\varepsilon_{eff} - 0.258)\left(\frac{w}{h} + 0.8\right)} \tag{10.21}$$

$$\varepsilon_{reff} = \frac{\varepsilon_r + 1}{2} + \frac{\varepsilon_r - 1}{2}\left(\frac{1}{\sqrt{1 + \frac{12h}{W}}}\right). \tag{10.22}$$

The width of the patch antenna

$$W = \frac{1}{2f_r\sqrt{\mu_0 \varepsilon_0}}\sqrt{\frac{2}{\varepsilon_r + 1}} = \frac{c}{2f_r}\sqrt{\frac{2}{\varepsilon_r + 1}}, \tag{10.23}$$

where ε_{reff} is the effective dielectric constant, ε_r is the dielectric constant of the substrate, h is the height of the dielectric substrate, and W is the width of the patch.

10.8.2 GAIN OF ANTENNA

The gain of a transmitting antenna can be defined as the "amount of efficiently conversion of input power into electromagnetic waves toward a particular direction." The gain of a receiving antenna can be defined as the "amount of efficiently conversion of electromagnetic waves received from a particular direction into microwave power." The gain of an antenna when the direction is not specified is measured in the main lobe of the antenna.

10.8.3 VSWR OF ANTENNA

The standing wave ratio (SWR) shows the mismatching between the load and the source. The SWR range is between 1 and infinity. The value of the voltage standing wave ratio (VSWR) should be between 1 and 2 for an efficient performance of an antenna.

VSWR can be defined as

$$\text{VSWR} = \frac{V_{max}}{V_{min}} = \frac{1+|\Gamma|}{1-|\Gamma|}, \quad (10.24)$$

where Γ is the reflection coefficient of the antenna.

10.8.4 ANTENNA IMPEDANCE

The input impedance of the antenna should properly match with the characteristic impedance of the transmission to achieve the maximum power transfer between the transmission line and an antenna. Impedance is a very important characteristic of an antenna. Improper matching of impedance leads to produce reflections and travel backs toward the energy source. This reflection of energy causes the reduction of overall system efficiency.

10.9 MICROSTRIP PATCH ANTENNA LOADED WITH METAMATERIAL

To verify the properties of metamaterial, first we simulate a patch antenna and find out its all parameters. Then we design a metamaterial for this antenna and measure the effects of metamaterial on the antenna.

This design presents a patch antenna loaded with a double-slit rectangle surrounded by four circle-shaped metamaterial structures. This antenna has been simulated at 1.8 GHz frequency by using CST software with reduced dimensions [20].

The parameters of the rectangular microstrip patch antenna with metamaterial are $W = 36.414837$ mm, $L = 28.2421$ mm, cut width = 4 mm, cut depth = 12mm, length of the transmission line feed = 30.3784 mm, with the width of the feed being 3 mm. The rectangular microstrip patch antenna designed on one side of the substrate with $\varepsilon_r = 4.3$ and the height from the ground plane $d = 1.6$ mm. The proposed design is based on "double-slit rectangle surrounded by four circles" shaping the metamaterial structure. The height of metamaterial from the ground plane is 3.314 mm and the substrate $\varepsilon_r = 4.3$.

Figure 10.4 shows the design of a patch antenna and Figure 10.5 shows the design and dimensions of metamaterial, in which dimensions of all circles are identical as well as dimensions of both slits are the same.

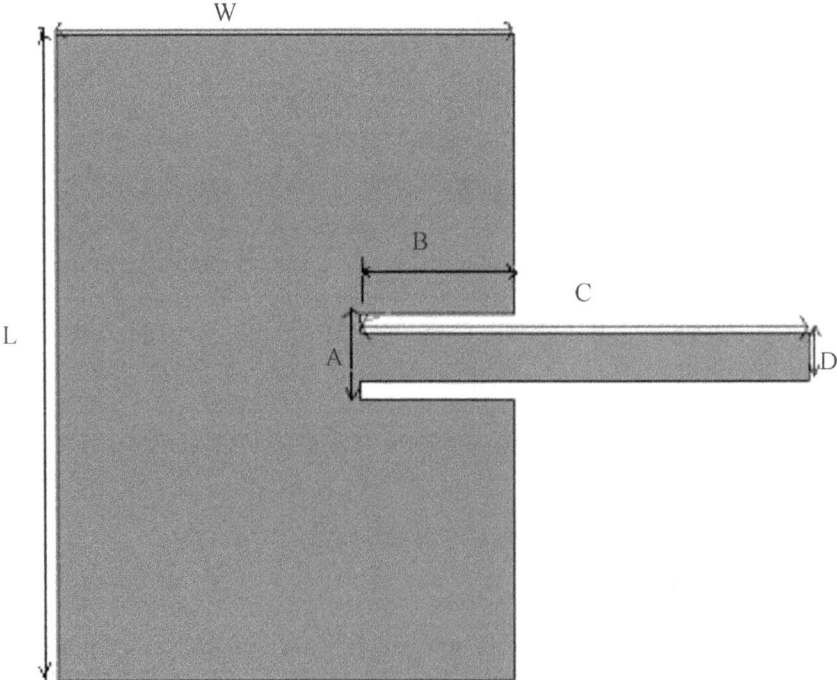

FIGURE 10.4 Design of rectangular microstrip patch antenna.

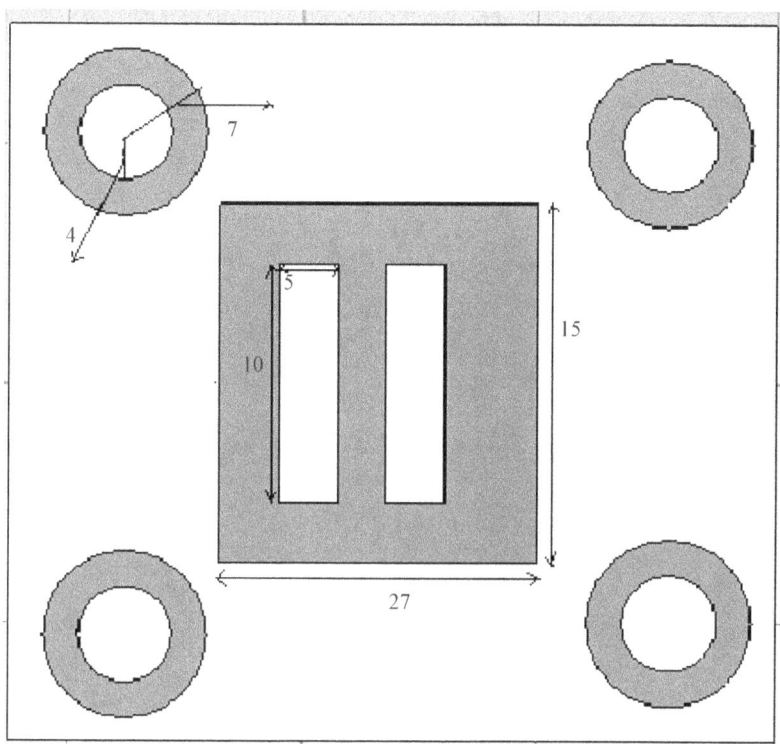

FIGURE 10.5 Structure of metamaterial.

Table 10.1 describes the specifications of designs of both the patch antenna without metamaterial and the patch antenna loaded with metamaterial. From Table 10.1, it is clear that metamaterial reduces the size of the microstrip patch antenna.

10.10 RESULTS OF PROPOSED PROTOTYPE

Figure 10.6 shows the return loss of −19.0801 dB and bandwidth of 31.3 MHz of the patch antenna without metamaterial. Figure 10.7 shows the return loss of −32 dB and the bandwidth of 34.4 MHz when the patch antenna loaded with metamaterial. Metamaterial is examined after designing and simulating the rectangular patch antenna. Metamaterial is placed between two waveguide ports on the left and right sides of the X-axis in order to calculate the S_{11} and S_{22} parameters. The wave was excited from the negative X-axis to the positive X-axis.

TABLE 10.1 Rectangular Microstrip Patch Antenna Specifications

Parameters	Dimensions of Patch Antenna for 1.8 GHz	Dimension of Patch Antenna for 1.8 GHz with Metamaterial	Unit
Dielectric constant (e_r)	4.3	4.3	–
Loss tangent (tan ∂)	0.02	0.02	–
Thickness (h)	1.6	1.6	mm
Operating frequency	1.8	1.8	GHz
Length (L)	39.4341	28.2421	mm
Width (W)	40.714	36.414837	mm
Cut width (A)	6	4	mm
Cut depth (B)	13.004	12	mm
Path length (C)	38.34744	30.3784	mm
Width of feed (D)	4	3	mm

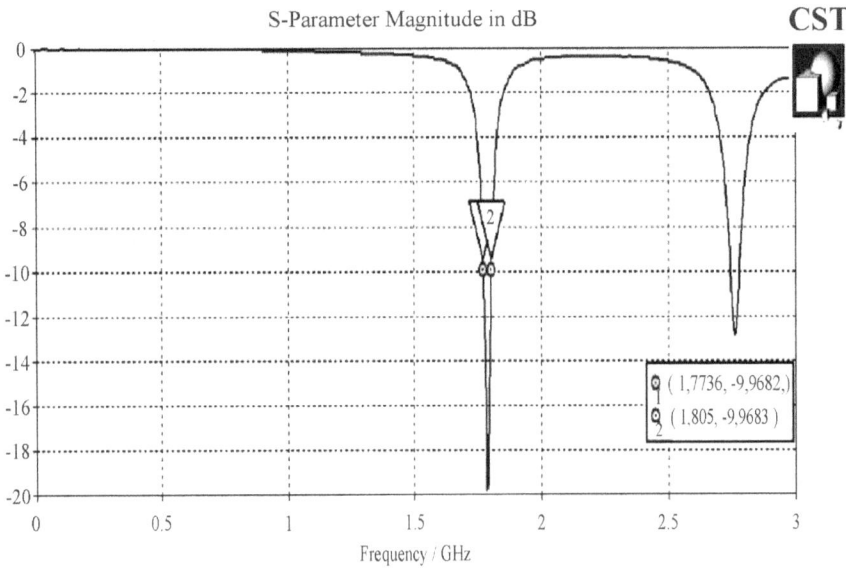

FIGURE 10.6 Simulation result of the rectangular microstrip patch antenna without metamaterial.

Figure 10.8 shows the smith chart of the rectangular microstrip patch antenna. The antenna is matched with the input impedance.

Figure 10.9 exhibits the gain of a rectangular microstrip patch antenna loaded with metamaterial. It can be understood from Figure 10.9 that the gain of 4.276 dB and radiation efficiency of −1.723 dB are obtained. The

Introduction to Metamaterials

graph shown in Figures 10.10 and 10.11 verify that metamaterial possesses double negative property or LHM. Figure 10.10 shows the graph between the frequency and permeability; it is seen from the graph that the value of permeability is negative. Similarly, Figure 10.11 shows the negative value of permittivity. Further Table 10.2 shows the comparison of the patch antenna with and without metamaterial [22].

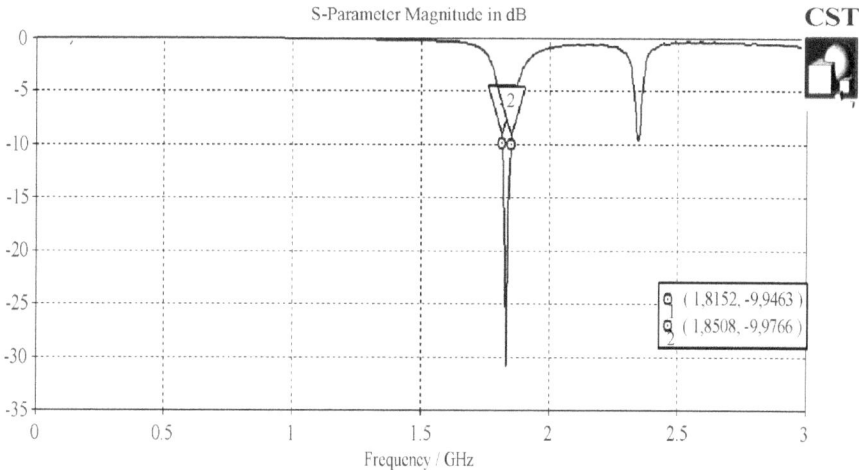

FIGURE 10.7 Simulation result of the rectangular microstrip patch antenna loaded with metamaterial.

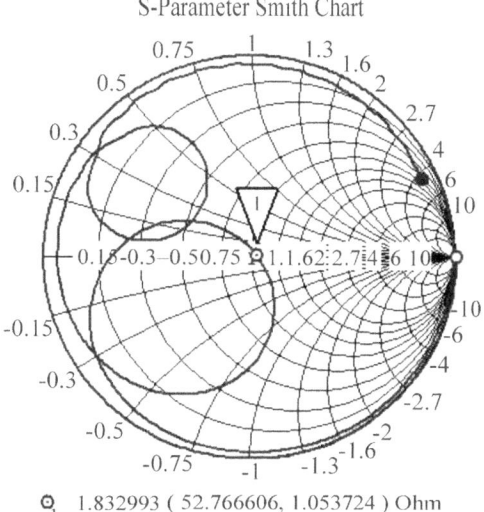

FIGURE 10.8 Smith chart of the rectangular microstrip patch antenna.

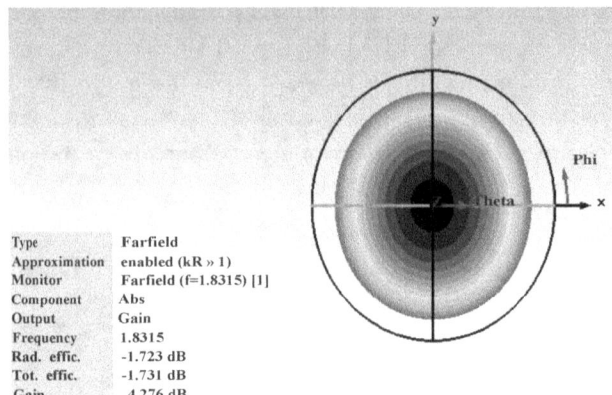

FIGURE 10.9 Gain of the proposed rectangular microstrip patch antenna loaded with metamaterial.

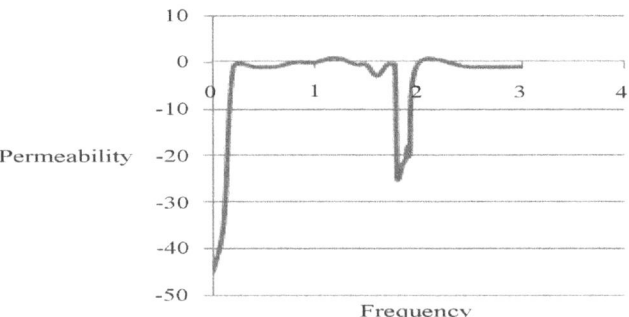

FIGURE 10.10 Graph between frequency and permeability.

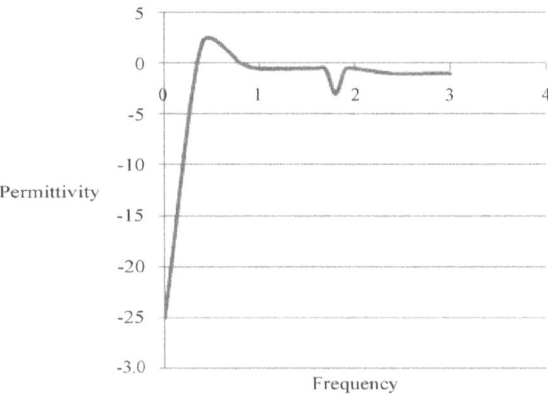

FIGURE 10.11 Graph between frequency and permittivity.

Introduction to Metamaterials

TABLE 10.2 Simulation Results Comparison

No.	Parameters	Without LH MTM (1.8 GHz)	With LH MTM (1.8 GHz)
1	Return loss (S11)	−19 dB	−32 dB
2	Bandwidth	31.3 MHz	34.4 MHz

10.11 FABRICATION AND MEASURED RESULT OF PROTOTYPE

Without metamaterial, the simulation result of the rectangular microstrip patch antenna has a return loss of −19.0801 dB and the bandwidth of 31.3 MHz, whereas it has a return loss of −32 dB and the bandwidth of 34.4 MHz when loaded with metamaterial. It is revealed that the incorporation of metamaterial with the patch antenna results in a greater increment (13.41%) in bandwidth and reduction in the return loss (67.711%) with a greater advantage of miniaturization of the patch antenna.

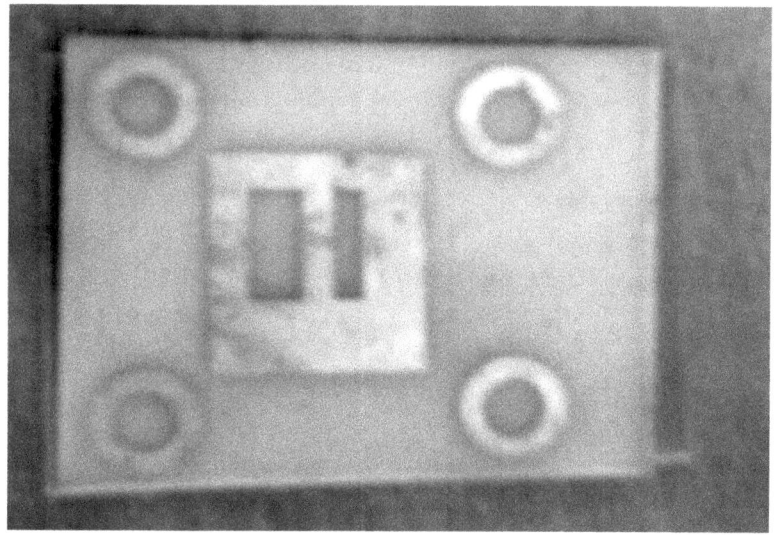

FIGURE 10.12 Fabrication of metamaterial.

The measured result of the proposed design shows a return loss of -22dB and a bandwidth of 30 MHz. All the measurements are made by the FS-314 spectrum analyzer, and readings are taken at the minimum hold condition as well as the constant condition of liquids. As far as the designed patch antenna with metamaterial is concerned, it successfully works at 1.8 GHz.

There is a difference between the simulated and measured results due to fabrication losses.

10.12 CONCLUSION

The conventional microstrip patch antenna has certain limitations in application because it is governed by the "right-hand rule" that determines the behavior of the electromagnetic wave. Metamaterial is a better alternative to enhance the application of the antenna.

Earlier investigation of the proposed design in chapter concludes that metamaterial incorporated with the microstrip antenna is useful to improve the performance of the antenna. Metamaterial enhanced the gain of the microstrip patch antenna and the reduced dimension of the antenna. With the incorporation of LHM, the return loss of the antenna also decreased and the bandwidth increased. Hence, LHM is useful for wideband applications.

Metamaterials are used to improve the performance of the MIMO antenna, microstrip antenna, and microwave filters. Metamaterials are widely applicable in microwave devices, wireless communication, acoustics, and optical physics.

KEYWORDS

- **left-handed material**
- **permittivity**
- **permeability**
- **split ring resonator**
- **thin wire**
- **refraction index**

REFERENCES

1. Veselago, V. G., "The electrodynamics of substances with simultaneously negative values of ε and μ," Sov. Phys.—Usp., Vol. 10, no. 4, pp. 509–514, 1968.

2. Pendry, J. B., "Negative refraction makes a perfect lens," Phys. Rev. Lett., Vol. 85, no. 18, pp. 3966–3969, 2000.
3. Pendry, J. B., Holden, A. J., Stewart, W. J., & Youngs, I., "Extremely low frequency plasmons in metallic mesostructures," Phys. Rev. Lett., Vol. 76, no. 25, pp. 4773–4776, 1996.
4. Pendry, J. B., Holden, A. J., Robbins, D. J., & Stewart, W. J., "Magnetism from Conductors and Enhanced Nonlinear Phenomena," IEEE Trans. Microw. Theory Tech., Vol. 47, no. 11, pp. 2075–2081, 2000.
5. Shelby, R. A., Smith, D. R., & Shultz, S., "Experimental verification of a negative index of refraction," Science, Vol. 292, 77–79, 2001.
6. Eleftheriades, G. V., & Balmain, K. G., Negative-Refraction Metamaterials: Fundamental Principles and Applications. Hoboken, NJ: Wiley-Interscience. 2005.
7. Engheta, N., & Ziolkowski, R. W., Metamaterials Physics and Engineering Explorations. Piscataway, NJ: Wiley-Interscience. 2006.
8. Hu, J., Yan, C.-S., & Lin, Q.-C. "New patch antenna with MTM cover," J. Zhejiang Univ. Sci. A—Appl. Phys. Eng., Vol. 7, no. 1, pp. 89–94, 2006.
9. Weng, Z.-B., Wang, N.-B., Jiao, Y.-C., & Rong-Guo, "The design of high gain omni directional monolope based on conformal meta-material cover." 7th International Symposium on Antennas, Propagation, & EM Theory, October 26–29, 2006, Guilin, China.
10. Erentok, A., Luljak, P. L., & Ziolkowski, R. W., "Characterization of a volumetric Meta-material realization of an artificial magnetic conductor for antenna application," IEEE Transactions on Antennas and Wireless Propagation, Vol. 53, no. 1, pp. 233–247, 2005.
11. Caloz, C., & Itoh, T., Electromagnetic Metamaterials Transmission Line Theory and Microwave Applications. Hoboken, NJ: John Wiley & Sons. 2006.
12. Jaksic, Z., Dalarsson, N., & Maksimovic, M., "Negative Refractive Index Metamaterials: Principles and Applications," Microw. Rev., Vol. 12, no. 01, pp. 36–49, 2006.
13. Szentpali, B. "Metamaterials: A new concept in the microwave technique." 6th International Conference on Telecommunications in Modern Satellite, Cable and Broadcasting Service, October 1–3, 2003. Serbia and Montenegro.
14. Wongkasem, N., & Akyurtlu, A., "Group Theory Based Design of Isotropic Negative Refractive Index Metamaterials," Prog. Electromagn. Res., Vol. 63, pp. 295–310, 2006.
15. Ziolkowski, R. W., "Wave propagation in media having negative permittivity and permeability," Phys. Rev. E, Vol. 64, no. 5, pp. 056625, 2001.
16. Cui, T. J., et al., "Study of lossy effects on the propagation of propagating and evanescent waves in left-handed materials," Phys. Lett., Vol. A323, no. pp. 484–494, 2004.
17. Ziolkowski, R. W., "Design, fabrication, and testing of double negative metamaterials," IEEE Trans. Antennas Wirel. Propag., Vol. 51, no. 7, p. 1516, 2003.
18. Wu, B.-I., Wang, W., Pacheco, J., Chen, X., Grzegorczyk, T., & Kong, J. A., "A study of using meta-material as antenna substrate to enhance gain," Prog. Electromagn. Res., Vol. 51, pp. 295–328, 2005.
19. Sharma, R., & Aghwariya, M. K., "Miniaturization of L-band rectangular patch antenna by using two rectangular slit," International Conference on Computational Intelligence and Communication Networks (CICN), 23–25 December 2016, Tehri, India.
20. Singhal, P. K., Garg, B., & Agrawal, N., "A high gain rectangular microstrip patch antenna using 'different C patterns' meta-material design in L-band," Adv. Comput. Tech. Electromagn., Vol. 1, pp. 1–5, 2012.

21. Sharma, R., & Singhal, P. K., "Miniaturized patch antenna loaded with meta-material for microwave sensor," Quantum Matter, Vol. 2, pp. 1–4, 2013.
22. Sharma, R., Aghwariya, M. K., & Singhal, P. K., "Design a patch antenna with meta-material for electromagnetic interference sensor," J. Power Electron. Power Syst., Vol. 3, no. 1, ISSN: 2249–863X, 2013.
23. Sharma, R., & Aghwariya, M. K., "Modified inverted fork patch antenna for microwave applications," Int. J. Eng. Res. General Sci., Vol. 3, no. 3, pp. 187–194, 2015.

Index

A

Adaptive array antenna, 212
Adaptive arrays, 101
Adaptive array smart antenna, 209
Adders, 35, 40–41
Adiabatic switching, 37
AlexNet network, 89, 91
Analog-FDMA, 218
AND gate, 34
ANOX gate, 35
Antennas, 206. *see also* nanoantenna
  aperture efficiency, 105–108
  characterization, 102–108
  classifications, 109–110
  CNT, 75–77
  cutting-edge electromagnetic, 75
  definition, 100
  directivity, 103–104
  diversity performance of, 3
  in free space, 4
  metallic, 78
  monolithic microwave integrated circuit (MMIC), 113–117
  ohmic efficiency, 104
  on-chip integration of, 74
  patch, 78, 100, 113–116
  planar, 100
  reflection coefficient, 104–105
  selection criteria of elements, 109–112
  smart (*see* smart antennas)
  substrate selection, 112–113
  superconducting, 78–79
  topologies, 108–109, 116
Aperture efficiency, 105–108
Arithmetic and logic units (ALUs), 35
Art-gallery-based coverage method, 201
Artificial intelligent agents, 150
Artificial material, 222
Artificial neural network (ANN), 84
  activation functions, 84–85
  hidden layer, 85–86
  input layer, 85
  neurons in, 85–86
  output layer, 86
  structure, 86
Average pooling, 88

B

Back-engendering topology, 95
Back-gate bias, 135–136
Back-gate voltage, 133–134
Back-propagation learning algorithms, 85
Back threshold voltage, 137–138
Backward wave propagation, 225–226
Base station (BS), 186
Benzocyclobutene (BCB), 116
Berkeley Short-channel IGFET Model, 73
Binary confusion matrix, 173
Binary disk sensing (BDS), 193
3-bit register, 46
Bonferroni–Dunn test, 179
Boolean coverage model, 193
BOR1 (body of revolution) Type 1 efficiency, 108
Bose, Sir Jagdish Chandra, 101

C

Camera sensor, 196
Carbon nanotube FET (CNTFET), 62, 69–70
Cassegrain reflector, 105
CDMA, 218
Cellular Telecommunications Industry Association (CTIA), 4–5
CNT antennas, 75–77
CNT dipoles, 77
CNT interconnect, 63–65
Complementary metal-oxide-semiconductor (CMOS), 32, 35, 53, 62
Computer vision, 84
Connectivity, 197
Convolution, 88
Convolutional neural networks (CNNs), 84, 86–89

facial features extracted by, 94
  motivation for, 87
  structure of, 87
Coplanar wire crossing, 37
Cover set-based approaches, 201
Cu/low-k interconnects, 62–63
Cutting-edge electromagnetic antennas, 75

D

Data classification, 93–94
  network structure, 94
  region, 95
Data position user proximity, 5–6
Data storage register, 46
Deep learning, 84–85, 89–93
Depth of field, 195
Digital signal processing (DSP), 206
Digital-TDMA, 218
Directional camera sensor, 195
Direction of arrival (DOA) estimation method, 209
Directivity of antennas, 103–104
Distributed Collaborative Camera Actuation Scheme based on Sensing Region Management (DCCA-SM), 198
D latches, 44–46
Double Feynman gate, 33
Double-negative (DNG) material, 222
Drain-induced barrier lowering (DIBL) effects, 135, 140
Duplex method, 219
  frequency division, 219
  time division, 219
Dynamic k-coverage, 199
Dynamic k-coverage scheduling scheme (DKCS), 199

E

Electromagnetic (EM) theory, 100
Ensemble decision tree (EDT), 172
Epsilon negative material, 222
Euclidean distance, 173, 193, 195
Event, 194
"Event Boundary (EB)" approach, 198
Event region, 194
EXclusive OR (XOR) Boolean function, 93

F

Fan-outs, 35
Fault tolerance, 53
Feedback, 35
Feed forward network structure, 95
Feynman gate, 33
Field encompassing techniques (FETs), 101
Field of view, 195
FinFET, 62, 72–73
FlexFET, 62, 72
Fredkin gate, 33
Friedman's statistic, 178
Friedman test, 178–179
Fringe scalar sensor, 196
Front-gate bias, 135–136
Front-gate voltage, 134–135
Front threshold voltage, 136–137, 141
Γ function, 154, 156

G

Garbage output, 34
Gate-all-around FET (GAAFET), 62, 73
Gestural commands, 150–151
Graph-based approaches, 199–200
Graphene, 65, 77
Graphene nanoantenna, 77–78
Graphene nanoribbons (GNRs), 66
  FET, 70–71
  interconnect, 65–67
  MOSFETs, 70–71
Green's functions and solutions, 126–132, 145–148
Grid-based working node (WN) choice method, 200

H

Half-power beamwidth (HPBW), 103
Hammerstad formula for fringing extension, 230
Human mind, 86
Hyperbolic function, 85

I

Identity function, 84
Illumination efficiency, 106
Impedance matching, 103
Incoherent environment, 149–151, 157, 176, 178, 180

Index 243

Industries Association's International Roadmap for Semiconductors (ITRS), 32
Inner and outer camera sensors, 194
Inner scalar sensor, 196
Insertion loss, 103
Interval Type-2 fuzzy set (IT2FS), 151, 155–157
IT2FS-based gesture-driven robot control system, 157–159
    DA and *DB* gesture, 167–168
    direction and speed calculation, 172
    DR and *DL* gesture, 163–166
    DS gesture, 161–162
    feature extraction, 159–161
    flowchart, 169
    parametric advantages of, 174–178
    performance of, 172–179
    recognition of direction of robot, 163–166
    recognition of gestural command, 171–172
    recognition of speed of robot, 167–168
    training and testing datasets, 170–171

J

JK latch, 44
Josephson-effect-based radiation detectors, 78

K

Khepera II, 153
Kinect sensor, 151–152, 175
K-nearest neighbor (kNN) classification, 172
K-sensors, 199

L

Latches, 44–46
Left-handed (LH) materials, 222, 224
    backward wave propagation, 225–226
    characteristics of, 224–227
    negative refraction, 224–225
    refractive index, 224
LeNet, 89
LeNet-5, 89
Levenberg–Marquardt algorithm induced neural network (LMA-NN), 173
L function, 154–155
Logical reversibility, 34

M

Machine learning, 84
Max pooling, 88
Maxwell, James Clerk, 100
Maxwell's equation, 100, 226
McCulloch–Pitts neuron, 92
Metallic antennas, 78
Metal–oxide–semiconductor field-effect transistors (MOSFETs), 121
Metamaterials, 222
    application of, 223
    fabrication of, 237
    features of, 227
    history of, 222–223
    left-handed (LH) materials, 224–227
    microstrip patch antennas loaded with, 231–238
    value of permittivity and permeability, 227–229
Microstrip patch antennas, 229–231
    frequency and permittivity, 236
    gain of, 231, 236
    impedance, 231
    loaded with metamaterial, 231–238
    rectangular, 234–235
    resonance frequency, 230
    Smith chart of, 235
    voltage standing wave ratio (VSWR), 231
Microwave integrated circuits (MIC), 101
Mobile handset planar inverted-F antenna (PIFA), 3
Mobile phone consumers, usage, 4
Modified LeNet Architecture, 90
Monolithic microwave integrated circuit (MMIC), 101–102
    advantages of, 102
    antennas, 113–117
    limitations of, 102
Moore's law, 33, 62
Multi-antenna systems in user proximity, study of performance of, 4–6
    channel capacity, 17–19
    data position, 5–6
    diversity parameters, estimation of, 7–15
    effective diversity gain (EDG), 14–15
    envelope correlation coefficient (ECC), 10–13
    human body phantom, 6

loss of power in user proximity, 21, 24
mean effective gain (MEG), 9–11
multiplexing efficiency (ME), 16–17
read position, 6
reflection coefficient of designed antenna, 7–8
SAR to peak location spacing ratio, 25–26
specific absorption rate (SAR), 22–25
total radiated power (TRP), 19–22
voice position, 5–6
Multibeam directional antenna, 209
Multihop sensor architecture, 188–189
Multilayer perceptron (MLP), 87
Multiple-input multiple-output antenna, 211
Multiple-input multiple output (MIMO) systems, 2, 5, 206
diversity and parameters of, 2–5
human body vicinity and performance, 3
performances of, 2–3
SAR of, 3–4
Multiple-input single-output antenna, 210
Multiplexer or data selector, 43
Multiuser beamforming, 210
Multi-walled CNTs (MWCNTs), 64–65
Mu-negative (MNG) material, 222

N

Nanoantenna, 74–75
graphene, 77–78
CNT, 76
Neocognitron, 93
Neural-based classifier, 93
Neural network structure, 94
Neurons, 85–86, 92
Neuroscience, 92
New gate, 35
Newton–Raphson method, 133
Nicolson-Ross-Wier method, 227
$N \times n$ reversible gate, 34
NOT gate, 34

O

Ohmic efficiency, 104
Omni-directional camera sensor, 195
OR gate, 34
Outer scalar sensor, 196

P

Patch antennas, 78
Peak location spacing ratio (SPLSR), 4
Peres gate, 33
Physical reversibility, 35
Planar antenna, 100
Poynting vector, 226
PPRG gate, 35
Priority-based target coverage approach, 200
Probability sensing coverage (PSC) model, 193–194
PRUG gate, 35

Q

QCA Pro tool, 49–50
Quality-based coverage approach, 200
Quantum-dot cellular automata (QCA), 32
circuits, 32–33
data processing and logical computations in, 32
Quantum-dot cellular automata (QCA) circuits, 36–39
applications and future aspects, 53–54
average leakage energy, 49
cell polarization in, 36–37
clocking in, 37
clocking zones in, 38
estimation of power dissipation, 49–51
fault tolerance of, 38
five-input majority gate of, 37
optimization of, 38
testing and fault characterization, 50–52

R

Radiation patterns, 103
Radio frequency (RF) energy, 206
RCQCA, 35
Read position user proximity, 6
Rectified Linear Unit activation function, 85
Redundancy cells (RCs), 199
Reflection coefficient, 104–105
Reflection coefficient of designed antenna, 7
Reflector antenna, 108
Register, 36, 46
Reversible circuits, 32–33
Reversible combinational circuits, 36

Reversible gates, 33
  fault characterization of, 52
  $n \times n$, 34
  quantum cost of, 53
Reversible latches, 35–36
Reversible logic circuit, 33–35, 54
  application-based, 35
  designing, 35–36
  reversible error-control circuits, 35
Reversible QCA circuits, 39–40, 54
  adder circuit, 40–41
  combinational circuits, 40–43
  comprehensive analysis of, 46–49
  multiplexer or data selector, 43
  sequential circuits, 44–46
  subtractor circuit, 42
Right-handed materials (RHMs), 222
RM gate, 33, 35
Robots, 150
RUG gate, 33, 35

S

Sayem gate, 33
Scalar count-based method, 197
Scalar count (SC), 196
Scalar premier (SP), 196
Scalar sensor, 196
Scheduling-oriented coverage method, 199
Sensing model relationships, 196
Sensing neighbors, 195
Sensing range, 194–195
Sensing region, 195–196
Sensing region management method, 198
Sensor architecture, 187–188
  multihop, 188–189
  single-hop, 188–189
  two-tier hierarchical cluster, 189–190
Sensor network
  data redundancy issue, 197–201
  definition, 185
  terminologies and definitions, 194–197
Sensor nodes, 186
Sensors, classification and applications of, 190–191
Sequential circuits
  latches, 44–46
  register, 46
Serial in serial out (SISO) shift register, 46

Shift register, 46
Sigmoidal function, 85
Silicon-on-insulator (SOI) metal–oxide–
    semiconductor field-effect transistors, 122
  back-threshold voltage shift, effects on, 142–143
  charge sharing phenomena, 141
  front-threshold voltage shift, effects on, 141–142
  fully depleted (FD), 123
  Green's functions and solutions, 126–132, 145–148
  model, 123–126
  surface potential distribution vs channel length, 138–139
  threshold voltages, 133–139
Single beam directional antenna, 209
Single-electron transistor, 67–68
Single-hop sensor architecture, 188–189
Single-input multiple-output antenna, 210
Single-input single-output (SISO) system, 207
Single user beamforming, 209
Single-walled CNTs (SWCNTs), 64–65
Small geometry effect, 141, 143
Smart antennas, 206
  advantages of, 214–217
  applications, 218–219
  area extension factor (AEF), 214
  base station reduction factor (BSRF), 215
  beamforming method, 213
  classification of, 208–210
  coverage area comparison, 213–214
  disadvantages of, 217–218
  DOA estimation, 212
  functions of, 212–214
  need for, 207
  range extension factor (REF), 214
  spectral efficiency improvement, 216–217
  system capacity improvement, 215–216
  types, 210–212
Snell's law, 225
Software development kit (SDK), 151
Spatial division multiple access (SDMA) system, 209
Spatial pooling, 88
Specific absorption rate (SAR), 3–4
Spillover efficiency, 106

Split ring resonator, 224
SR latch, 44
Standing wave ratio (SWR), 231
Static k-coverage, 199
Stride, 88
Subsampling, 88
Subthreshold CMOS, 62
Subtractors, 35, 42
Sum pooling, 88
Superconducting antenna, 78–79
Superconducting nanowire single-photon detectors, 79
Support vector machine (SVM) classifier, 172
Switched beam smart antenna, 208, 212

T

Target region, 196
Terahertz (THz) field, 101
Time-varying EM fields, 100
T latch, 36, 45–47
Toffoli gate, 33
Total radiated power (TRP), 4
TQCA gate, 35
Transistor-less circuits, 32
Transistor size, 62
Tri-gate transistors, 71–72
Triple-gate FET, 62
TSG gate, 33, 35
Tunnel field effect transistor (TFET), 74
Two-tier hierarchical cluster, 189–190
Type-1 fuzzy sets (T1FS), 153–154
Type 1 fuzzy-system-based classifier (T1FS), 172

U

Ultra-sensitive optical detection property, 79
Unbalanced fed dipole antenna, 3
User proximity
  data position, 5–6
  performance of an antenna, 3
  read position, 6
  simulation set-up, 4–5
  total radiated power (TRP) and loss of power, 4
  voice position, 5–6

V

Very large-scale integration (VLSI) circuit, 61–62, 65, 121–122
Visual information, 83
Voice position user proximity, 5–6
Voltage standing wave ratio, 103
Voltage standing wave ratio (VSWR) of antenna, 231

W

Wireless sensor network (WSN), 185–187
  advantages of, 187
  area coverage, 192
  barrier coverage, 192
  coverage models, 192–194
  data-centric approaches, 186
  energy-harvesting system architecture, 187
  limitations of, 187
  target coverage, 191

X

Xbox 360, 152

For Product Safety Concerns and Information please contact our EU
representative GPSR@taylorandfrancis.com
Taylor & Francis Verlag GmbH, Kaufingerstraße 24, 80331 München, Germany

www.ingramcontent.com/pod-product-compliance
Lightning Source LLC
Chambersburg PA
CBHW071633220526
45469CB00002B/593